Adjuvant Therapy of CANCER

VIII

Adjuvant Therapy of CANCER

VIII

Proceedings of the
Eighth International Conference on the
Adjuvant Therapy of Cancer

Scottsdale, Arizona
March 1996

EDITED BY

***Sydney E. Salmon,* M.D.**

Regents Professor of Medicine
Section of Hematology and Oncology
Department of Internal Medicine
Director, Arizona Cancer Center
University of Arizona College of Medicine
Tucson, Arizona

Lippincott - Raven
PUBLISHERS
Philadelphia • New York

Developmental Editor: Eileen Jackson
Production Manager: Janet Greenwood
Production Editor: Molly Connors
Production Service: Berliner Inc.
Printer/Binder: Maple Press

ISBN: 0-397-58443-1
ISSN: 1040-5089

---

9 8 7 6 5 4 3 2 1

Contributors

David J. Adelstein, m.d., The Cleveland Clinic Foundation, Cleveland, Ohio

Frederick R. Ahmann, m.d., Associate Professor of Medicine and Surgery, Hematology/Oncology and Urology, Arizona Cancer Center, The University of Arizona, Tucson, Arizona

David S. Alberts, m.d., Section of Hematology and Oncology, Arizona Cancer Center, The University of Arizona, Tucson, Arizona

D. Aldrighetti, Istituto Scientifico S. Raffaeleh, Milan, Italy

Frederick Ames, m.d., Department of Surgical Oncology, University of Texas, M.D. Anderson Cancer Center, Houston, Texas

D. Amoroso, Istituto Nazionale per la Ricerca sul Cancro, Genova, Italy

Karen H. Antman, m.d., Professor of Medicine, Columbia University, New York, New York

Susan Ashley, m.d., Breast Cancer Unit, Royal Marsden Hospital, Sutton, Surrey, United Kingdom

Lina Asmar, ph.d., Department of Breast Medical Oncology, University of Texas M.D. Anderson Cancer Center, Houston, Texas

L. Ayash, m.d., Dana-Farber Cancer Institute, Boston, Massachusetts

G. Bacci, m.d., Department of Oncology, Istituti Ortopedici Rizzoli, Bologna, Italy

Joseph S. Bailes, m.d., Physician Reliance Network, Dallas, Texas

Laurence H. Baker, d.o., Professor of Medicine, Director for Clinical Research, Comprehensive Cancer Center, University of Michigan, Ann Arbor, Michigan

Raymond T. Bartus, Medical Affairs and Pharmacology, Alkermes, Inc., Cambridge, Massachusetts

E. H. Bernicker, m.d., Department of Medical Oncology, The University of Texas M.D. Anderson Cancer Center, Houston, Texas

D. Berry, ph.d., Karmanos Cancer Institute, Detroit, Michigan

F. Bertucci, m.d., Unité d'Oncologie Médicale, Institut Paoli-Calmettes, Marseille, France

J. Bitran, m.d., University of Chicago, Chicago, Illinois

Ronald Blum, m.d., New York Univesity Medical Center, New York, New York

F. Boccardo, m.d., Servizio di Oncologia Medica II, Istituto Nazionale per la Ricerca sul Cancro, Genova, Italy

Gianni Bonadonna, m.d., Division of Medical Oncology, Istituto Nazionale Tumori, Milan, Italy

Daniel Booser, m.d., Department of Breast Medical Oncology, The University of Texas M.D. Anderson Cancer Center, Houston, Texas

Ernest Borden, m.d., University of Maryland Cancer Center, Baltimore, Maryland

C. Boshoff, St Bartholomew's and The Royal London School of Medicine and Dentistry, St Bartholomew's Hospital, London, United Kingdom

A. Brach del Prever, m.d., 3rd Pediatric Clinic, University of Torino, Turin, Italy

Cristino Brambilla, m.d., Division of Medical Oncology, Istituto Nazionale Tumori, Milan, Italy

Aman U. Buzdar, m.d., Professor of Medicine, Deputy Chairman, Department of Breast Medical Oncology, The University of Texas M.D. Anderson Cancer Center, Houston, Texas

J. Camerlo, m.d., Unité d'Oncologie Médicale, Institut Paoli-Calmettes, Marseille, France

M.A. Cappiello, m.d., Unité d'Oncologie Médicale, Institut Paoli-Calmettes, Marseille, France

Susan Carlin, b.a., Southwest Oncology Group Statistical Center, Seattle, Washington

James R. Cassady, m.d., Chairman, Department of Radiation Oncology, Lahey Clinic, Burlington, Massachusetts

C. Chabannon, m.d., ph.d., Département de Thérapie Génique et Unité de Transplantation et de Thérapie Cellulaire, Institut Paoli-Calmettes, Marseille, France

Alexander Chan, m.d., Department of Radiation Oncology, Tom Baker Cancer Centre, Calgary, Alberta, Canada

Ellen Chase, B.S., Arizona Cancer Center, The University of Arizona, Tucson, Arizona

A. Comandone, m.d., Department of Oncology, San Giovanni Vecchio Hospital, Torino, Italy

D. Cowen, m.d., Département de radiothérapie, Institut Paoli-Calmettes, Marseille, France

Steve Dahlberg, m.s., Southwest Oncology Group Statistical Center, Seattle, Washington

Roger Dansey, m.d., Karmanos Cancer Institute, Detroit, Michigan

P. Delia, Istituto di Clinica Oncologica dell'Università di Messina, Messina, Italy

C. De Sanctis, Cattedra di Ginecologia Oncologica dell'Università di Torino, Turin, Italy

Kapil Dhingra, m.d., Department of Breast Medical Oncology, The University of Texas M.D. Anderson Cancer Center, Houston, Texas

Eleni Diamandidou, m.d., Department of Breast Medical Oncology, The University of Texas M.D. Anderson Cancer Center, Houston, Texas

James Dignam, ph.d., NSABP Biostatistician, Department of Biostatistics, University of Pittsburgh Graduate School of Public Health, School of Medicine, Pittsburgh, Pennsylvania

D. Donati, Arcispedale S. Anna, Ferrara, Italy

James H. Doroshow, m.d., City of Hope National Medical Center, Duarte, California

Lawrence H. Einhorn, m.d., Indiana University Medical Center, Indianapolis, Indiana

A. Elias, m.d., Dana-Farber Cancer Institute, Boston, Massachusetts

Peter J. Elliott, Alkermes, Inc., Medical Affairs and Pharmacology, Cambridge, Massachusetts

Marc S. Ernstoff, m.d., University of Pittsburgh Medical Center, Pittsburgh, Pennsylvania

A. Farris, Cattedra di Oncologia Clinica dell'Università di Sassari, Sassari, Italy

Laura Ferrari, m.d., Division of Medical Oncology, Istituto Nazionale Tumori, Milan, Italy

S. Ferrari, m.d., Department of Oncology, Istituti Ortopedici Rizzoli, Bologna, Italy

Lynn G. Feun, m.d., University of Miami School of Medicine, Miami, Florida

Bernard Fisher, m.d., Scientific Director, National Surgical Adjuvant Breast and Bowel Project (NSABP), Distinguished Service Professor, University of Pittsburgh, School of Medicine, Pittsburgh, Pennsylvania

Richard I. Fisher, m.d., Loyola University, Stritch School of Medicine, Maywood, Illinois

Lawrence E. Flaherty, m.d., Wayne State University Medical Center, Detroit, Michigan

Emil Frei, III, m.d., Director, Dana Farber Cancer Institute, Boston, Massachusetts

Dava J. Garcia, b.s., Section of Hematology and Oncology, Arizona Cancer Center, The University of Arizona, Tucson, Arizona

D. Genre, m.d., Unité d'Oncologie Médicale, Institut Paoli-Calmettes, Marseille, France

F. GENTA, Cattedra di Ginecologia Oncologica dell'Università di Torino, Turin, Italy

O. GERACI, Istituto di Clinica Oncologica dell'Università di Messina, Messina, Italy

G. GRAVIS, M.D., Unité d'Oncologie Médicale, Institut Paoli-Calmettes, Marseille, France

DANIEL M. GREEN, M.D., Division of Hematology/Oncology, Department of Pediatrics, Children's Hospital of Buffalo, Department of Pediatrics, School of Medicine and Biomedical Sciences, University at Buffalo, State University of New York, Department of Pediatrics, Roswell Park Cancer Institute, Department of Pediatrics, Buffalo, New York

D. GRISWALD, M.D., Dana-Farber Cancer Institute, Boston, Massachusetts

THOMAS M. GROGAN, M.D., Arizona Cancer Center, The University of Arizona, Tucson, Arizona

JOHN J. GROUS, Medical Affairs and Pharmacology, Alkermes, Inc., Cambridge, Massachusetts

EVAN M. HERSH, M.D., Section of Hematology and Oncology, Arizona Cancer Center, The University of Arizona, Tucson, Arizona

FRANKIE A. HOLMES, M.D., Department of Breast Medical Oncology, The University of Texas M.D. Anderson Cancer Center, Houston, Texas

W. K. HONG, M.D., Department of Medical Oncology, The University of Texas M.D. Anderson Cancer Center, Houston, Texas

GABRIEL N. HORTOBAGYI, M.D., Department of Breast Medical Oncology, The University of Texas M.D. Anderson Cancer Center, Houston, Texas

G. HOUVENAEGHEL, M.D., Département de Chirurgie Oncologique, Institut Paoli-Calmettes, Marseille, France

WILLIAM J.M. HRUSHESKY, M.D, Professor of Medicine and Microbiology/Immunology, Albany Medical College, Professor of Chemical Engineering, Rensselaer Polytechnic Institute, Professor, Department of Pharmaceutics, Albany College of Pharmacy, Professor, Department of Biomedical Sciences, School of Public Health, State University of New York at Albany, Senior Attending Oncologist, Stratton VA Medical Center, Albany, New York

J. INGLE, M.D, Mayo Clinic, Rochester, Minnesota

INTACC (INTERGRUPPO NAZIONALE TERAPIA ADIUVANTE CARCINOMA COLON, NATIONAL INTERGROUP OF ADJUVANT THERAPY FOR COLON CANCER), c/o Istituto Nazionale per la Ricerca sul Cancro, Genova, Italy

L. IRTELLI, Cattedra di Oncologia Medica dell'Università "G. D'Annunzio" di Chieti, Chieta, Italy

JOHN A. KANIS, M.D., WHO Collaborating Centre for Metabolic Bone Diseases, Department of Human Metabolism & Clinical Biochemistry, University of Sheffield Medical School, Sheffield, United Kingdom

David Kelsen, M.D., Professor of Medicine, Cornell University, Chief, Gastrointestinal Oncology Service, Department of Medicine, Memorial Sloan-Kettering Cancer Center, New York, New York

F. R. Khuri, M.D., Department of Medical Oncology, The University of Texas M.D. Anderson Cancer Center, Houston, Texas

John M. Kirkwood, M.D., Director, Melanoma Center, University of Pittsburgh Medical Center, Pittsburgh, Pennsylvania

Jared Klein, M.D., Karmanos Cancer Institute, 110 East Warren Avenue, Detroit, Michigan

Kenneth J. Kopecky, Ph.D., Southwest Oncology Group Statistical Center, Seattle, Washington

J. Kugler, M.D., Mayo Clinic, Rochester, Minnesota

Michael LeBlanc, Ph.D., Southwest Oncology Group Statistical Center, Seattle, Washington

Thierry Le Chevalier, M.D., Department of Medicine, Institut Gustave-Roussy, Villejuif, France

S. M. Lippman, M.D., Department of Medical Oncology, The University of Texas M.D. Anderson Cancer Center, Houston, Texas

M. Liquori, Istituto Nazionale per la Ricerca sul Cancro, Genova, Italy

A.M. Mancini, M.D., 3rd Pediatric Clinic, University of Bologna, Bologna, Italy

D. Maraninchi, M.D., Unité d'Oncologie Médicale, Institut Paoli-Calmettes, Marseille, France

Eugene V McCloskey, M.D., WHO Collaborating Centre for Metabolic Bone Diseases, Department of Human Metabolism and Clinical Biochemistry, University of Sheffield Medical School, Sheffield, United Kingdom

Marsha McNeese, M.D., Department of Radiotherapy, The University of Texas M.D. Anderson Cancer Center, Houston, Texas

M. Mercuri, M.D., Department of Oncology, Istituti Ortopedici Rizzoli, Bologna, Italy

M. Mesiti, Istituto di Clinica Oncologica dell'Università di Messina, Messina, Italy

Frank L. Meyskens, Jr., M.D., Director, UCI Clinical Cancer Center, University of California at Irvine, Orange, California

Thomas P. Miller, M.D., Hematology/Oncology, Room 1957, Arizona Cancer Center, The University of Arizona, Tucson, Arizona

Angela Moliterni, M.D., Division of Medical Oncology, Istituto Nazionale Tumori, Milan, Italy

Angela Morris, R.N., Department of Breast Medical Oncology, The University of Texas M.D. Anderson Cancer Center, Houston, Texas

Robert D. Noyes, m.d., University of Utah Medical Center, Salt Lake City, Utah

R.T.D Oliver, St Bartholomew's and The Royal London School of Medicine and Dentistry, St Bartholomew's Hospital, London, United Kingdom

P. Pacini, Policlinico Careggi, Florence, Italy

Alexander H.G. Paterson, m.d., Tom Baker Cancer Centre, Department of Medicine, Calgary, Alberta, Canada

F. Penault-Llorca, m.d., Laboratoire d'Anatonomo-pathologie, Institut Paoli-Calmettes, Marseille, France

William P. Peters, m.d., ph.d., President and Chief Executive Officer, Karmanos Cancer Institute, Detroit, Michigan

Piero Picci, m.d., Direttore, Laboratorio di Ricerca Oncologica, Istituti Ortopedici Rizzoli, Bologna, Italy

M. Pollak, m.d., Department of Oncology, Jewish General Hospital, Montreal, Quebec, Canada

Trevor Powles, m.d., Breast Cancer Unit, Royal Marsden Hospital, Sutton, Surrey, United Kingdom

P. Richardson, m.d., Dana-Farber Cancer Institute, Boston, Massachusetts

Olivier Rixe, m.d., Department of Medicine, Institut Gustave-Roussy, Villejuif, France

A. Rubagotti, Istituto Nazionale per la Ricerca sul Cancro, Istituto di Oncologia dell'Università, Genova, Italy

Howard Rockette, ph.d., Professor and Acting Chairman, Department of Biostatistics, University of Pittsburgh, Pittsburgh, Pennsylvania

G. Rulli, Laboratorio di Ricerca Oncologica, Istituti Ortopedici, Rizzoli, Italy

Sydney E. Salmon, m.d., Director, Arizona Cancer Center, The University of Arizona, Tucson, Arizona

G. Schieppati, Ospedale Generale Provinciale, Saronno, Italy

Ann Schott, m.d., Comprehensive Cancer Center, University of Michigan, Ann Arbor, Michigan

T. Scotto, Cattedra di Oncologia Clinica dell'Università di Sassari, Sassari, Italy

S. Eva Singletary, m.d., Department of Surgical Oncology, The University of Texas M.D. Anderson Cancer Center, Houston, Texas

John W. Smith, II, m.d., University of Michigan Medical Center, Ann Arbor, Michigan

Thomas Smith, m.d., Morristown Memorial Hospital, Morristown, New Jersey

Vernon Sondak, m.d., Surgical Oncology, University of Michigan Medical Center, Ann Arbor, Michigan

Catherine M. Spier, m.d., Arizona Cancer Center, The University of Arizona, Tucson, Arizona

Alison T. Stopeck, m.d., Section of Hematology and Oncology, Arizona Cancer Center, The University of Arizona, Tucson, Arizona

Myla Hunt Strawderman, Dana-Farber Cancer Institute, Boston, Massachusetts

Eric Strom, m.d., Department of Radiotherapy, The University of Texas M.D. Anderson Cancer Center, Houston, Texas

V. Suman, m.d., Mayo Clinic, Rochester, Minnesota

B. A. Teicher, ph.d., Associate Professor of Medicine, and Radiation Therapy, Dana-Farber Cancer Institute, Boston, Massachusetts

Monica Terenziani, m.d., Division of Medical Oncology, Istituto Nazionale Tumori, Milan, Italy

Richard Theriault, d.o., Department of Breast Medical Oncology, The University of Texas M.D. Anderson Cancer Center, Houston, Texas

A. Tienghi, m.d., Department of Oncology, Santa Croce Hospital, Ravenna, Italy

Ralph J. Tuthill, m.d., The Cleveland Clinic Foundation, Cleveland, Ohio

Pinuccia Valagussa, ph.d., Istituto Nazionale Tumori, Milan, Italy

P. Viens, m.d., Unité d'Oncologie Médicale, Institut Paoli-Calmettes, Marseille, France

E. Villa, Istituto Scientifico S. Raffaele, Milano, Milan, Italy

Ronald Walters, m.d., Department of Breast Medical Oncology, The University of Texas M.D. Anderson Cancer Center, Houston, Texas

C. Wheeler, m.d., Dana-Farber Cancer Institute, Boston, Massachusetts

Maria A.Witjaksono, m.d., Department of Breast Medical Oncology, The University of Texas M.D. Anderson Cancer Center, Houston, Texas

Norman H. Wolmark, m.d., Allegheny General Hospital, Division of Surgical Oncology, Pittsburgh, Pennsylvania

Alfred Wong, m.d., f.r.c.p. (c), Department of Medical Oncology, Tom Baker Cancer Centre, Calgary, Alberta, Canada

Vance Wright-Browne, m.d., Department of Breast Medical Oncology, The University of Texas M.D. Anderson Cancer Center, Houston, Texas

Milvia Zambetti, m.d., Division of Medical Oncology, Istituto Nazionale Tumori, Milan, Italy

H. Zmerly, m.d., Department of Oncology, Istituti Ortopedici Rizzoli, Bologna, Italy

Preface

The purpose of adjuvant therapy of cancer is to increase the efficacy of primary surgery, radiation, or chemotherapy in order to more effectively treat the primary tumor while eradicating or suppressing the growth of occult micrometastases of cancer. To date, adjuvant approaches have been focused primarily on cancers known to be at high risk for early metastasis. Adjuvant approaches have generally used cytotoxic, endocrine, or biologic agents. A variety of approaches to reduce toxicity has made the administration of adjuvant therapy more acceptable. In the future, our adjuvant armamentarium may also include agents to open pharmacologic sanctuaries, overcome drug resistance, and, in the long run, utilize genetic therapy, which focuses on the underlining lesions in the diseases we call cancer.

The concept of adjuvant therapy of cancer is by no means new; evaluation of this approach for improving the effectiveness of cancer management was initiated in a systematic fashion about two decades ago. The initial chapter in this volume provides some historical background on these conferences and tries to look into the near future. Use of primary chemotherapy (or "neoadjuvant chemotherapy") often permits evaluation of the clinical chemosensitivity of the patient's tumor prior to major surgical intervention. Presumably, micrometastases will display similar chemosensitivity to that manifested by the primary tumor. When drugs are administered with the neoadjuvant approach, they provide the potential of reducing the extent of local surgery or radiotherapy, culminating in a better cosmetic result and functional recovery of the patient.

Over the years, and as documented in the eight volumes in this series, the promise of applying adjuvant therapy to increase long-term survival has been clearly translated into a reality for an increasing number of tumor types. These international conferences on adjuvant therapy of cancer were established by the Arizona Cancer Center in order to stimulate and disseminate conceptual and practical knowledge that makes the initial treatment of the cancer patient more effective. In that context, this series of publications from the proceedings of the Conference on the Adjuvant Therapy of Cancer has proven to be a central reference for this field, in large part due to rapid publication through the use of desktop publishing techniques. In order to facilitate speedy publication, the submitted manuscripts are subjected to only minimal editing. In view of their brevity, the papers in this volume should be considered to be extended abstracts rather than complete reports. For the current volume, Lippincott-Raven Publishers has worked closely with us to maintain the rapid publishing schedule achieved at our last conference. For this eighth conference (held in Scottsdale, Arizona on March 13–16, 1996) we were pleased to have participation of over 360 clinical investigators and practicing oncologists from more than 43 states and 18 countries. Relevant scientific advances in cancer biology and genetics as well as in adjuvant therapy were reported at this eighth conference. Advances in adjuvant therapy in sarcoma, melanoma, and non-Hodgkin's lymphoma and more effective adjuvant therapy for colorectal cancer were some of the new features reported at this meeting. The final chapter in this volume, by Drs. Anne Schott and Lawrence Baker, provides a superb overview on the proceedings of this conference.

Selection of invited and competitive speakers for the conference was achieved with the assistance of an outstanding scientific advisory board, comprised of Drs. Gianni Bonadonna, Lawrence Einhorn, Emil Frei III, Bernard Fisher, Vincent T. DeVita, Jr., and Norman Wolmark. I also want to acknowledge the excellent conference logistics coordinated by Ms. Patty Sundberg, and thank my long-time colleague at the Arizona Cancer Center, Dr. David S. Alberts, for agreeing to serve as co-chair for this conference. Finally, I want to express my heartfelt thanks to my wife, Joanie, for her unflagging support of my efforts during these eight conferences and during our life together; she has continued to remain my lifelong companion and best friend.

Sydney E. Salmon, M.D.
March 1996

Contents

I: Scientific Overview and Perspectives

1. Adjuvant Therapy of Cancer: Past, Present, and Future 3
Sydney E. Salmon

2. Gene Transfer into Tumor Cells *In Vitro* and *In Vivo:* Potential for Adjuvant Therapy of Cancer 9
Alison T. Stopeck and Evan M. Hersh

3. Development of RMP-7: A Novel Bradykinin Agonist That Increases Delivery of Chemotherapeutics to Gliomas 19
John J. Grous, Peter J. Elliott, and Raymond T. Bartus

4. Late Effects of Adjuvant Chemotherapy for the Treatment of Cancer in Children and Adolescents 33
Daniel M. Green

5. Use and Coverage of Novel Cancer Agents in Managed Care 51
Joseph S. Bailes

II: Airway Tumors

6. Advances in the Biological Study, Prevention, and Therapy of Head and Neck Cancer 59
E. H. Bernicker, F. R. Khuri, S. M. Lippman, and W. K. Hong

7. Adjuvant Chemotherapy of Non–Small-Cell Lung Cancer 71
Olivier Rixe and Thierry Le Chevalier

III: Breast Cancer

Large-Scale Adjuvant Trials

8. Update of the Milan Cancer Institute Studies in Operable Breast Cancer 77
Gianni Bonadonna, Pinuccia Valagussa, Angela Moliterni, Milvia Zambetti, Monica Terenziani, Laura Ferrari, and Cristina Brambilla

9. Recent Findings from Three NSABP Clinical Trials Evaluating Systemic Adjuvant Therapy in Patients with Primary Breast Cancer and Negative Axillary Nodes 83
Bernard Fisher and James Dignam

10. Impact of FAC-Adjuvant Therapy on Mortality of Early Breast Cancer: Long-Term Results of the M. D. Anderson Cancer Center Studies — **93**
Aman U. Buzdar, Gabriel N. Hortobagyi, S. Eva Singletary, Frankie A. Holmes, Richard Theriault, Ronald Walters, Kapil Dhingra, Daniel Booser, Angela Morris, Lina Asmar, Vance Wright-Browne, Eleni Diamandidou, Maria A.Witjaksono, Eric Strom, Marsha McNeese, and Frederick Ames

11. CMF Versus Tamoxifen Plus Goserelin as Adjuvant Treatment of ER-Positive Pre-Perimenopausal Breast Cancer Patients: Preliminary Results of an Ongoing Italian Breast Cancer Adjuvant Study Group (GROCTA) Trial — **101**
F. Boccardo, A. Rubagotti, D. Amoroso, M. Liquori, M. Mesiti, O. Geraci, P. Delia, E. Villa, D. Aldrighetti, F. Genta, C. De Sanctis, L. Irtelli, D. Donati, P. Pacini, A. Farris, T. Scotto, G. Schieppati, and other participants in the GROCTA, National Institute for Cancer Research, Genoa, Italy

High-Dose Chemotherapy

12. High-Dose Chemotherapy with Stem Cell Protection: Tandem, Sequence, and Phenylalanine Mustard Studies — **111**
Emil Frei III, J. Bitran, L. Ayash, A. Elias, D. Griswald, B. Teicher, P. Richardson, and C. Wheeler

13. High-Dose Chemotherapy for High-Risk Primary Breast Cancer — **117**
William P. Peters, Roger Dansey, Jared Klein, and D. Berry

14. High–Dose-Intensity Doxorubicin–Cyclophosphamide with rh-GCSF and Peripheral Blood Stem Cells: Outpatient Adjuvant Treatment for Premenopausal Patients with Breast Carcinoma. — **123**
P. Viens, D. Genre, G. Gravis, M.A. Cappiello, J. Camerlo, D. Cowen, F. Bertucci, G. Houvenaeghel, F. Penault-Llorca, C. Chabannon, and D. Maraninchi

Biologic Observations and Potential Clinical Relevance

15. Breast Cancer, Surgery, and the Menstrual Cycle — **133**
William J. M. Hrushesky

16. Rationale for Combined Antiestrogen–Somatostatin Analogue Therapy of Breast Cancer — **145**
M. Pollak, J. Ingle, V. Suman, and J. Kugler

17. Clodronate as an Adjuvant to Hormone and Chemotherapy in Patients with Breast Cancer — **153**
Alexander H. G. Paterson, John A. Kanis, Trevor Powles, Eugene V. McCloskey, and Susan Ashley

18. Breast Cancer Roundtable 163
Emil Frei III (Chair), Karen Antman, Bernard Fisher, William P. Peters, Sydney E. Salmon, and Pinuccia Valagussa, with audience participation

IV: Gastrointestinal Cancer

19. Adjuvant Therapy of Upper Gastrointestinal Tract Cancers 173
David Kelsen

20. Adjuvant Therapy for Carcinoma of the Colon and Rectum: Review of the NSABP Clinical Trials 183
Norman H. Wolmark, and Bernard Fisher

21. 5-Fluorouracil Plus Levamisole with or without 6-S-Leucovorin as Adjuvant Treatment of Resected Colon Cancer 193
The INTACC (Intergruppo Nazionale Terapia Adiuvante Carcinoma Colon)

22. A Prospective Comparison of Fluorouracil/Folinic Acid versus Levamisole/Fluorouracil as Adjuvant Therapy after Resection of Stage III Colon Carcinoma 199
Alfred Wong and Alexander Chan

V: Gynecologic and Genitourinary Cancer

23. Adjuvant Therapy of Ovarian Cancer—Is There Reason for Optimism? 207
David S. Alberts and Dava J. Garcia

24. A Review of the Neoadjuvant and Adjuvant Treatment of Prostate Cancer 217
Frederick R. Ahmann

25. Adjuvant Trials in Bladder Cancer: Scientific Background, Review, and New Directions 227
R. T. D. Oliver and C. Boshoff

26. Adjuvant Concepts in Testicular Cancer 239
Lawrence H. Einhorn

VI: Lymphoma, Melanoma and Sarcoma

27. CHOP Plus Radiotherapy Is Superior to CHOP Alone for Adjuvant Therapy of Resected Localized Unfavorable Non-Hodgkin's Lymphoma: A Southwest Oncology Group Study 245
Thomas P. Miller, Steve Dahlberg, James R. Cassady, David J. Adelstein, Catherine M. Spier, Thomas M. Grogan, Susan Carlin, Ellen Chase, Michael LeBlanc, and Richard I. Fisher

28. Adjuvant Therapy of High-Risk Melanoma: The Role of High-Dose Interferon α-2b **251**
John M. Kirkwood, Myla Hunt Strawderman, Marc S. Ernstoff, Thomas Smith, Ernest Borden, and Ronald Blum

29. Is Interferon-γ Detrimental? Results of a Southwest Oncology Group Randomized Trial of Adjuvant Interferon-γ versus Observation in Melanoma **259**
Vernon K. Sondak, Kenneth J. Kopecky, John W. Smith II, Evan M. Hersh, Robert D. Noyes, Ralph J. Tuthill, Thomas P. Miller, Lynn G. Feun, James H. Doroshow, Lawrence E. Flaherty, and Frank L. Meyskens, Jr., for the Southwest Oncology Group

30. The Recent Experience at the Rizzoli Institute in the Treatment of Osteosarcoma **273**
P. Picci, G. Bacci, S. Ferrari, A. Brach del Prever, A. Tienghi, A. Comandone, A. M. Mancini, H. Zmerly, G. Rulli, and M. Mercuri

31. Adjuvant Therapy of Sarcomas of Bone and Soft Tissue **279**
Karen H. Antman

VII: Conference Summary

32. Adjuvant Therapy of Cancer VIII: Concluding Perspectives **289**
Anne Schott and Laurence H. Baker

Adjuvant Therapy of CANCER

VIII

I

Scientific Overview and Perspectives

Adjuvant Therapy of Cancer VIII, edited by Sydney E. Salmon. Lippincott–Raven Publishers, Philadelphia © 1997.

1

Adjuvant Therapy of Cancer: Past, Present, and Future

Sydney E. Salmon

It seems like only yesterday, but it was 20 years ago when we at the Arizona Cancer Center decided to organize the First International Conference on Adjuvant Therapy of Cancer. Adjuvant therapy generally refers to systemic therapy administered around the time that the initial local treatment is given for cancer. The objective of adjuvant therapy is to eradicate or suppress occult micrometastases and thereby to attempt to increase the cure rate. Occult micrometastases are now recognized as the major cause of failure of cancer treatment for many apparently localized cancers. For the first conference (March 3–5, 1977) we invited to Tucson a group of investigators who were active in preclinical or clinical explorations of adjuvant therapy (1). We assumed that the conference would attract an audience of 80–100, and were we surprised when 500 registrants showed up! Fortunately the hotel had a larger meeting room than the one we'd booked! Some of the topics addressed at our first conference are shown in Table 1-1.

One concept that was explored concerned tumor stem cells as the seeds of metastasis. At that time, my group had just developed a human tumor colony or tumor stem cell assay technique to evaluate clonogenic tumor cells in a patient's tumor biopsy and conduct predictive drug sensitivity testing (2). That technology has since become available for clinical use. However, the technique is no better than available drugs, and often shows drug resistance to commonly used agents. Predictions of drug resistance in this assay have proven remarkably accurate, and therefore the assay gives a better idea of what drugs not to use than which ones to use for a given patient. The relevance of the initial tumor burden to the development of metastasis and death was clearly shown in a mouse model of breast cancer developed by Schabel (3). When

TABLE 1-1. Focal Points of the First International Conference on Adjuvant Therapy of Cancer (March 5–7, 1977)

- Concepts: tumor stem cells, micrometastasis, kinetic analysis
- Positive results in animal models
- Initial breast cancer trial reports from NSABP, Milan
- No mature positive trials in adult oncology
- Positive trials in childhood cancers such as Wilm's tumor
- High degree of enthusiasm (despite limited data)!

surgery was performed on small tumors, most animals survived and surgery was curative. With increasing tumor size at the time of surgery, more animals died of metastatic disease. Skipper and Schabel extrapolated from mice to women with breast cancer and related node positivity and its effects on relapse-free survival to a predicted tumor burden at the time of local surgery (Figure 1-1) (4). Their analysis provided scientific rationale for use of systemic chemotherapy as an adjuvant to local therapy for cancer. Preclinical tests of adjuvant chemotherapy were performed by this group in animal models (Figure 1-2). In a number of dramatic examples in mice the survival of tumor controls, as well as of mice receiving chemotherapy alone, surgery alone, or the combination of surgery plus chemotherapy, underscored the dramatic improvement in survival that adjuvant chemotherapy could have when treating a minimal micrometastatic tumor cell burden after surgery. Similar results have since been achieved clinically for some, but far from all, human cancers at high risk of metastasis.

Another important consideration that we recognized to be important even at that time was dose intensity. In that early era, many were exploring "low-dose chemotherapy" with the view that if there are fewer tumor cells present, then less chemotherapy would be needed and treatment could be less intense. However, by applying Gompertzian growth kinetics to model growth after surgery in minimal residual ER-negative breast cancer (Figure 1-3) we predicted shorter intervals between adjuvant courses (greater dose intensity) could make the difference between success and failure (5). Maturing trials of high-dose chemotherapy with autologous hematopoietic stem cell rescue are currently testing this hypothesis.

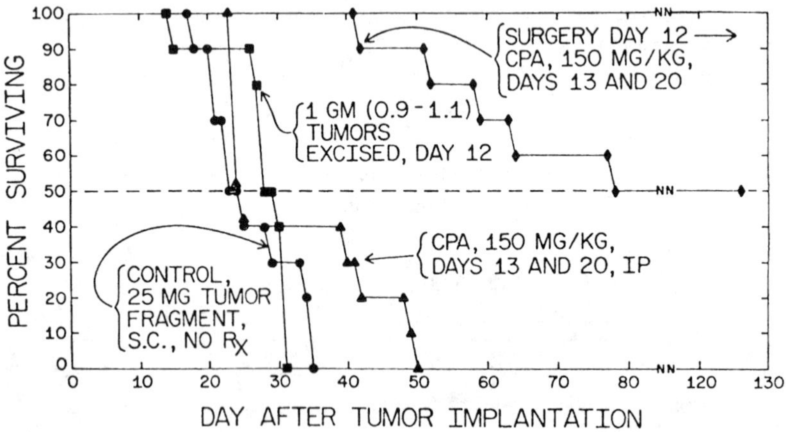

Figure 1-1. Hypothesized relationship between lymph node status, prognosis, and residual tumor burden after surgery for women with stage I or II primary breast cancer who have undergone mastectomy and axillary node dissection. The numbers of residual tumor cells calculated to be present are based on an assumed median doubling time of 40 days. (Reproduced with permission from reference 4.)

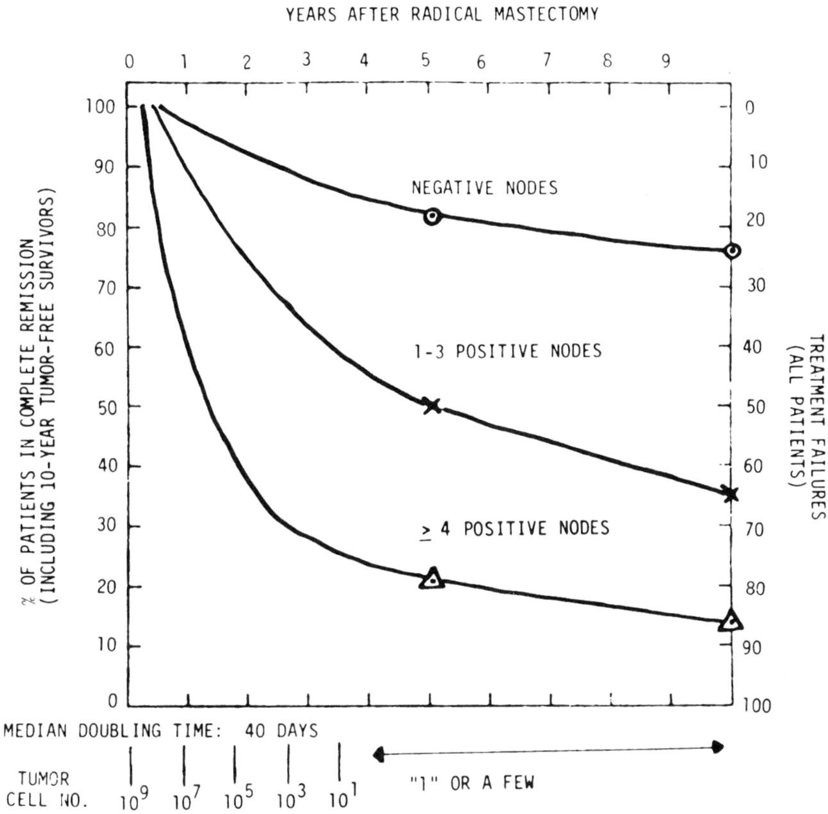

Figure 1-2. Curative adjuvant chemotherapy of micrometastases in Lewis lung carcinoma in BDF[1] mice with surgical removal of the primary tumor (no cures); treatment with cyclophosphamide (CPA) on days 1 and 8 after surgery (no cures); and surgery followed by the same schedule of CPA (50 % cured). Analogous results were obtained in murine breast and colon cancer and melanoma using other chemotherapeutic agents after surgery. (Reproduced with permission from reference 3.)

ADJUVANT THERAPY IN THE LAST QUARTER OF THE 20th CENTURY

In the 1970s there were only a few major drugs or drug classes that could be considered for use in adjuvant therapy. These included fluorouracil, methotrexate, cyclophosphamide, the vinca alkaloids, doxorubicin and, cisplatin. Most of the adjuvant trials involving the latter two agents did not begin until the late 1970s. In the 1980s there were several new innovations reported for adjuvant therapy. These included anti-endocrine agents such as tamoxifen (6), the implementation of high-dose chemotherapy with stem cell rescue, and the concept of so-called neoadjuvant therapy (7), wherein chemotherapy was given prior to surgery. In this setting, the local surgery could perhaps be considered as the adjuvant. Additionally, radiation

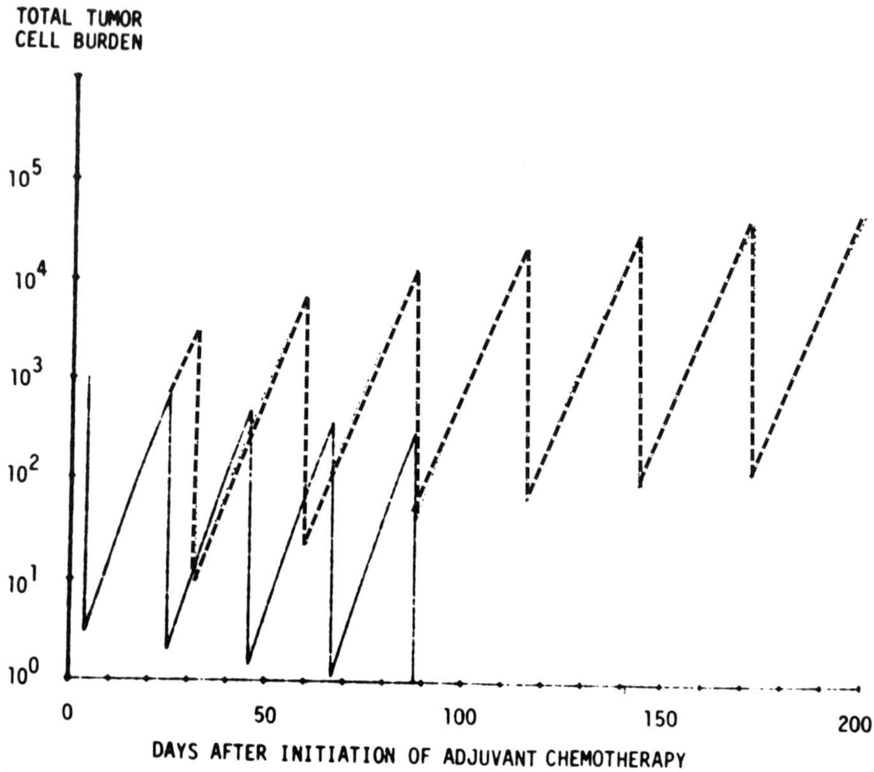

Figure 1-3. Gompertzian kinetic model examining the effect of dose intensity on the outcome of adjuvant chemotherapy for residual micrometastases after surgery in primary breast cancer. Each perpendicular line on the tumor growth curve reflects a tumor cell kill of 99.7% with each course of chemotherapy. In this specific model, tumor cells could be eradicated with an every-3-week schedule after 5 courses of therapy, but cures could not be obtained when the same doses of chemotherapy were given every 4 weeks irrespective of the number of courses. (Reproduced with permission from reference 5.)

therapy was increasingly used as an essential component of local therapy as its use could significantly reduce the extent of surgery and improve cosmetic effects and patient acceptance while still maintaining the beneficial effects of local therapy.

Multimodality therapy had finally come of age, and the various major treatment modalities (surgery, radiation therapy, chemotherapy, biotherapy) were no longer being given in the order in which they were discovered, but rather in the sequence or combination that appeared to work best. In the 1990s, stereotactic radiosurgery and 3D conformal therapy have been added to the standard armamentarium in a number of major cancer centers.

In the 1990s other kinds of new agents received wider use and are already impacting on adjuvant therapy. These include bone marrow toxicity-reducing agents such as granulocyte-colony-stimulating factor, granulocyte-macrophage-stimulating factor, and erythropoietin. Thrombopoietin may soon be added to this group. Other agents such as amifostine to reduce renal toxicity, and dexrazoxane to reduce cardiac toxicity have also been approved for clinical use. Potent anti-emetics such as ondansetron or granisetron have made many of the available cytotoxic drugs more acceptable to patients. Currently in clinical trial are second-generation chemosensitizers, which appear to block *p*-glycoprotein-mediated multidrug resistance in certain neoplasms and the first fledgling efforts in gene therapy, which are intended to either alter the tumor or the host's immune response to the tumor. Several important new classes of chemotherapy drugs, including the taxoids and the camptothecans, are being increasingly studied and efforts are being made to define their role in adjuvant therapy. After decades of experimentation, novel drug formulations or modifications of existing drugs have appeared in the clinic. These include liposomal formulations for intravenous use, or other special formulations for local drug delivery. Progress is being seen in the use of monoclonal antibody-radionuclide conjugates as "smart bombs" to incorporate into multimodality therapy. The pace of progress is quickening; some of these advances in the 1980s and 1990s will become part of standard therapy before the year 2000.

THE FUTURE

In my concluding remarks, I thought I should try to look ahead at least a little bit into the 21st century. We have been in the era of molecular biology for the past 20 years and are now transitioning into the era of molecular genetics of cancer. For the first time, we are beginning to gain major insights on specific structural abnormalities that lead to cancer, such as the mutations in the *BRCA1* gene, which greatly increase the risk of developing breast or ovarian cancer. Cancer is a disease of molecular genetics, and one for which genetic approaches to diagnosis, prevention, and therapy will become increasingly important. Understanding both the structure and function of normal and mutated oncogenes and tumor suppressor genes has a high probability of leading to entirely new forms of cancer treatment that are extraordinarily difficult to envision today. Nonetheless, I'll make a few predictions on therapeutic advances for the early 21st century. These are summarized in Table 1-2.

Technologies are now being developed to rapidly detect specific genetic mutations in key genes such as *BRCA1* and *p53*. The next challenge will be to develop

TABLE 1-2. Adjuvant Therapy of Cancer in the Early 21st Century?

- Detect and eliminate cells with altered genes such as *BRCA1* or *p53*
- Block expression of oncogenes (e.g., with antisense)
- Block intracellular signaling in preneoplastic and neoplastic cells
- Repair damaged tumor suppressor genes or replace their products with functional gene products
- Convert tumor cells to normal cells

techniques to eliminate cells with seriously damaged tumor suppressor genes from the body. Methods will also be needed to block expression of oncogenes—such as with the use of antisense compounds that are just now entering phase I clinical trials. The major signaling pathways that are preferentially used in cancer as compared to normal cells are being identified and a search is on for new pharmacologic agents that will selectively inhibit these pathways in cancer cells. A more difficult task will be to repair damaged tumor suppressor genes, which perhaps will be better achieved with gene product replacement therapy, wherein the normal gene product is administered much as hormonal replacement is administered in hormone-deficient states. Early evidence supporting this approach has just recently been suggested for the *BRCA1* gene and its product. The most difficult step of all may be to convert tumor cells to normal cells. While early efforts to accomplish this objective have used "differentiating agents," a solution to this problem may seem further away but nonetheless not an outrageous idea in the era of molecular genetics of cancer. Thus, it would appear that we now stand on the threshold of a new era in cancer therapy, in which new treatment paradigms will be struck. Most likely, the terms "adjuvant therapy" and "neoadjuvant therapy" will remain relevant to cancer treatment, but may need to make room for entirely new approaches based on molecular genetics.

It will be our task as clinicians to take the steps needed to convert such futuristic ideas into standard medical practices for diagnosis and cure of patients with cancer, and to prevent development of cancer whenever possible. The essential step in translation of new knowledge and new agents from the bench to the bedside is the clinical trial, and we must also ensure that the mechanisms to conduct such trials and to make therapeutic advances are not blocked by the changing environment we see emerging in health care delivery.

REFERENCES

1. Salmon SE, Jones SE, eds. Adjuvant therapy of cancer. Amsterdam: Elsevier/North Holland Biomedical Press, 1977.
2. Salmon SE, Hamburger AW, Soehnlen BS, et al. Quantitation of differential sensitivity of human-tumor stem cells to anticancer drugs. N Engl J Med 1978;298:1321.
3. Schabel FM Jr. Concepts for treatment of micrometastases developed in murine systems. Am J Roentgenol 1976;126:500.
4. Skipper H, Schabel FM Jr. Quantitative and cytokinetic studies in experimental tumor systems. In: Holland JF, Frei E III, eds. Cancer medicine, 2nd ed. Philadelphia: Lea and Febiger, 1977.
5. Salmon SE. Kinetic rationale for adjuvant chemotherapy of cancer. In: Salmon SE, Jones SE, eds. Adjuvant therapy of cancer. Amsterdam: Elsevier/North Holland Biomedical Press, 1977, p 15.
6. Baum M. Prospects for the future in the management of carcinoma of the breast: The biological fall out from clinical trials. In: Jones SE, Salmon SE, eds. Adjuvant therapy of cancer IV. Orlando: Grune & Stratton, 1984, p 321.
7. Frei E III, Clark JR, Miller D. The concept of neoadjuvant chemotherapy. In: Salmon SE, ed. Adjuvant therapy of cancer. Orlando: Grune & Stratton, Inc., 1987.

Adjuvant Therapy of Cancer VIII, edited by Sydney E. Salmon. Lippincott–Raven Publishers, Philadelphia © 1997.

2

Gene Transfer into Tumor Cells *In Vitro* and *In Vivo*: Potential for Adjuvant Therapy of Cancer

Alison T. Stopeck and Evan M. Hersh

Over 135 gene therapy protocols have been approved in the United States, with approximately 750 patients enrolled in these trials to date (1). The majority of these protocols are aimed at treating or furthering our understanding of cancer through various approaches. Pro-drug activating enzymes capable of activating drugs such as gancyclovir into cellular toxins are being introduced into cancer cells. MDR genes are being transferred into hematopoietic stem cells to protect against chemotherapy-induced myelosuppression. Wild-type tumor suppressor genes are being delivered into tumor tissue expressing mutated or inactivated suppressor genes in the hope of restoring normal growth regulation. Marker genes that confer neomycin resistance are being transferred into bone marrow and peripheral blood stem cells prior to re-infusion to determine the origin of recurrent disease.

A major area of interest is gene therapy or gene administration as a method of cancer immunotherapy. Three approaches are currently being used. For example, cytokine genes are being introduced into effector cells to increase their cytotoxicity. The interferon-γ or TNF genes have been transferred into tumor-infiltrating lymphocytes (TIL) to increase cell-mediated cytotoxicity (2). Effector cells can also be transfected with T-cell receptors engineered with a specificity of choice. A current clinical trial employs effector lymphocytes modified to express a T-cell receptor with reactivity to HIV GP120. A second approach is to introduce genes into tumor cells which increase their immunogenicity. This is the most common approach currently in human clinical trials, and typically involves the transfer of cytokine genes or genes of co-stimulatory molecules, such as B7.1 or B7.2, into tumor cells. A third approach is to encode the genes for tumor-specific antigens into appropriate delivery systems. This allows immunostimulatory genes to be directly introduced into muscle or antigen-presenting cells for generation of specific anti-tumor cytotoxic effects.

GENETICALLY MODIFIED TUMOR VACCINES

Much of the animal work and current clinical trials are focused on developing genetically modified tumor cell vaccines. Previous vaccine trials utilizing non-specific immunostimulants or poorly immunogenic tumor cells have produced disappointing results (3,4). Theoretically, by specifically stimulating the immune system to produce long-lasting anti-tumor immunologic memory, genetically modified tumor cell vaccines will lead to improved success.

Genetically modified tumor cell vaccines can be divided into two broad categories. In the first approach, tumor cells are removed from the patient, the gene of interest is transferred into the tumor cells and the now genetically modified tumor cells are reintroduced into the patient as a vaccine. This method allows for selection of tumor cells expressing high quantities of the transferred gene prior to reintroduction into the patient. The technical difficulties of establishing short-term tumor cultures, time required for generating and selecting sufficient numbers of genetically modified tumor cells, and cost and morbidity of the required surgeries for tumor procurement limit the applicability of this *in vitro*/*in vivo* approach.

In the *in vivo* method, genes of interest are directly introduced into the tumor by intratumoral injection. Specific tumor immunity may also be generated through direct intramuscular injection of plasmids expressing cloned tumor antigens. For example, Ulmer et al. have induced specific anti-influenza CTL responses in mice after intramuscular injection of naked plasmid DNA encoding an influenza gene (5). This approach eliminates much of the cost and time constraints of the *in vitro*/*in vivo* approach, but is limited by inefficient transfection techniques and poor expression of the transferred gene *in vivo*.

LESSONS FROM ANIMAL MODELS

Both of these vaccine approaches using genetically modified tumor cells have been studied extensively in murine models. Multiple cytokines including interleukin-1, interleukin-2, interleukin-4, interleukin-6, interleukin-7, interleukin-10, interleukin-12, GM-CSF, and interferon-γ have been transferred into murine tumor cell lines (6–8). Generally, these cytokine-modified tumor cells are less tumorogenic and produce specific CTL responses against unmodified or wild-type tumor cells. Vaccination with genetically modified tumor cells has also produced rejection of wild-type tumor cells on re-challenge and occasional regressions of pre-existing tumors when tumor burden is limited at the start of the vaccination protocol.

Animal studies have also suggested areas that need further study. For example, the most effective cytokine at producing specific anti-tumor immunologic responses varies depending on experimental design, mouse strain, and tumor cell line used. Only mice with small tumor burdens are cured after treatment with genetically modified tumor cell vaccines. Transferring multiple genes into tumor cells is sometimes, but not always, more effective than single-gene transfections (9,10). Gene transfection efficiencies, *in vitro* growth conditions, host immune function, and tumor procurement are easily optimized in murine tumor models, but not in human cancer patients. The immediate environment of the tumor may effect host immune response. Orthotopically implanted tumors may be more resistant to vaccine therapy than subcutaneously implanted tumors (11). Thus, animal models have provided the "proof of principle": tumor cells can be genetically modified to produce host CTL responses against unmodified tumor cells that lead to slowed progression or disease regression of wild-type tumor. Unfortunately, animal studies cannot adequately model the complexity and heterogeneity of human cancers and cancer patients. Well designed and executed phase I/II clinical trials are necessary for understanding the biology, immunology, and therapeutic potential of genetically modified tumor cell vaccines in patients.

HUMAN CLINICAL TRIALS

We have been involved in three gene therapy trials to date involving direct intratumoral gene injection (Table 2-1). All of these trials have used cationic lipid to carry plasmid DNA into tumor cells. Our first trial, sponsored by Vical Inc. (San Diego, CA), involved the treatment of patients with metastatic melanoma with Allovectin-7, a formulation of cationic lipid, DMRIE/DOPE, combined with plasmid DNA encoding the major histocompatibility gene (MHC), HLA-B7, and the β_2-microglobulin gene. The premise of the trial was based on previous animal and human studies conducted by Gary Nabel et al. (12,13). In these studies, Nabel's group demonstrated that introduction of an allogeneic histocompatibility antigen directly into a murine tumor *in vivo* reduced tumor growth and prolonged mouse survival (13). Importantly, allogeneic MHC gene transfer resulted in specific immunity against wild type, unmodified tumor cells. In their first published human trial using this approach, five patients with metastatic melanoma were treated with intratumoral injection of the allogeneic MHC gene, HLA-B7 (12). In all five patients, gene expression of the plasmid was observed. In two patients, cellular cytotoxicity against parental tumor developed, and in one patient, tumor regression occurred at both injected and non-injected tumor sites. Nabel's group hypothesized that expression of the allogeneic MHC antigen on tumor cells stimulated an allogeneic immune response, triggering a cytokine cascade and anti-tumor responses against unmodified as well as gene-modified tumor cells.

In our phase I clinical trial at the Arizona Cancer Center, 17 HLA-B7 negative patients with accessible metastatic melanoma nodules were treated with intratumoral gene injection of Allovectin-7 (14). All patients had failed prior therapy for metastatic melanoma, had a performance status of 70% or greater, normal hematologic and

TABLE 2-1. Clinical Trials of Plasmid DNA in a Cationic Lipid Vector (DMRIE/DOPE)

First Author	Gene	Tumor Type	Evaluable/ Entered	Gene Expressed	Objective Tumor Shrinkage
Nabel	HLA-B7	Melanoma	5/5	5	1
Nabel	HLA-B7	Melanoma	10/10	9	2
Stopeck	HLA-B7	Melanoma	14/17	13	7
Vogelzang	HLA-B7	Melanoma	14/16	12	0
Rubin	HLA-B7	Colon	15/16	12	0
Stopeck	IL-2	Various	24	TE	1

blood chemistry parameters, and a normal lymphocyte proliferative response *in vitro* to the mitogen PHA. The protocol was approved by the Human Subjects Committee of Arizona Health Sciences Center, the Biological Safety Committees of the University of Arizona and Vical, Inc., the Recombinant Advisory Committee of the National Institutes of Health, and the Food and Drug Admininstration.

Eleven men and six women were treated with intratumoral Allovectin-7. Twelve patients received a single dose of 10, 50, or 250 μg plasmid DNA formulated with cationic lipid. Five patients received two or three gene injections with 10 μg plasmid DNA at 2-week intervals. The same nodule was re-treated in patients who received multiple injections. Tumor sites injected included lymph nodes, lung nodules, liver nodules, and skin nodules. All gene injections were given in the outpatient setting. Fourteen patients underwent the required post-therapy biopsies and 6 week observation period and were thus considered evaluable. Median follow-up post-gene injection was 6.5 months, with minimum and maximum follow-up of 6 weeks and 22 months, respectively.

The only toxicities observed were directly related to complications of biopsy or gene injection procedures. These included pain requiring narcotics in 4 patients, pneumothorax in 2 patients, and hematoma or hemorrhage in 5 patients. Expression of the plasmid at the DNA (PCR analysis), mRNA (RT-PCR analysis), or protein (FACs or immunohistochemical analysis) level was found in 93% of patients' tumors post-gene injection. Half of the patients developed immune reactivity to HLA-B7 as evidenced by the ability of their lymphocytes to kill HLA-B7-positive peripheral blood lymphocytes in a cytotoxicity assay. Increased numbers of CD4- or CD8-positive lymphocytes were seen in post–gene-therapy tumor biopsies in 5 patients.

Seven of the 14 evaluable patients had a 25% or greater decrease in the size of their injected nodule. No significant regressions were seen in any non-injected metastatic sites. Three of the 7 patients who had regression in injected lesions have continued to do well. As the protocol contained a provision for re-treatment in responding patients with 10 μg plasmid DNA injections, all 3 of these patients have received further gene injections. One patient, with a single site of disease, initially had an 87% reduction in her tumor size after her first gene injection. She has received two additional injections and is without clearly definable residual tumor by CT scan 22 months from her initial therapy. The other 2 patients who have received re-treatment to lung nodules have had >50% reductions in their lesions and have not developed additional disease sites. The median survival of our 14 evaluable patients is 8.1 months, which compares favorably to survival rates reported in large series of patients with metastatic melanoma. Various parameters including site of injection, previous therapies, tumor burden, number of metastatic sites, performance status, success of gene transfer, CTL generation, and TIL infiltration post therapy were compared in responding and non-responding patients. No parameter appeared to correlate with response to gene therapy, though the limited number of patients in each group precluded statistical analysis or conclusions to be drawn.

Concurrent with our study, the University of Chicago and Mayo Clinic conducted identical trials involving intratumoral injection of Allovectin-7 in patients with metastatic renal cell (15) and colorectal carcinoma (16), respectively. Similar molecular, immunologic, and safety data were obtained in these studies involving 29 additional patients. No objective responses were seen in any tumor nodules. Nabel's group have also treated an additional 10 melanoma patients with this approach and 2 have responded (personal communication). Phase II trials with multiple injections of Allovectin-7 at the 10 μg DNA dose are currently underway in several centers involving patients with metastatic melanoma, renal cell carcinoma, colorectal cancer, breast cancer, and lymphoma.

Our center in collaboration with Scott and White Clinic in Temple, Texas has an ongoing phase I trial involving intratumoral injection of plasmid DNA encoding the interleukin-2 gene with cationic lipid (Leuvectin). Patients with all tumor types were eligible for this trial with similar inclusion/exclusion criteria as above. A total of 24 patients were treated at weekly intervals with plasmid DNA doses ranging from 10 to 300 μg. Patients received up to 12 injections with plasmid DNA doses up to 300 μg without significant systemic toxicities. Side effects were limited to mild flu-like symptoms noted in several patients approximately 2–4 days after gene injection. Gene expression data are not yet available, but only one clinical response has been observed in a patient with metastatic melanoma.

These early clinical trials involving direct intratumoral gene injection with a cationic lipid are important first steps in the development of gene-therapy-based cancer treatment. They provide evidence of biologic activity including induction of specific CTLs and systemic immunity. Clinical responses with associated clinical benefit have been seen in several patients. Furthermore, plasmid DNA gene expression has been documented in the majority of treated nodules up to 8 weeks after gene injection (17). No significant systemic toxicity including induction of autoimmune disease or anti-double-stranded DNA antibodies has been seen in any of the 88 patients treated with intratumoral plasmid DNA injections.

These human trials have also suggested areas that need to be improved and explored. Little is known about the pharmacokinetics of intratumoral gene injections. The optimal schedule, DNA dose, and duration of therapy need to be defined. Studies are needed to understand the roles of tumor burden, host immunocompetence, and tumor microenvironment in response to specific antitumor immunotherapy. As tumors have evolved multiple mechanisms to escape immunologic detection including down-regulating MHC molecules (18–20) and secreting immunosuppressive cytokines (IL-10 and TGF-β) (21,22), several strategies may be required to cure metastatic disease. For example, multiple genes may be simultaneously delivered or gene delivery may be coupled with systemic immunorestorative therapy and low-dose IL-2 or interferon γ to optimize host T-cell recognition of tumor antigens.

Alternative routes of gene delivery are also being explored. While gene expression was seen in the majority of our patients' post–gene-therapy biopsies, less than 10% of tumor cells expressed the transferred HLA-B7 gene at the protein level. The results of current clinical trials involving retroviral mediated gene transfer and selection should help clarify the role increased gene expression will play in improving antitumor immunologic responses. Intraperitoneal, intravenous, or intra-arterial plasmid gene delivery may also improve gene expression over direct intratumoral injection by increasing the volume of distribution of the plasmid. One patient with pulmonary metastases has been treated safely with intravenous administration of plasmid DNA mixed with cationic lipid (23). Molecular biology techniques will also lead to improvements in gene delivery and expression as vectors, promoter constructs, and gene targeting are areas of active research.

IN VITRO STUDIES

Our own *in vitro* work has concentrated on optimizing methods for rapid delivery of genetically modified tumor cell vaccines using cationic lipid vectors. By using fresh tumor cells established in culture for a minimal number of days, we hope to avoid the delay and costs required in retroviral transduction and selection methods. Our initial studies with a reporter gene, *E. coli* β-galactosidase, established the CMV promoter to be superior to an RSV promoter in transfecting short-term cultures of primary human tumor cells *in vitro*. The cationic lipid used was a mixture of DMRIE (1,2-dimyristyloxypropyl-3-dimethyl-hydroxyethyl ammonium bromide) and DOPE (dioleoyl-phosphadylethanolamine) supplied by Vical, Inc. Additional studies concentrated on transfecting primary human tumors with a plasmid encoding the interleukin-2 gene as this plasmid is currently in human clinical trials at our institution.

A total of 33 fresh or short-term cultured primary tumor cells have been transfected with cationic lipid and plasmid DNA containing the IL-2 gene driven by a CMV promoter. All transfections have resulted in IL-2 production above background as measured by an ELISA assay. Median values of IL-2 production have ranged from 5–95 IU/ml/10^6 cells depending on tumor type (Table 2-2). Tumor cell lines identically transfected produced 1000-fold more IL-2 by ELISA assay. Biologic activity of secreted IL-2 from transfected tumor cells was measured in several different assay systems. IL-2-transfected primary tumor cells stimulated lymphocyte proliferation *in vitro* comparable to that obtained with recombinant IL-2. LAK cell activity could also be induced in peripheral blood lymphocytes (PBLs) cultured with IL-2-transfected fresh tumor cells. Importantly, PBLs from patients could be stimulated by their own IL-2-transfected tumor cells to show cytotoxic activity against their autologous tumor cells.

TABLE 2-2. Transfection of Tumor Cells with the IL-2 Gene in a Cationic Lipid Vector (DMRIE/DOPE)

Tumor Type	Number	IL-2 IU/ml Median	IL-2 IU/ml Range
Ovarian	12	9.45	23.7–2653
Melanoma	10	86.7	2.9–794.4
Lung	2	5.0	2–8
Colon/Adeno Ca	4	18.6	2–49
Renal	2	40.7	32.5–49
Other	3	75.6	1.4–85.2

As preparation of clinical vaccines requires freezing and irradiating tumor cells, experiments were performed to ensure that these manipulations would not affect IL-2 production. Transfected tumor cells in short-term culture continued to produce IL-2 up to 2 weeks after irradiation with 8000 rad. Freezing and thawing the cells either before or after transfection did not affect IL-2 production significantly.

Our goal is to obtain tumor tissue during clinically indicated surgical debulking or resection; process the tumor for short-term culture through enzymatic digestion; transfect the tumor cells within several days; and irradiate and freeze the gene-modified tumor cells in appropriate aliquots for future vaccination protocols. Our *in vitro* experiments using DMRIE/DOPE cationic lipid and DNA plasmid encoding the IL-2 gene suggest this approach is feasible.

ADJUVANT GENE THERAPY

The goal of adjuvant cancer therapy is to eliminate residual micrometastatic disease and thereby prevent or delay future recurrence of the tumor. Adjuvant therapy should also be non-toxic as many candidate patients are cured of their disease without additional treatment. Unlike conventional chemotherapy or hormonal therapy, genetically modified tumor cell vaccines have virtually no associated toxicities. Immunotherapy is designed to produce specific anti-tumor immunity with long-lasting cellular memory to prevent future recurrences. Additionally, animal models suggest that specific active immunotherapy will be most effective early in disease when the patient's immune system is intact, tumor burden is low, and the tumor's anti-inflammatory and immunosuppressive effects are minimal. Thus, the cancer patient most likely to benefit from genetically modified tumor cell vaccines is the adjuvant patient with only micrometastatic disease and preserved immune function.

An obstacle to the use of genetically modified tumor cell vaccines in the adjuvant setting is tumor availability for gene transfer and immunization. Many vaccinations may be required to produce specific anti-tumor immunity, particularly if gene transfer efficiencies remain low. Difficulties in *ex vivo* propagation of tumor cells also limit the number of cells available as immunogens. Several malignancies, including ovarian, breast, and colorectal, require surgical resection or debulking as their initial therapy. This provides an early opportunity to process tumor cells into genetically modified tumor cell vaccines for administration to the patient after surgical recovery or adjuvant chemotherapy. Genetically modified tumor cell vaccines could also be readily prepared in hematological malignancies, such as acute leukemias and lymphomas. Patients could have their malignant cells harvested and processed at disease presentation for immunization after chemotherapy-induced remission is achieved.

The increasing number of tumor-associated antigens being discovered and cloned could be used as specific immunogens in vaccination protocols (24–26). Plasmids encoding tumor-associated antigens could be constructed for use in patients with the matching malignancy. For example, patients with resected melanoma at high risk of relapse secondary to regional lymph node involvement could receive intramuscular vaccination with one or several DNA plasmid encoding genes for melanoma-associated antigens such as MAGE-1, tyrosinase, or gp100.

Tumor-associated antigens often need to be presented in the context of self-HLA proteins for recognition by T lymphocytes (24,25). Autologous cell vaccines could be genetically engineered using easily obtainable and propagated cells such as fibroblasts or endothelial cells. Several investigators have proposed obtaining skin biopsies from cancer patients to establish fibroblasts in culture for *in vitro* gene transfer and *in vivo* gene delivery. Genes for immunostimulatory cytokines would be transferred into fibroblasts for vaccination with autologous tumor cells (27). Paracrine release of cytokines from the transfected fibroblasts are sufficient to induce antitumor immune responses in murine melanoma models (28). Lotze et al. have recently initiated a trial in melanoma patients using this approach and IL-4 transfected autologous fibroblasts (29).

The use of easily obtainable and transfectable autologous cells may be ideal for gene therapy approaches to immunotherapy. For example, several genes encoding immunostimulatory cytokines such as IL-2 or interferon-γ, co-stimulatory molecules such as B7, and specific tumor-associated antigens such as MAGE-1 could be simultaneously transfected into autologous fibroblasts or endothelial cells to create stronger immunogens for HLA-A1 positive patients with melanoma. Similarly, optimized antigen-presenting cells capable of inducing specific and potent host antitumor responses could be constructed for many malignancies.

The initial phase I/II cancer trials by necessity were initiated in patients with late metastatic disease and large tumor burdens. The results obtained from these studies suggest that gene therapy is safe and can induce specific immune responses. Animal data strongly suggest cancer vaccines will be most effective in patients with low tumor burden and preserved immune function. Thus, the true test of immunotherapy involving gene transfer or gene therapy approaches will most likely occur in cancer patients treated in the adjuvant setting.

REFERENCES

1. Unterhuber R. Germany playing “catch-up” in gene therapy. Nature Med 1996;2:136.
2. Hwu P, Rosenberg SA. The genetic modification of T cells for cancer therapy: An overview of laboratory and clinical trials. Cancer Detect Prevent 1994;18:43.
3. Morton DL, Foshag LJ, Hoon DSB, Nizze JA, Waner LA, et al. Prolongation of survival in metastatic melanoma after active specific immunotherapy with a new polyvalent melanoma vaccine. Ann Surg 1992;216:463.
4. Dalgleish AG. Cancer vaccines. Eur J Cancer 1994;30A:1029.
5. Ulmer J, Donnelly J, Parker S, et al. Heterologous protection against influenza by injection of DNA encoding a viral protein. Science 1993;259:1745.
6. Colombo MP, Forni G. Cytokine gene transfer in tumor inhibition and tumor therapy: Where are we now? Immunol Today 1994;15:48.
7. Pardoll DM. Cancer vaccines. Immunol Today 1993;14:310.
8. Gilboa E, Lyerly HK. Specific active immunotherapy of cancer using genetically modified tumor vaccines. Biol Ther Cancer Updates 1994;4:1.
9. Dranoff G, Jaffee E, Lazenby A, et al. Vaccination with irradiated tumor cells engineered to secrete murine granulocyte-macrophage colony-stimulating factor stimulates potent, specific, and long-lasting anti-tumor immunity. Proc Natl Acad Sci USA 1993;90:3539.
10. Rosenthal FM, Cronin K, Bannerji R, Golde DW, Gansbacher B. Augmentation of antitumor immunity by tumor cells transduced with a retroviral vector carrying the interleukin-2 and interferon-γ cDNAs. Blood 1994;83:1289.
11. Vieweg J, Rosenthal F, Bannerji R, et al. Immunotherapy of prostate cancer in the Dunning rat model: Use of cytokine gene-modified tumor vaccines. Cancer Res 1994;54:1760.

12. Nabel GJ, Nabel EG, Yang ZY, et al. Direct gene transfer with DNA-liposome complexes in melanoma: Expression, biologic activity, and lack of toxicity in humans. Proc Natl Acad Sci USA 1993;90:11307.
13. Plautz GE, Yang ZY, Wu BY, Gao X, Huang L, Nabel GJ. Immunotherapy of malignancy by *in vivo* gene transfer into tumors. Proc Natl Acad Sci USA 1993;90:4645.
14. Hersh EM, Akporiaye E, Harris D, Stopeck AT, Unger EC, Warneke JA. Phase I study of immunotherapy of malignant melanoma by direct gene transfer. Hum Gene Ther 1994;5:1371.
15. Vogelzang NJ, Sudakoff G, McKay S, Lesting T, Stahl S. A phase I study of intra-lesional (IL) gene therapy in metastatic renal cell cancer (RCC). Proc Am Soc Clin Oncol 1995;14:242. [Abstr.]
16. Rubin J, Charboneau JW, Reading CC, Galanis E, Pitot HCIV, Kovach JS. Phase I study of immunotherapy of hepatic metastasis of colorectal carcinoma by direct gene transfer. Proc Am Soc Clin Oncol 1995;14:228. [Abstr.]
17. Akporiaye ET, Schluter S, Harris DT, et al. Expression of intratumorally injected HLA-B7 gene: Results from a phase I clinical trial. Proc Am Assoc Cancer Res 1995;36:220. [Abstr.]
18. Restifo NP, Esquivel F, Kawakami Y, et al. Identification of human cancers deficient in antigen processing. J Exp Med 1993;177:262.
19. Vegh Z, Wang P, Vanky F, Klein E. Selectively down-regulated expression of major histocompatibility complex class I alleles in human solid tumors. Cancer Res 1993;53:2416.
20. D'Urso CM, Wang A, Cao Y, Takate R, Zeff RA, Ferrone S. Lack of HLA class I antigen expression by cultured melanoma cells FO-1 due to a defect in β_2 microglobulin gene expression. J Clin Invest 1991;87:284.
21. Chen Q, Daniel V, Maher DW, Hersey P. IL-10 is produced by melanoma cells and may have a role in immunosuppression mediated by melanoma. Int J Cancer 1994;56:1.
22. Rozman T, Elliott L, Brooks W. Modulation of T-cell function by gliomas. Immunol Today 1991;12:370.
23. Nabel EG, Yang Z, Miller D, et al. Safety and toxicity of catheter gene delivery to the pulmonary vasculature in a patient with metastatic melanoma. Hum Gene Ther 1994;5:1089.
24. Transversari C, van der Bruggen P, Luescher IF, et al. A nonapeptide encoded by human gene MAGE-1 is recognized on HLA-A1 by cytolytic T lymphocytes directed against tumor antigen MZ2-E. J Exp Med 1992;176:1453.
25. Brichard V, Van Pel A, Wolfel T, et al. The tyrosinase gene codes for an antigen recognized by autologous cytolytic T lymphocytes on HLA-A2 melanomas. J Exp Med 1993;178:489.
26. Bakker AB, Schreurs MW, de Boer AJ, et al. Melanocyte lineage-specific antigen gp100 is recognized by melanoma-derived tumor-infiltrating lymphocytes. J Exp Med 1994;179:1005.
27. Veelken H, Jesuiter H, Mackensen A, et al. Primary fibroblasts from human adults as target cells for *ex vivo* transfection and gene therapy. Hum Gene Ther 1994;5:1203.
28. Tahara H, Zeh HJ, Storkus WJ, et al. Fibroblasts genetically engineered to secrete interleukin-12 can suppress tumor growth and induce antitumor immunity to a murine melanoma *in vivo*. Cancer Res 1994;54:182.
29. Lotze MT, Rubin JT, Carty S, et al. Gene therapy of cancer: A pilot study of IL-4-gene modified fibroblasts admixed with autologous tumor to elicit an immune response. Hum Gene Ther 1994;5:41.

Adjuvant Therapy of Cancer VIII, edited by Sydney E. Salmon. Lippincott–Raven Publishers, Philadelphia © 1997.

3

Development of RMP-7: A Novel Bradykinin Agonist That Increases Delivery of Chemotherapeutics to Gliomas

John J. Grous, Peter J. Elliott, and Raymond T. Bartus

OVERVIEW

The presence of a highly selective blood-brain barrier (BBB) and blood-brain tumor barrier (BBTB) precludes chemotherapeutic agents from achieving therapeutic levels at target tissue sites in malignant glioma. Biomodulation of the BBB and BBTB with the bradykinin agonist RMP-7 has been demonstrated in animal models of glioma. RMP-7 is a synthetic bradykinin nonapeptide with specificity for β_2 bradykinin receptors on brain endothelial cells. Binding to and stimulation of these receptors result in a transient relaxation of tight junctions of the BBB and BBTB, resulting in increased diffusion from vascular spaces to the brain and brain tumor. RMP-7 administered both intra-arterially and intravenously to rat models of implanted glioma has shown selective uptake into tumor of a variety of water-soluble drugs and biologics, including the chemotherapeutic carboplatin. Efficacy studies in rat glioma models adding RMP-7 to carboplatin administration produces a doubling of chemotherapeutic levels to tumor and in survival, compared to that achieved with carboplatin alone. Preclinical and human clinical trials have shown an excellent safety profile of RMP-7, with mild vasodilation as the major adverse experience (warmth and flushing). Initial imaging trials with SPECT ^{99m}Tc DTPA and Ga-68 EDTA PET in patients with malignant glioma have shown an increase in permeability of tumor and brain-surrounding tumor.

Clinical trials are underway with RMP-7 added as an adjunct to both the intravenous and intra-arterial delivery of carboplatin to patients with recurrent malignant glioma.

BACKGROUND

The Blood-Brain Barrier

Hydrophilic substances are inhibited from freely diffusing from the blood into the brain by tightly arranged endothelial cells that comprise the BBB (1). The BBB is characterized by lack of fenestrations, lack of pinocytic activity and the presence of tight junctions between the endothelial cells comprising brain capillaries. While the regulation of these tight junctions is not fully elucidated, recent studies have shown that both luminal and abluminal surfaces of the endothelial cells possess a variety of peptide receptors that are linked to conventional, intracellular second messengers (2). This implies that modification of signal transduction that effects biologic activity within and between the endothelial cells, might regulate the integrity of the tight junctions and hence BBB permeability.

Bradykinin as an Endogenous Permeabilizer

Recent data suggest that one peptide in particular, bradykinin, can permeabilize the BBB to facilitate passage of compounds to the brain or brain tumors which are normally excluded by the vascular barriers (3–6). Bradykinin is a nonapeptide derived from the high-molecular-weight kininogen precursor by the proteolytic activity of kallikreins. Once released, bradykinin acts on constitutive β_2 receptors which have been implicated in a number of physiological responses including acute pain, hyperalgesia, edema, hypotension, and increased vascular permeability (7,8). Cleavage of the C-terminal arginine gives rise to a biologically active octapeptide (desArg^9-bradykinin) which acts selectively on β_1 receptors. These β_1 receptors are induced under conditions of an inflammation and a pathology and have been implicated in mediating chronic pain, inflammation, collagen protein synthesis, and cell proliferation (9).

RMP-7 as a Selective Bradykinin Agonist

RMP-7 is also a nonapeptide designed as a bradykinin β_2 agonist with greater β_2 receptor selectivity and plasma stability (10–12). These features were conferred by the substitution of three unnatural amino acids into the bradykinin sequence and substitution of the peptide bond between amino acids 8 and 9 with a reduced chemical bond (Figure 3-1).

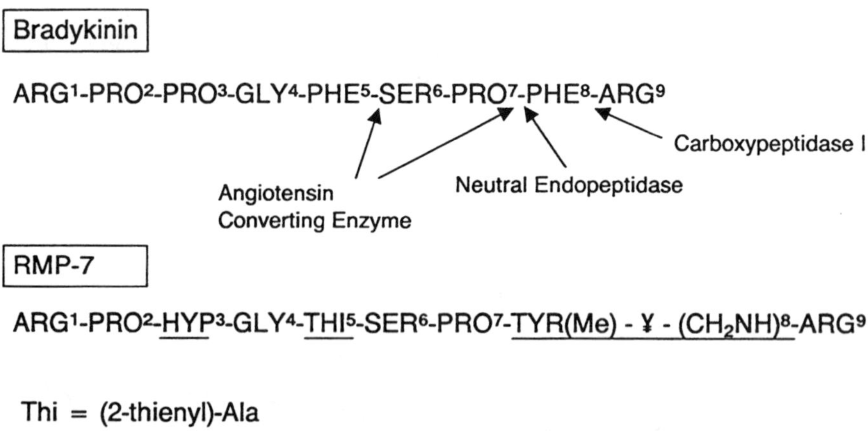

Figure 3-1. Amino acid sequence of bradykinin and RMP-7 highlighting major proteolytic sites. Note that RMP-7 contains three substituted unnatural amino acids and one reduced peptide bond to increase its selectivity for β_2 receptors and to enhance its half-life.

While exact cellular mechanisms through which RMP-7 opens the tight junctions have not been completely elucidated, it has been clearly established as a β_2 agonist. Moreover, the selectivity of RMP-7 for β_2 receptors has been demonstrated in that RMP-7 exhibited affinity for the guinea pig ileum β_2-binding sites, with an IC_{50} of approximately 50 nM, but exhibited no affinity for angiotensin II, neurotensin, vasopressin, and neurokinin binding sites (up to 100 μM). RMP-7 also increased turnover of the intracellular second messenger, phosphatidylinositol, in a concentration-dependent manner with an EC_{50} of approximately 30–50 nM. Additionally, RMP-7 (1 μM) elicited an equivalently robust increase in cytosolic calcium levels, manifested as a transient peak (persisting for approximately 1 minute), followed by a sustained plateau (persisting for several minutes). Peak calcium levels were increased by RMP-7 by greater than 10-fold above basal levels, while plateau levels were elevated 2-fold. Finally, the β_2 selective antagonist HOE-140 blocked RMP-7's effects in both assays while the β_1 selective antagonist, desArg^{10}-HOE-140, was ineffective. These data offer direct evidence that RMP-7 is a potent and selective β_2 agonist, inducing conventional bradykinin intracellular second messenger responses following β_2 receptor activation (12).

Similarly to bradykinin, RMP-7 also permeabilizes the BBB. Furthermore, detailed experiments using electron microscopy have shown that RMP-7 permeabilizes the mouse BBB by opening the tight junctions between endothelial cells (13). Corroborating data for RMP-7's ability to permeabilize other vascular barriers has recently been obtained in rat brain tumors (12,14–16,16a), and guinea pig retina and lens epithelium (17).

RESEARCH WITH RAT GLIOMA MODELS

RMP-7 Selectively Permeabilizes the BBTB

Numerous studies have been performed with RMP-7 using rat glioma models. In these studies cells from tumor lines are implanted into the brain and uptake of radiolabeled compounds is measured using quantitative autoradiography. Because RMP-7 is currently being developed as an adjunctive therapy to treat gliomas in combination with carboplatin, the majority of the preclinical studies have used radiolabeled carboplatin. This typically involves implanting RG2 gliomas into the striatum and 1 week later, administering RMP-7 or vehicle in combination with ^{14}C-carboplatin (though other cell lines, such as D74 and RT2, have also been used). Quantitative autoradiography of the radioactivity within coronal sections is subsequently evaluated with the assistance of an image analysis system, with uptake of carboplatin expressed as the unidirectional transfer constant, *Ki*. By independently defining the location of the tumor within each coronal section (using standard histologic methods), we are able to characterize and distinguish the effects of RMP-7 in both brain tumor and non tumor (i.e., brain tissue) regions.

These studies consistently demonstrated that intracarotid RMP-7 could reliably enhance the uptake of carboplatin into the tumor area by approximately 100%. Moreover, the brain tissue proximal to (e.g., < 2 mm), but clearly outside, the tumor mass was similarly affected. Finally, brain distal to tumor was affected progressively less with increasing distance from the tumor (Figure 3-2, top). Together, these findings encourage the use of RMP-7 as an adjunctive to enhance delivery of carboplatin to tumors, for the most robust effects were observed in tumor-associated tissue, with relatively little effect seen in distal healthy brain. Thus, the results from this animal glioma model predict that increased delivery of carboplatin should occur in and near the tumor where it is needed, with much less effect in healthy brain

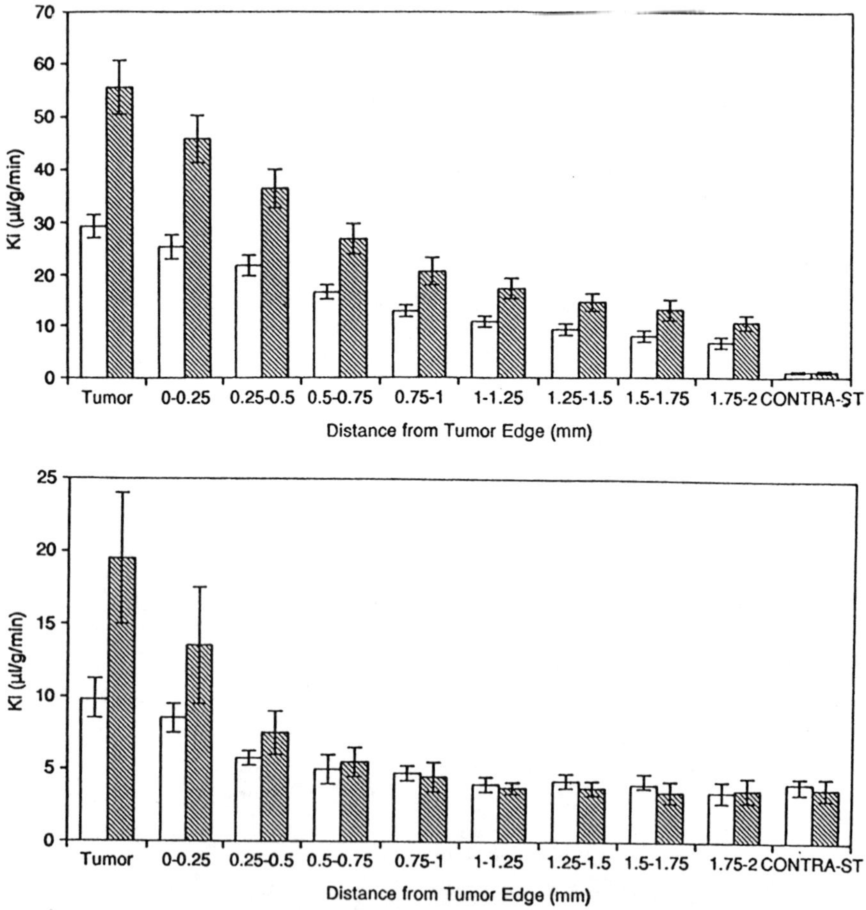

Figure 3-2. Topographic profile of carboplatin (Top) and 70 kDa dextran (bottom) uptake in tumor and brain-surrounding tissue at increasing 0.25mm bands from the tumor edge following intracarotid infusion of either vehicle (open bars) or RMP-7 (1.5 µg/kg; hatched bars). Columns represent mean ± sem. Contra-ST = contralateral striatum. Note that (i) both labeled compounds permeate tumor-associated tissue under vehicle conditions, (ii) the tumor uptake effect is greater with RMP-7, (iii) the effects of RMP-7 are selective for tumor and tumor-associated brain tissue, and (iv) the topographic effects of dextran drop off more rapidly than carboplatin, distal to the tumor.

where delivery of the chemotherapeutic is undesirable. Furthermore, the fact that brain proximal to but outside the tumor was robustly affected offers hope that RMP-7 might provide therapeutic effects against gliomas that have infiltrated from the tumor mass into adjacent brain parenchyma.

Intravenous and Intracarotid RMP-7 Dose-Response Functions

Studies infusing intravenous RMP-7 into tumor-bearing rats have produced results similar to those achieved with intracarotid RMP-7. While both routes display a dose-response function, a higher dose range is required by the intravenous route, while the maximal effect achieved is not quite as great (Figure 3-3). This difference in effective dose range is logical, given the higher concentrations of RMP-7 that can be achieved at the brain capillary target sites when RMP-7 is infused directly into the internal carotid artery, as opposed to a vein. Thus, different clinical considerations will likely weigh the somewhat greater effects that might be anticipated with intracarotid infusions of RMP-7 versus the greater cost, risks, and inconvenience associated with intracarotid infusions.

In studies with animal models, very few side effects were observed with either the intravenous or intracarotid route. Transient hypotension (and compensatory tachycardia) were clearly the most consistent effects seen, being most prominent at the highest doses. In a recent series of studies, the BBB permeability effects have been empirically dissociated from the hypotensive effects (18). The fact that RMP-7 exhibits a clear dose-response function and is void of adverse side effects offers further encouragement that it can be used safely and effectively in the clinical setting.

Enhanced Uptake for Range of Molecular Weight Compounds

Studies with RMP-7 have shown that it can increase the uptake of many different compounds into tumor and surrounding brain tissue. For example, another chemotherapeutic, methotrexate, has previously been shown to penetrate the tumor more effectively when administered at the same time as RMP-7 (14). Additional studies have shown that RMP-7 not only is able to increase the uptake of 70 kDa dextran into the tumor area, but that the selectivity for the tumor relative to healthy brain is even greater with this relatively large compound (Figure 3-2, bottom) (12,14,16).

The effects with 70 kDa dextran predict that the permeability to many relatively large therapeutic agents might be enhanced with RMP-7. In fact, this has recently been confirmed with IFN-γ, TNF-α, and IL-2 (20) (see Figure 3-4). Finally, a recent report demonstrated that high doses of bradykinin were able to increase the penetration of a herpes viral vector into the border of a rat glioma (19). This observation, coupled with RMP-7's demonstrated advantages over bradykinin in permeabilizing the blood tumor barrier (21), offers promise that RMP-7 may provide an even more effective means of enhancing delivery of gene therapy vectors to gliomas.

Text continues on page 26

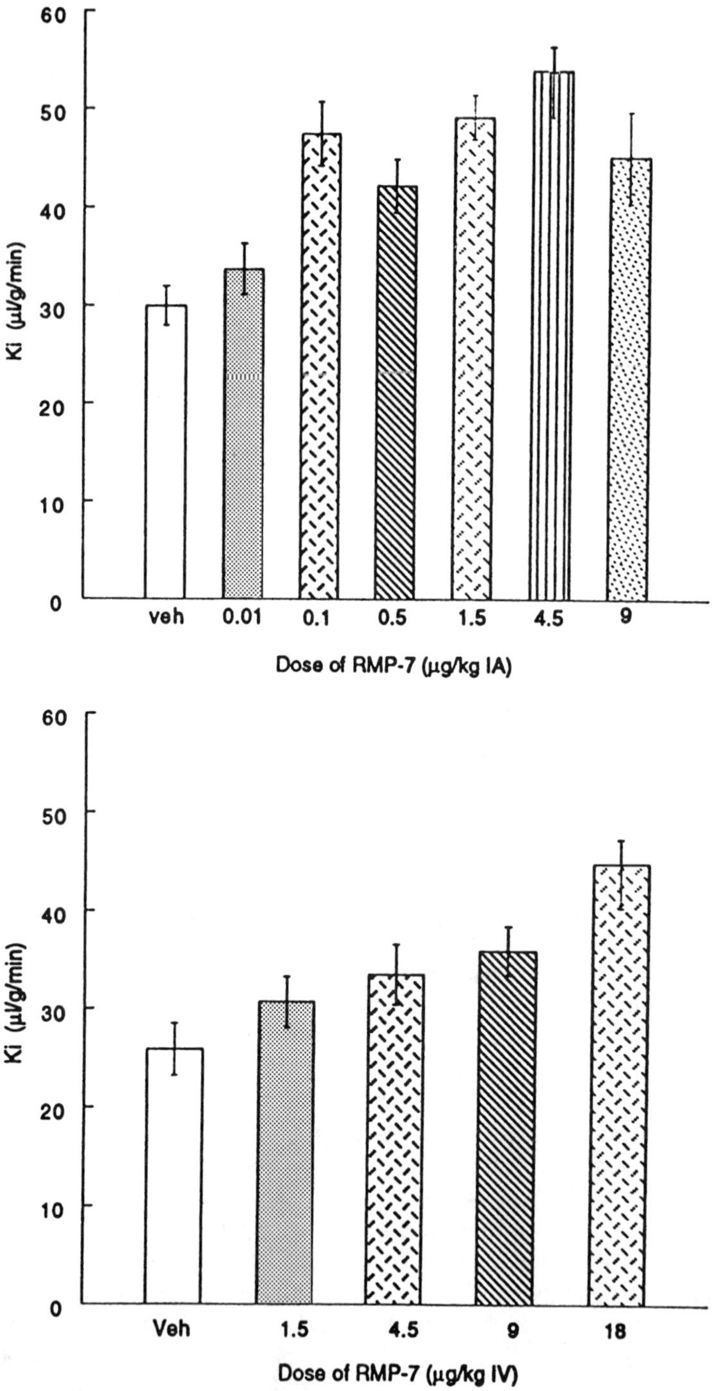

Figure 3-3. Uptake of carboplatin into brain tumor after intracarotid (top) or intravenous (bottom) infusion of vehicle (open bars) or various doses of RMP-7 (solid and hatched bars). Columns represent mean ± SEM.

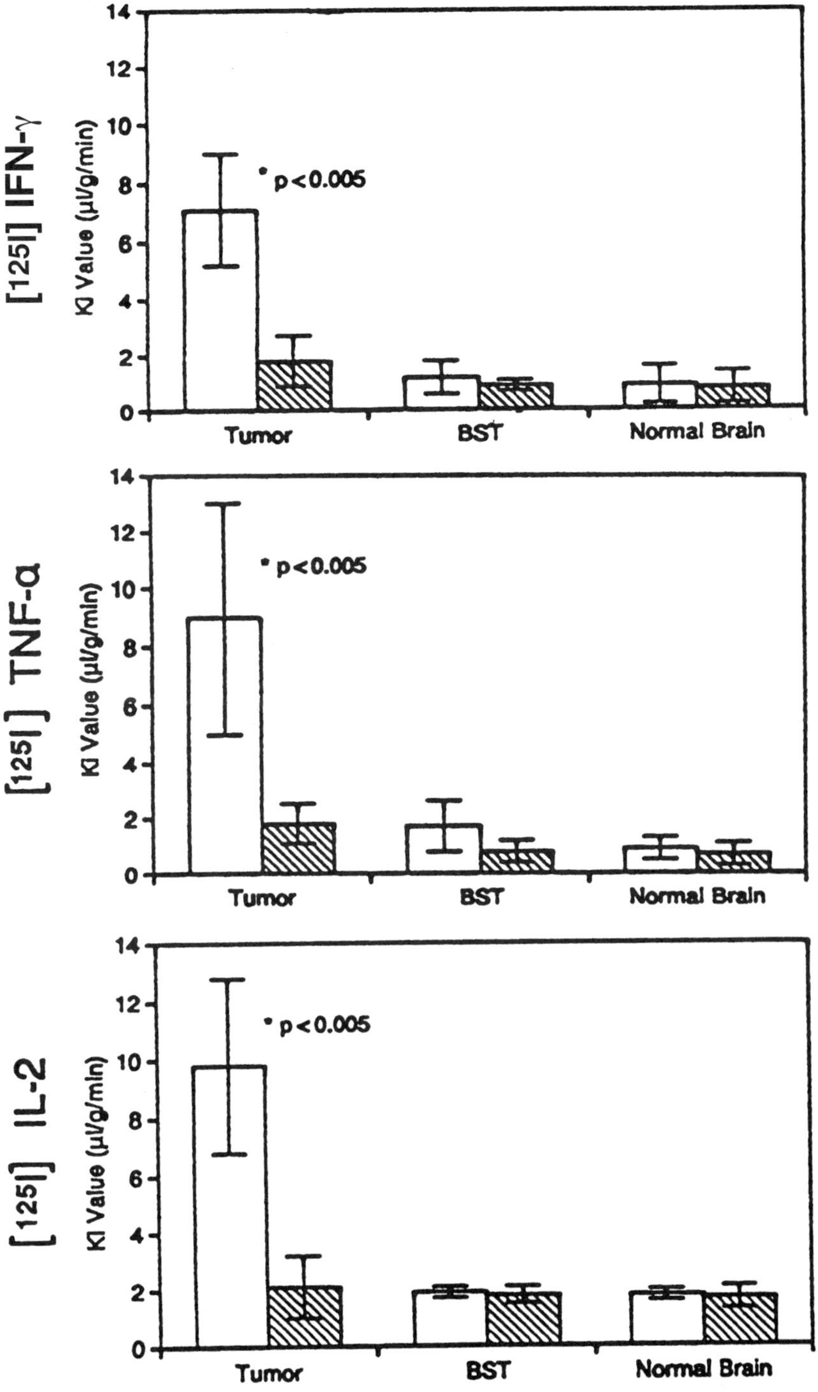

Figure 3-4. Uptake of various cytokines into tumor and brain after intracarotid infusion of vehicle (open bars) or RMP-7 (1.5 µg/kg; hatched bars). Columns represent mean ± SEM. IFN-γ = Interferon-γ; TNF-α = Tumor Necrosis Factor-α; IL-2 = Interleukin-2.

In Vivo Evidence for a β_2 Receptor Mechanism of Action

Recent *in vivo* studies have begun to elucidate the mechanism of action of RMP-7. These studies have corroborated and extended previous *in vitro* studies that demonstrated that RMP-7 acts as a selective β_2 agonist, exhibiting no binding to β_1 bradykinin receptors or several other classes of peptide receptors (15). In the RG2 model, co-administration of HOE-140 (a selective β_2 antagonist) completely blocked the BBB permeability effects of RMP-7, while co-administration of a selective β_1 antagonist did not affect the permeability changes induced by RMP-7. Additionally, co-administration of the H_1/H_2 histamine antagonists (cimetidine and mepyramine) failed to reduce RMP-7's effects on BBB permeability (16a). These data demonstrate that the changes in BBB permeability induced by RMP-7 are mediated specifically through β_2 receptors, with little or no contribution of either β_1 or histamine receptors.

RMP-7 Safely Permeabilizes Barrier

A number of studies with RMP-7 argue that when RMP-7 permeabilizes the BBB, no apparent toxicity or serious pathologic risks are incurred. Thousands of rats with gliomas have been studied using light microscopy and autoradiography with no evidence of edema or other neuropathologic signs noted. This is consistent with other evaluations using electron microscopy in mice (13) and ultrafast CT scans in dogs (13a) which also failed to detect any neuropathologic effects of RMP-7.

There exist many reasons why RMP-7 seems relatively innocuous to the brain and vascular system. One likely reflects the manner in which it acts. First, we have shown that RMP-7 permeabilizes the BBB via stimulation of endogenous β_2 receptors at very low concentrations. Thus, contrary to many other methods of permeabilizing the barrier, RMP-7's actions are mediated through a natural receptor-based system, itself being an analog of a natural, endogenous ligand. Secondly, as discussed earlier, the more robust effects of RMP-7 are in vessels within or near the tumor, with considerably smaller effects on vessels within healthy brain. This selectivity to tumor-associated tissue offers less opportunity for chemotherapeutics to affect normal brain function or morphology. Similarly, even in the brain areas proximal to tumor where RMP-7 is effective, the increased permeation seems limited to smaller molecular weight substances, making it unlikely that permeation of larger compounds, serum proteins, virus, etc. would be able to penetrate healthy brain.

Another reason for RMP-7's safety likely involves the fact that modulation of the BBB via bradykinin receptors induces a relatively transient effect, apparently persisting for only as long as the receptors are occupied by agonists (12,14). Thus, when administration of RMP-7 is terminated, the barrier is restored within minutes. Moreover, this β_2 receptor system is autoregulated, in that desensitization or tachyphylaxis occurs with continuous infusion of bradykinin or RMP-7 (5,12). This phenomenon makes it very unlikely that RMP-7-induced permeabilization of the barrier can create vasogenic edema. Spontaneous restoration of the barrier occurs within approximately 30 minutes of RMP-7 stimulation (5,12), whereas in order for vasogenic edema to occur, the barrier must be compromised for hours (Rapoport, personal communication).

Finally, the multiple classical toxicology studies required of RMP-7 prior to testing in humans have failed to reveal any serious toxicity or neuropathology. These tests have included both single and multiple administrations of RMP-7, alone and in combination with carboplatin and other therapeutic agents. In many instances, these studies have included the testing of doses many times higher than the pharmacologically active dose range (Table 3-1). These formal toxicology studies, combined with our pharmacologic and pharmacodynamic studies in normal rats, mice, and dogs, as well as tumor-bearing rats, demonstrated the wide safety margin provided by this approach to permeabilizing the BBB.

TABLE 3–1. Summary of the Safety/Toxicology Studies Conducted with RMP–7, Wherein No Significant Toxicologic or Pathologic Effects Were Observed

RMP-7 (max dose tested)

- Acute RMP-7 in mouse (53 mg/kg), rat (20 mg/kg), and dog (300 ng/kg)
- 2 Week daily RMP-7 in rat (5 mg/kg) and dog (300 ng/kg)
- 13 Week daily RMP-7 in rat (5 mg/kg) and dog (100 ng/kg)

RMP-7 and Carboplatin (max dose tested of each respectively)

- Acute RMP-7/carboplatin in mouse (5 mg/kg; 120 mg/kg) and rat (1 mg/kg; 50 mg/kg)
- 4 Week RMP-7/carboplatin in dog (100 ng/kg; 15 mg/kg, weekly)
- 4 Week neurotox RMP-7/carboplatin in rat (1 mg/kg; 20 mg/kg, weekly)
- 24 Week chronic toxicokinetic RMP-7/carboplatin in rat (2 μg/kg; 40 mg/kg, monthly)
- Acute intracarotid neurotox RMP-7/carboplatin in swine (750 ng/kg; 50 mg/pig), and rat (1 mg/kg; 50 mg/kg)

Traditional Studies

• Repro/development	Embryotoxicity	Rat/rabbit
• Genetic toxicology	Ames mutation	*S. typhimuium*
	In vitro cytogenetics	Human lymphocytes
	Mouse lymphoma mutation	L5178Y cells
	Micronucleus	Mouse
• Special toxicology	Immunogenicity (DTH, Ab)	Rabbit
	Sensitization/anaphylaxis	Guinea pig
• Safety pharmacology	Cardiovascular	Rat, dog, swine
	Intracranial pressure	Dog

Survival Effects of RMP-7 Combined with Carboplatin

Intracarotid infusions of RMP-7 have recently been shown to increase the survival in an RG2 model beyond what is achieved with carboplatin alone (Figure 3-5). Under saline (and other control conditions) rats with striatal RG2 tumors normally die within 30 days of implantation, with fewer than 10% surviving. However, two doses of 10 mg of carboplatin at days 5 and 7 following implantation increased the proportion of rats surviving from 10% to 40%. When combined with RMP-7, the same doses of carboplatin further increased surviving rats to 70%—a statistically significant difference (16). These data suggest that the effects of RMP 7 on barrier permeability measured as changes in *Ki* (i.e., uptake constant) can be reflected in more meaningful physiologic assessments; in this case, endpoints consistent with a positive therapeutic response.

SUMMARY: PRECLINICAL RESEARCH

The *in vitro* and *in vivo* data reviewed in this chapter provide the empirical foundation that supports the clinical development of RMP-7 as an adjunctive treatment for human gliomas. The results of several published studies demonstrate that both

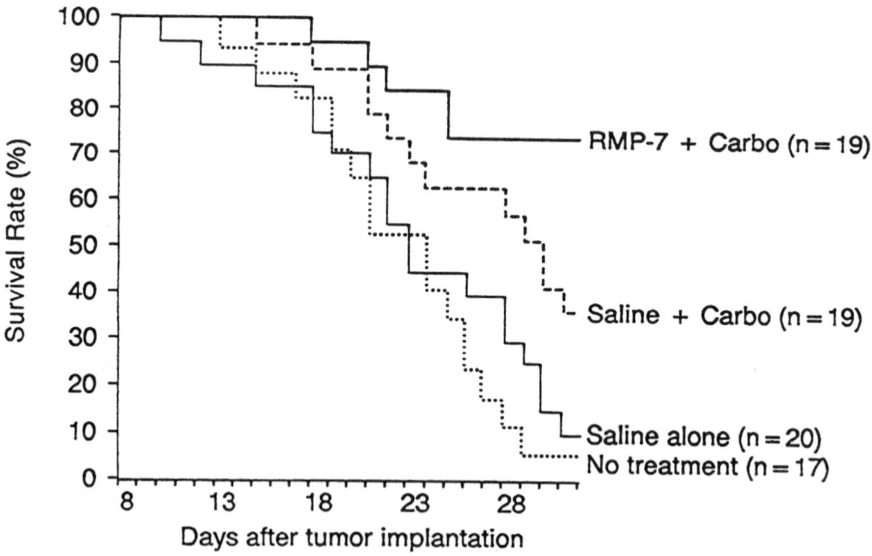

Figure 3-5. Effect of intracarotid RMP-7 (1.5 μg/kg) and carboplatin on the survival of RG2-glioma-bearing rats when agents were administered on days 5 and 7, post-tumor implantation. Carboplatin (10 mg/kg) alone exhibited a modest increase in survival (37%) compared to controls (<10%). Rats given a combination of RMP-7 and carboplatin had a significantly higher survival rate (74%).

bradykinin and RMP-7 can permeabilize the BBB and related BBTB. Moreover, RMP-7 shows particular promise as a treatment for gliomas because it exhibits: (i) a wide safety margin, with minimal side effects, (ii) selectivity for the brain tumor and adjacent brain tissue, (iii) the ability to increase permeability to a range of compounds with varying molecular weights, (iv) effectiveness in various rat glioma models, (v) effectiveness with both intracarotid as well as intravenous administration, and (vi) ability to enhance survival when combined with carboplatin. Collectively, these data indicate that RMP-7 represents a unique and potentially valuable approach to treating human gliomas and offers objective reasons to be encouraged about ongoing clinical trials.

HUMAN TRIALS

Safety Profile of RMP-7

RMP-7 has been administered to over 400 human subjects including normal volunteers and patients with malignant glioma, HIV, and AIDS. The maximum tolerated dose from Phase I testing is 300 ng/kg intravenously or intra-arterially over 10 minutes. RMP-7 has been well tolerated and safe. Mild vasodilation, manifested as warmth, flushing, and mild erythema, has been the most consistent adverse experience at doses of 300 ng/kg and above. Other adverse events at the 300 ng/kg dose occurring at greater than 10% frequency in patients with malignant glioma, possibly or probably related to RMP-7 include (in decreasing order): vasodilation, nausea, mild headache, abdominal cramping, vomiting, pain, mild increase in heart rate, and asthenia. All adverse experiences have been temporally associated with the infusion, and resolve immediately thereafter (22). There have been no cumulative side effects or toxicity with multiple doses. There has been no evidence of inflammatory effects, edema, hypotension, or bronchoconstriction. No clinically significant changes in physical, neurological, ophthalmologic, pulmonary, urinary, and cardiac parameters has been seen.

Increased Permeability in Human Gliomas

Patients with malignant glioma were studied with SPECT (single positron emission computed tomography) imaging with ^{99m}Tc DTPA at baseline and subsequently with RMP-7. SPECT images were obtained at baseline (60 minutes), and with RMP-7 added intravenously immediately after baseline and at 24 hours. Kinetic modeling and quantitation of BBB permeability were done showing permeability surface products over regions of interest corresponding to glioma. A significant increase in permeability was seen in the areas corresponding to glioma after RMP-7 administration with no changes measured in normal brain regions (23).

In another study, Ga-68 EDTA PET was used for quantitative determination of tumor tissue permeability. Dynamic PET scans, with and without intra-arterial RMP-7, were performed for nine patients with recurrent malignant glioma. Changes between the results of the two scans were used to assess the effect of the drug. MRI was also performed to provide anatomic correlation. The transport constant from plasma to tissue (*Ki*) that was related to BBB permeability was estimated using a two-compartment model. Whole tumor *Ki* increased by 46% with RMP-7 (24,25).

RMP-7 and Carboplatin for Recurrent Malignant Glioma

Primary brain tumors occur at an incidence of 17,000 per annum in the United States. The majority of these are tumors derived from glial or astrocytic cells, with approximately half being high-grade histologies of anaplastic astrocytoma and glioblastoma multiforme. These tumors are highly infiltrative at presentation, making the majority of surgical resections incomplete and cures rare. Standard therapy includes tumor debulking either with craniotomy and surgical resection, or gamma knife, followed by involved field irradiation. Adjuvant chemotherapy with a nitrosourea confers a 10% survival advantage at 1 year. Prognostic factors for malignant glioma include age (< or > 45 years), histology (astrocytoma vs. glioblastoma multiforme), performance status, and extent of resection. Treatment of recurrent gliomas includes all of the above modalities. Active chemotherapeutic agents in the recurrent setting include the nitrosoureas (CCNU and BCNU), procarbazine, and platinum compounds (cisplatin and carboplatin) (26–28). In addition, the interferons have shown some activity (29–31).

Phase I studies of patients with recurrent malignant glioma treated monthly with intravenous RMP-7 (300 ng/kg) and carboplatin at AUCs of 3–7 using the Calvert formula (31a) revealed safe tolerability of the combination with no increase in carboplatin toxicity and no change in carboplatin pharmacokinetics (32).

A multicenter phase II trial is underway comparing intravenous carboplatin and RMP-7 versus carboplatin and placebo for patients with progressive, recurrent malignant glioma, in a prospective, randomized, double-blind study. The hypothesis is that RMP-7 will allow planned dose intensity of carboplatin across the BBTB and translate into a clinical advantage in one or more of the endpoints. The trial, initiated in March 1995, will accrue 80 evaluable patients who have received two cycles of treatment. The study drug is given at the end of the carboplatin infusion (every 4 weeks) to overlap the *Cmax* of systemic carboplatin. Assessments include safety, clinical status, tumor area and volume, quality of life using the FACT-BR, functional independence measure (FIM) (33), and a neuropsychological battery of cognitive tests (34,35). The primary endpoint is time to tumor progression; secondary measures include response rates and time to change(s) in the other assessments. Other features include: the use of a blinded neuropsychology tester; safety committees; central pathology review; monthly MRI, clinical, quality of life, FIM, and neuropsychological assessments; and population pharmacokinetics of carboplatin.

Additionally, intra-arterial administration of RMP-7 and carboplatin is under investigation in a smaller multicenter phase II open-label trial. RMP-7 (300 ng/kg) and carboplatin (600 mg fixed dose) will be given supra-ophthalmically every 4 weeks to 45 patients with recurrent, malignant glioma. Assessments and endpoints are similar to the intravenous trial.

Synopsis

RMP-7 offers promise as a new, adjunctive modulator of brain tumor permeability and chemotherapy delivery. A strong empirical foundation of effectiveness and safety has been established in an extensive series of preclinical tests including rodent models of glioma. Tests in humans have confirmed the excellent safety margin of RMP-7, and have demonstrated it is well tolerated. Recent studies in human glioma patients indicate RMP-7 enhances permeation of imaging/contrast agents to the tumor area. Initial trials with carboplatin are currently underway with both intravenous and intra-arterial administration. RMP-7 in combination with other therapeutics awaits development.

ACKNOWLEDGMENTS

The authors would like to acknowledge that the toxicology work presented in this paper was carried out by Dr. Gary Riley, Dr. Carl LeBel, and Norman Kim and the pharmacological studies were performed by Dr. Neil Hayward, Reginald Dean, Dana Blunt, Michael Huff, Pamela Snodgras, Trish Nagle, Calvin Kim, and Christine Pien. We would also like to thank Dr. Keith Black for his insight and assistance in helping establish the uptake methods. Finally, we would like to thank Connie DiStefano for her assistance in typing this manuscript.

REFERENCES

1. Brightman MW, Hori M, Rapoport SI, Reese TS, Westergaard E. Osmotic opening of tight junctions in cerebral endothelium. J Comp Neurol 1973;152:317.
2. Betz AL. An overview of the multiple functions of the blood-brain barrier. In: Frankenheim J, Brown R, eds. Bioavailability of drugs to the brain and the BBB, vol 120. Rockville, MD, 1992, p 54.
3. Raymond JJ, Robertson DM, Dinsdale HB. Pharmacological modification of bradykinin induced breakdown of the blood brain barrier. Can J Physiol Pharmacol 1986;13:214.
4. Wahl M, Unterberg A, Whalley ET, et al. Effects of bradykinin on cerebral hemodynamics and blood-brain barrier function. In: Edvinsson L, et al., eds. Peptidergic mechanisms in the cerebral circulation. Chichester: Norwood, 1987, p 166.
5. Inamura T, Black KL. Bradykinin selectively opens blood-tumor barrier in experimental brain tumors. J Cereb Blood Flow Metab 1994;14:862.
6. Nomura T, Inamura T, Black KL. Intracarotid infusion of bradykinin selectively increases blood-tumor permeability in 9L and C6 brain tumors. Brain Res 1994;658:62–66.
7. Regoli D, Barabe JJ. Pharmacology of bradykinin and related kinins. Pharmacol Rev 1980;32:1.
8. Bhoola KD, Figuerroa CD, Worthy K. Bioregulation of kinins: Kallikriens, kininogens, and kinases. Pharmacol Rev 1992;44:1.
9. Hall J. Bradykinin receptors: Pharmacological properties and biological roles. Pharm Ther 1992;56:131.
10. Doctrow SR, Abelleira SM, Curry LA, et al. The bradykinin analog RMP-7 increases intracellular free calcium levels in rat brain microvascular endothelial cells. J Phar Exp Ther 1994;271:229.
11. Straub JA, Akiyama A, Parmar P. *In vitro* plasma metabolism of RMP-7. Pharmaceut Res 1994;11:1673.
12. Bartus RT, Elliott PJ, Hayward NJ, Matsukado K, Black KL. Bradykinin permeation of the BBB: evidence for a sensitive autoregulated, receptor-mediated system. Immunopharmacol 1996;33: 270–278.
13. Sanovich E, Bartus RT, Friden PM, Dean RL, Le HQ, Brightman MW. Pathway across blood-brain barrier opened by the bradykinin agonist, RMP-7. Brain Res 1995;705:125.
13a. Fike JR, Gobbel GT, Nakagawa M, Mesiwala BS, Seilhan TM. Effect of bradykinin agonist RMP-7 on normal and abnormal blood-brain barrier. Am Assoc Neurol Surg 1994 Ann Mtg, San Diego, CA, April 13, 1994. [Abstr.]

14. Inamura T, Nomura T, Bartus RT, Black KL. Intracarotid infusion of RMP-7, a bradykinin analog: A method for selective drug delivery to brain tumors. J Neurosurg 1994;81:752.
15. Elliott PJ, Hayward NJ, Huff MR, Nagle TL, Black KL, Bartus RT. Unlocking the blood-brain barrier: a role for RMP-7 in brain tumor therapy. Exp Neurol 1996;141:214–224.
16. Matsukado K, Inamura T, Nakano S, Fukui M, Bartus RT, Black KL. Enhanced tumor uptake of carboplatin and survival in glioma-bearing rats by intracarotid infusion of bradykinin analog, RMP-7. Neurosurg 1996;39:125–134.
16a. Elliott PJ, Hayward NJ, Dean RL, Blunt DG, Bartus ET. Intravenous RMP-7 selectively increases uptake of carboplatin into rat brain tumors. Cancer Research 1996;56:3998–4005.
17. Elliott PJ, Mackic JB, Graney WF, Bartus RT, Zlokovic BV. RMP-7, a bradykinin agonist, increases permeability of blood-ocular barrier in the guinea pig. J Invest Opth Vis Sci 1995;36:2542.
18. Elliott PJ, Hayward NJ, Dean RL, Bartus RT. Dissociation of blood-brain barrier permeability and the hypotensive effects of the bradykinin β_2 agonist, RMP-7. Immunopharmacol 1996;33:205–208.
19. Rainov NG, Zimmer C, Chase M, et al. Selective uptake of viral and monocrystalline particles delivered intra-arterially to experimental brain neoplasms. Human Gene Therapy 1995;6:1543.
20. Nakano S, Matsukado K, Black KL. Enhanced cytokines delivery and intercellular adhesion molecule 1 (ICAM-1) expression in glioma by intracarotid infusion of bradykinin analog, RMP-7. In press 1996; Cancer Research.
21. Black KL. Biochemical opening of the blood-brain barrier. Adv Drug Deliv Rev 1995;15:37.
22. Grous JJ, Prados MD, Hochberg FH, Schold C. Safety profile of RMP-7 in patients with recurrent malignant glioma. 7th Canadian Neuro-Oncology Mtg Abstr, Montreal, Quebec, Canada, May 29–31, 1996.
23. Shao L, Alavi A, Lattanand D, Loessner A, Graney W. Dynamic modeling to measure changes in blood brain barrier with SPECT-Tc-DTPA imaging following the RMP-7 injection. Society of Nuclear Medicine, 42nd Annual Mtg Abstr, Minneapolis, MN, June 12–15, 1996.
24. Cloughesy T, Black K, Grous JJ, et al. Ascending dose, intra-arterial RMP-7 and carboplatin are safe and tolerable in recurrent malignant glioma patients. ASCO Annual Mtg Abstr, Philadelphia, PA, May 18–21, 1996.
25. International Conference on Computer-Aided Design and Computer Graphics, Computer-Aided design and computer graphics: fourth International Conference on Computer-Aided Design and Computer Graphics 1995.
26. Yung WKA, Mechtler L, Gleason MJ. Intravenous carboplatin for recurrent malignant glioma: A phase II study. J Clin Oncol 1991;9:860.
27. Warnick RE, Prados MD, et al. A phase II study of intravenous carboplatin for the treatment of recurrent gliomas. J Neuro-oncol 1994;19:69.
28. Dodion P, Sanders C, Georges P, Yvon K. *In vitro* chemosensitivity of brain tumors to cisplatin and its analogues, iproplatin and carboplatin. Cancer Chemother Pharmacol 1988;22:80.
29. Moynihan TJ, Grossman SA. The role of chemotherapy in the treatment of primary tumors of the central nervous system. Cancer Invest 1994;12:88.
30. Lesser GJ, Grossman S. The chemotherapy of high-grade astrocytomas. Semin Oncol 1994;21:220.
31. Black PM. Brain tumors. New Engl J Med 1991;324:1471.
31a. Calvert AH, Newell DR, Gumbrell S, et al. Carboplatin dosage: Prospective evaluation of a simple formula based on renal function. J Clin Oncol 1989;7:1748.
32. Siddik ZH, Grous JJ, Chang S, et al. Pharmacokinetics of carboplatin and RMP-7 in patients with recurrent malignant glioma. ASCO Annual Mtg Abstr, Philadelphia, PA, May 18–21, 1996.
33. Linacre JM, Heinemann AW, et al. The structure and stability of the functional independence measure. Arch Phys Rehabil 1994;75:127.
34. Meyers CA, Weitzner MA. Neurobehavioral functioning and quality of life in patients treated for cancer of the central nervous system. Cur Opin Oncol 1995;7:197.
35. Aiken RD. Quality-of-life issues in patients with malignant gliomas. Semin Oncol 1994;21:273.

Adjuvant Therapy of Cancer VIII, edited by Sydney E. Salmon. Lippincott–Raven Publishers, Philadelphia © 1997.

4

Late Effects of Adjuvant Chemotherapy for the Treatment of Cancer in Children and Adolescents

Daniel M. Green

The treatments for various types of cancer diagnosed during childhood or adolescence have become increasingly successful with the advent of planned multimodality treatment administered by specialists in pediatric surgery, pediatric radiation therapy, and pediatric oncology. Prior to the mid 1960s, many forms of childhood cancer were associated with a uniformly fatal outcome. The improvement in the survival percentages for pediatric patients with the common types of cancer, including acute lymphoblastic leukemia, Hodgkin's disease, non-Hodgkin's lymphoma, and Wilms tumor, has been dramatic (Table 4-1). Approximately one-half of all children with cancer will now survive their disease for at least five years following diagnosis, with most of these surviving continuously free of disease into adulthood (1,2).

The distribution of diagnoses among 5-year survivors of childhood cancer, which will differ in only minor ways from the distribution of diagnoses among newly identified patients, will include many children treated successfully for acute lymphoblastic leukemia, Hodgkin's disease, various types of bone cancer, Wilms tumor, soft tissue sarcomas, and some types of brain tumors. The treatments received by these groups define the spectrum of organ specific complications which may be anticipated in those treated successfully.

The population of long-term survivors of pediatric cancer is growing. The number of survivors of childhood cancer in the United States population was estimated to be 125,000 in 1990, or approximately 1 in 1000 persons between the ages of 15 and 45 years (3). These former patients are now completing their primary and secondary educations, and are making decisions regarding additional education, employment, marriage, and reproduction. Many former patients have concerns regarding their past medical history, and how their previous diagnosis of cancer and the treatment they received may affect their educational achievement, employment, reproductive potential, and life span. Adverse effects of treatment on organ function may influence career and life-style choices. Barriers to obtaining adequate health and life insurance as well as the known mutagenic and carcinogenic effects of cancer therapy may impact on the decision of the former childhood cancer patient to marry and have natural children. Frequently these former patients continue their medical follow-up through their pediatrician, internist, or obstetrician, and direct their questions to these professionals.

TABLE 4-1. Comparison of 5-Year Survival Percentages in Patients Less Than 15 Years of Age at Diagnosis

Diagnosis	1967–1973*	1974–1976**	1977–1979**	1980–1982**	1983–1990**
Acute lymphoblastic leukemia	18%	53%	67%	70%	73%
Acute myeloblastic leukemia	0%	14%	26%	23%	28%
Brain tumors	45%	54%	56%	55%	60%
Hodgkin disease	78%	78%	83%	91%	90%
Non-Hodgkin lymphoma	24%	44%	50%	62%	70%
Sympathetic nervous system	42%	52%	52%	52%	57%
Soft tissue sarcomas	44%	61%	68%	65%	71%
Kidney tumors	65%	74%	77%	86%	88%
Bone tumors	28%	54%	52%	54%	59%

*SEER Registry, 1967–1973 (1).

**SEER Registry, 1973–1990 (2).

In this article we will review the reported research in these areas, emphasizing those outcomes related primarily to the administration of combination chemotherapy to children and adolescents.

CENTRAL NERVOUS SYSTEM

Treatment of the brain with radiation therapy can result in substantial long-term morbidity. Although the proportion of children with acute lymphoblastic leukemia who are exposed to central nervous system radiation therapy is decreasing, with the recognition that intrathecal chemotherapy administered every 8 weeks during the first year after diagnosis is an equally effective form of therapy (4), there is concern that prolonged intrathecal therapy may produce central nervous system damage.

Abnormalities in computed tomographic (CT) scans of the head were identified in approximately one-fifth of patients treated with intrathecal and high-dose intravenous methotrexate without maintenance intrathecal chemotherapy (5). The structural abnormalities identified in the CT scans raised the possibility that abnormal central nervous system function might be demonstrated. In one prospective study of patients randomized to treatment with 2400 cGy cranial irradiation or high dose intravenous methotrexate, a significant decline in the mean full scale IQ of irradiated patients, compared to unirradiated patients, was demonstrated when the patients were evaluated 42 months after diagnosis (6). However, another prospective evaluation of patients randomized to central nervous system prophylaxis with either 1800 cGy cranial irradiation or high-dose intravenous methotrexate revealed no differences in the results on 16 standardized memory measures between patients receiving one of the two treatments (7), although serial evaluation of these patients demonstrated decreased scores between tests performed at the time of diagnosis and those obtained after prolonged follow-up in both treatment groups, suggesting that a common factor, such as the disease or school absence, may be responsible for some of the abnormalities noted by others (8). The results of these studies suggest that intensive systemic and intrathecal therapy produce adverse effects on central nervous system function.

Most former childhood cancer patients appear to have normal intellectual function, as estimated by their educational achievement. Kelaghan et al. reported the results of an evaluation of educational achievement of 2283 survivors of childhood and adolescent cancer, and compared the outcomes to those of 3261 sibling controls (9). There were no differences between the former patients with a diagnosis other than central nervous system tumor and the sibling controls when achievement was evaluated using the percentage of subjects who completed eighth grade, the percentage who completed 12th grade, the percentage who entered college or the percentage who completed 4 years of college. These findings are similar to those reported by others (10). By contrast, a significantly lower percentage of patients with central nervous system tumors completed high school compared to their siblings (77% vs. 83%) (9).

These patients should be followed closely for evidence of post-treatment central nervous system dysfunction. Early evaluation for neuropsychological dysfunction should be performed to facilitate placement in enrichment or alternative programs.

HEART

The heart may be damaged by radiation therapy and several chemotherapeutic agents. The anthracycline antibiotics, daunorubicin and doxorubicin, cause a dosage-related cardiomyopathy. Von Hoff et al., in a study of 3941 patients whose treatment included doxorubicin, reported that the cumulative risk of congestive heart failure was correlated with the age of the patient, the total anthracycline dosage administered, and the schedule of drug administration employed (11). The study by Von Hoff et al. suggested that children had a decreased risk of cardiomyopathy compared with adults at any given cumulative doxorubicin dosage. However, others suggested that the risk of cardiomyopathy was increased in children (12,13), particularly those who received mediastinal irradiation (14) or irradiation that included the lower part of the heart (15,16).

Chemotherapeutic regimens that include an anthracycline are being employed with increasing frequency for the treatment of children with Hodgkin's disease, with the goal of avoiding the serious adverse effects of conventional radiation therapy methods on bone and soft tissue growth, and are an integral part of the chemotherapeutic regimens employed for the treatment of patients with acute myelogenous leukemia, T-cell acute lymphoblastic leukemia, T-cell non-Hodgkin's lymphoma, osteosarcoma, Ewing sarcoma, stages III and IV Wilms tumor, neuroblastoma, and advanced embryonal rhabdomyosarcoma. In one study of patients treated with combined modality therapy for Hodgkin's disease which included low dose mediastinal irradiation and doxorubicin, the ejection fraction, determined using gated nuclear angiocardiography, was decreased in 2 of 14 patients treated (17).

Most early studies of anthracycline cardiac toxicity evaluated the frequency of congestive heart failure during or shortly after the completion of treatment. However, pathological data obtained from serial endomyocardial biopsies demonstrated that histological evidence of myocardial damage could be identified after cumulative doses of anthracycline as low as 45 mg/m^2 (18). The histological findings suggested that anthracycline administration might impair the growth potential of the left ventricular myocardium. Continued somatic growth would eventually result in an insufficient left ventricular mass, with resulting excessive afterload and depressed function. Left ventricular function and/or afterload was abnormal in almost 60% of 97 patients evaluated 1–15 years (median: 6.4 year) after completion of therapy for acute lymphoblastic leukemia that included doxorubicin (19). The onset of congestive heart failure may be many years after the completion of therapy (20–22), and is occasionally precipitated by a physiological stress, such as pregnancy (23) or vigorous exercise (24), or life-style, such as increased alcohol consumption (22). Sudden death, presumably due to arrhythmia, has been reported in anthracycline-treated patients with no antecedent history of cardiac abnormality (24). Girls are at increased risk to develop late left ventricular dysfunction (25,26).

There are insufficient data available to recommend one or more specific tests of cardiac function as routine follow-up for patients previously treated with cardiotoxic therapy. However, patients with a previous history of congestive heart failure or decreased left ventricular function at the completion of chemotherapy appear to be a greater risk of late congestive heart failure and/or sudden death. Those who plan to become pregnant or to initiate vigorous physical training should undergo a thorough preliminary non-invasive cardiac evaluation.

LUNGS

Pulmonary toxicity is a recognized side effect of chemotherapeutic agents, including several alkylating agents and bleomycin. 1,3-Bis(2-chloroethyl)-1-nitrosourea (BCNU), employed previously in treatment regimens for patients with Hodgkin's disease, non-Hodgkin's lymphoma, acute lymphoblastic leukemia, and brain tumors, and at present as a component of chemotherapy regimens preceding autologous bone marrow transplantation, causes interstitial pneumonitis with pulmonary fibrosis, the frequency of which is correlated with the total dosage of drug administered (27). The onset of symptoms is usually during the period of drug treatment, but has been reported as long as 17 years after cessation of treatment (28).

Bleomycin is used for the treatment of germ cell tumors and Hodgkin's disease in children and adolescents and can cause pneumonitis (29). The frequency of pulmonary toxicity is correlated with the cumulative dosage received (30). The administration of oxygen in high concentrations, such as during general anesthesia, may cause fulminant respiratory failure in patients previously treated with bleomycin (31). This complication is not observed when the oxygen concentration is maintained below 25% and fluid balance is carefully monitored (32).

Routine screening of pulmonary function of asymptomatic patients previously treated with chemotherapeutic agents with known pulmonary toxicity is not indicated. However, such patients should be questioned regularly regarding decreases in exercise tolerance, shortness of breath, etc. because these symptoms may signify the onset of clinically significant pulmonary disease. Pulmonary function testing should be performed to determine the severity of pulmonary functional impairment. At the present time no specific therapeutic intervention for chemotherapy induced pulmonary fibrosis is available.

KIDNEYS

Nephrotoxicity has been reported following administration of several chemotherapeutic agents including *cis*-diamminedichloro-platinum(II) (DDP), BCNU, 1-(2-chloroethy1)-3-(4-methylcyclohexyl)-1-nitrosourea (methyl-CCNU), ifosfamide, and methotrexate.

DDP is an essential component of most curative combination chemotherapy regimens for osteosarcoma, neuroblastoma, and germ cell tumors. Renal function, as measured by the creatinine clearance and effective renal plasma flow, decreased approximately 25% in patients treated for testicular cancer with the combination of DDP, vinblastine, and bleomycin (33,34), a regimen that is employed frequently for the treatment of pediatric patients with malignant germ cell tumors. There was no evidence of recovery of renal function 6 weeks (33) or 24 months (35) after the completion of this treatment. Further deterioration of renal function may be observed (36). Others reported the occurrence of renal salt-wasting nephropathy, characterized by orthostatic hypotension, volume depletion, low aldosterone levels, and low or undetectable renin levels with profound hyponatremia in 10% of 70 patients after cumulative DDP dosages of 200–600 mg/square meter (median: 300 mg/m^2) (37).

There have been no studies of glomerular or tubular function in long-term survivors of osteosarcoma, neuroblastoma, or germ cell tumors treated during childhood or adolescence with DDP-containing regimens. However, the data available from studies of adults treated with these agents do not suggest that impairment of renal function will either first become apparent or progress during the follow-up period after treatment is completed if renal function was normal at the end of therapy.

Nitrosoureas have been used for the treatment of some children with brain tumors, Hodgkin's disease, non-Hodgkin's lymphoma, and acute lymphoblastic leukemia and in preparative regimens for solid tumor patients undergoing autologous bone marrow transplantation. Impaired renal function has been reported rarely in patients who received BCNU (38), but progressive renal failure has been reported in several patients following treatment with methyl-CCNU (39). This complication should be rare in survivors of childhood cancer who are no longer treated with methyl-CCNU, and rarely treated with BCNU.

Ifosfamide, an alkylating agent structurally related to cyclophosphamide which has been employed with increasing frequency in combination chemotherapy regimens for the treatment of osteosarcoma, Ewing's sarcoma, and advanced embryonal rhabdomyosarcoma, produces nephrotoxicity, which is potentiated by prior therapy with DDP (40), after approximately 5% of courses (41). Both proximal and distal tubular defects have been reported in children treated with ifosfamide, with the damage of sufficient severity in some children to produce clinical rickets (42–44). The frequency of Fanconi's syndrome following treatment with ifosfamide is approximately 5%, and is more common in patients previously treated with cisplatinum or carboplatinum (43,44), and in those with pre-existing impairment of renal function.

Patients who have received nephrotoxic therapy should have regular evaluation of blood pressure and renal function. Tubular function should be monitored in patients previously treated with ifosfamide or DDP.

BLADDER

Cystitis may occur following treatment with oxazaphosphorine alkylating agents. Cyclophosphamide is a component of most chemotherapy programs for pediatric patients with soft tissue and Ewing's sarcomas, many of whom also receive bladder irradiation. Jayalakshmamma and Pinkel reported that the frequency of bladder toxicity was 34% (17/50) among patients treated with pelvic irradiation and cyclophosphamide, compared with 8.3% (5/60) among those who received extrapelvic irradiation and cyclophosphamide. Nine of the 17 patients who received pelvic irradiation and cyclophosphamide had chronic or intermittent bladder toxicity, whereas all patients who developed bladder toxicity but had not received pelvic irradiation had transient bladder toxicity (45).

Hemorrhagic cystitis was diagnosed in 7.9% (25/134) of children with acute lymphoblastic leukemia who received weekly cyclophosphamide as part of their treatment.

Cystitis occurred after a median cyclophosphamide dosage of 10.1 g (range: 2.0–27.6 g), but was not correlated with the cumulative cyclophosphamide dosage. Cystitis was more frequent among black (16%, 6/31) than white (7.1%, 20/283) patients (46). Hemorrhagic cystitis was reported in 13.2% (21/159) of patients who received cyclophosphamide for the treatment of a malignant disease. Two-thirds of the patients had urgency, frequency, and/or dysuria, but the remainder were asymptomatic (47). Pathologic examination of bladders from patients treated with cyclophosphamide revealed that the severity of fibrosis correlated with the total dosage of cyclophosphamide administered. Twenty-five percent (10/40) of children had bladder fibrosis. Only five of those with fibrosis had a positive past history of hemorrhagic cystitis. Bladder fibrosis was more common in those patients who had received a cumulative cyclophosphamide dosage that exceeded $5 g/m^2$ (48).

The occurrence of hemorrhagic cystitis following the administration of cyclophosphamide or chemically related alkylating agents is due to the presence of acrolein, a product of the conversion of cyclophosphamide to an active alkylating agent, in significant concentration in the urine (49). Cystitis can be prevented by maintaining adequate hydration, encouraging frequent emptying of the bladder, and administering agents such as MESNA which can bind covalently to acrolein.

GONADAL FUNCTION

Damage to the male and female reproductive systems caused by cancer therapy may result in infertility or hormonal dysfunction (50).

Ovarian function was evaluated in women following treatment with combination chemotherapy (Table 4-2). These studies, performed on women following treatment with MOPP or MVPP, demonstrated the sensitivity of the older patient to the gonadal toxicity of such therapy, whether three or six cycles were administered. Younger women have a lower frequency of amenorrhea following treatment with one of these combinations. Although these studies identified older women as having an increased risk of developing ovarian failure after combination chemotherapy, they should not be interpreted as showing that younger women do not incur subclinical ovarian damage from such treatment. Premature menopause is well documented in childhood cancer survivors (56). Prolonged follow-up will be necessary to determine if these young women enter menopause prematurely or suffer other effects from this treatment.

Loss of ovarian function following chemotherapy administration is associated with significant changes in libido and sexual function (57). Recovery of ovarian function is unlikely if menstrual periods do not return within 3 months after cessation of treatment (58).

Chapman and Sutcliffe reported that permanent amenorrhea did not occur in six women, aged 18–31 years, who received an oral contraceptive during the period of treatment with MVPP. These authors attributed the lack of amenorrhea to suppression of ovarian function by the oral contraceptive agent, but the study subjects were in an age group known to have a lower frequency of post-therapy amenorrhea (59). Whitehead et al. were unable to demonstrate a protective effect of oral contraceptive administration among women treated with MVPP (54).

TABLE 4-2. Frequency of Amenorrhea Following Treatment with Combination Chemotherapy

Author	Frequency of Amenorrhea	Follow-Up (months)
Chapman (51)		10–78
30–51 years	84% (21/25)	
< 30 years	31% (5/16)	
Schilsky (52)		24–168
< 25 years	20% (3/15)	
> 25 years	89% (8/9)	
Andrieu (53)		
16–30 years		
3 cycles	3% (1/31)	
6 cycles	9% (1/11)	
31–45 years		
3 cycles	61% (11/18)	
6 cycles	62% (5/8)	
Whitehead (54)	39% (17/44)	6–120
King (55)	55% (10/18)	6–120

Ovarian function was evaluated in patients treated with drug combinations that did not include procarbazine. Green et al. reported normal ovarian function in 100% (6/6) of women treated for non-Hodgkin's lymphoma with a cyclophosphamide containing drug combination (60). Siris et al. reported that pubertal progression was adversely affected in 5.8% (1/17) of patients treated before puberty, compared to 33.3% (6/18) of patients treated during puberty or after menarche. However, the administration of cyclophosphamide did not correlate with the abnormal pubertal progression observed in these patients (61).

Combination chemotherapy that includes an alkylating agent and procarbazine causes severe damage to the testicular germinal epithelium (Table 4-3). Chapman et al. evaluated 64 men following completion of six cycles of MVPP chemotherapy. Twenty-six of 27 (96.2%) were azoospermic when evaluated 0–12 months after the completion of therapy. Sixteen of 19 (84.2%) of those evaluated 37–48 months after treatment were azoospermic, suggesting that recovery of spermatogenesis in this population of patients was infrequent (65). Forty-seven men with Hodgkin's disease were evaluated in a prospective study of the effect of MVPP on testicular function. All men were azoospermic or had ejaculates which contained low numbers of non-motile sperm after the beginning of the third cycle of chemotherapy (66). Azoospermia occurs less frequently following treatment with two, rather than six, cycles of MOPP (67).

TABLE 4-3. Frequency of Azoospermia after Combination Chemotherapy

Author	Treatment Regimen	Frequency of Azoospermia	Follow-Up
DeVita (62)	MOPP	60% (6/10)	NA
Asbjornsen (63)	M(O/V)PP, COPP	87% (5/6)	12–29 months
Sherins (64)	MOPP	100% (6/6)	NA
Chapman (65)	MVPP	83% (54/64)	1–62 months
Chapman (66)	MVPP	100% (14/14)	NA
da Cunha (67)	MOPP		
2 cycles		0% (0/7)	
6 cycles		90% (9/10)	
King (55)	MVPP	70% (14/20)	2–120 months
Charak (68)	COPP	100% (92/92)	1–17 years
Clark (69)	MVPP	93% (14/15)	NA
	ChlVPP/EVA	95% (21/22)	NA
Viviani (70)	MOPP	86% (18/21)	4–67 months
	ABVD	0% (0/13)	2–80 months

Roeser compared the toxicity of a drug combination that did and did not contain procarbazine. Six of 6 (100%) men became azoospermic following treatment with MOPP. One patient recovered spermatogenesis, whereas the remaining 5 men were azoospermic when evaluated 6–54 months after diagnosis. Ten additional men were treated for non-Hodgkin's lymphoma with cyclophosphamide, vincristine, and prednisone. All had an elevated serum FSH level when treatment was completed. However, evaluations 13–24 months after therapy demonstrated that 70% (7/10) of these men had normal serum FSH levels, with 4 of the 7 having evidence of spermatogenesis in semen samples (71). The combination of doxorubicin, bleomycin, vinblastine, and DTIC produces oligo- or azoospermia frequently during the course of treatment. However, recovery of spermatogenesis occurs frequently after treatment is completed, in contrast to the experience reported following treatment with MOPP (Table 4-3) (70).

Sherins et al. suggested that the prepubertal testis was less sensitive than the postpubertal testis to damage by MOPP chemotherapy (64). Two groups of investigators reported that damage to the prepubertal testis cannot be identified until the patient enters puberty, if the frequency of testicular damage is estimated by the presence of an elevated serum FSH level. Green et al. obtained serial serum FSH levels from 3 patients treated with chemotherapy for Hodgkin's's disease prior to puberty. The FSH levels remained normal until pubarche, at which time abnormally high levels were found (72). A similar FSH pattern was reported in 1 patient studied by Whitehead et al. (73). Shafford confirmed the high incidence of azoospermia among males following treatment during childhood or adolescence with the combination of chlorambucil, vinblastine, procarbazine, and prednisone (74), a finding consistent with data reported for adult males treated with the same combination (75).

Testicular function has been evaluated in patients following treatment with combination chemotherapy for acute lymphoblastic leukemia during childhood. Basal serum FSH and LH levels were normal in 32 prepubertal boys evaluated, whereas 3/8 (37.5%) early pubertal and 2/4 (50%) late pubertal subjects had raised basal serum FSH levels. The tubular fertility index of the prepubertal subjects was 49%, suggesting that significant tubular damage was present despite the normal serum gonadotropin levels (76). The factors which influenced the severity of testicular damage, as estimated by the tubular fertility index, were the total dose of cyclophosphamide, administration of a cumulative dose of cytosine arabinoside that exceeded 1 g/m^2, and the length of time between the cessation of treatment and testicular biopsy (77).

Blatt et al. reported normal testicular function in 14 boys treated for ALL with therapy that did not include either cyclophosphamide or intravenous cytosine arabinoside, emphasizing the importance of the agents employed in determining the gonadal toxicity of a combination chemotherapy program (78).

Most chemotherapeutic agents are mutagenic, with the potential to cause germ cell chromosomal injury. Possible results of such injury include an increase in the frequency of genetic diseases and congenital anomalies in the offspring of successfully treated pediatric and adolescent cancer patients.

Several early studies of the offspring of patients treated for diverse types of childhood cancer identified no effect of previous treatment on pregnancy outcome and no increase in the frequency of congenital anomalies in the offspring (79–81). However, a study of offspring of patients treated for Wilms tumor demonstrated that the birthweight of children born to women who had received abdominal irradiation was significantly lower than that of children born to women who had not received such irradiation (82), a finding that was confirmed in several subsequent studies (83–85).

Prior studies of offspring of childhood cancer survivors were limited by the size of the population of offspring and the number of former patients who had been exposed to mutagenic therapy. Several recent studies that attempted to address some of these limitations did not identify an increased frequency of major congenital malformations (81,86,87), genetic disease (81), or childhood cancer (88,89) in the offspring of former pediatric cancer patients.

In general, the studies of pregnancy outcome following treatment with chemotherapeutic agents are reassuring with respect to the possible increased occurrence of congenital malformations or genetic diseases in the offspring. However, the number of exposed patients available for study is still small, and the follow-up of those offspring who have been identified is short, precluding definitive statements regarding the risk of cancer in the offspring.

SECOND MALIGNANT TUMORS

The occurrence of second malignant neoplasms is a devastating reality of successful treatment for some types of childhood cancer. The reported cumulative frequency of second malignant tumors was 3.7–12.1% at 25 years after diagnosis (90–95). These series differed in the time period during which the patients were treated, the completeness of follow-up, and the treatment exposures experienced by the patients (Table 4-4). One series identified radiation therapy as the most significant factor associated with the risk of a second malignant tumor (90), although radiation therapy was shown in three pediatric cohort studies to have no effect on the risk of a second cancer (93–95). Case-control studies have documented a clear relationship between prior therapeutic irradiation and the occurrence of sarcomas of bone (96), tumors of the brain and nervous system (97), and thyroid cancer (98).

Alkylating agents are employed in the treatment of children and adolescents with Hodgkin's disease, non-Hodgkin's lymphoma, T-cell acute lymphoblastic leukemia, osteosarcoma, Ewing sarcoma, neuroblastoma, and some brain tumors. Prior treatment with an alkylating agent increased the risk of developing bone cancer (96) or leukemia (99) as an SMN, or any SMN (100). Recently the alkylating agent BNCU was shown not only to increase the risk of SMNs, as predicted by previous studies, but also to be associated with SMNs within the central nervous system (95). Prior treatment with more than 20 g of cyclophosphamide is associated with a substantial increase in the risk of developing carcinoma of the bladder (101).

The epipodophyllotoxins, etoposide and teniposide, employed for the treatment of patients with acute lymphoblastic leukemia, Ewing's sarcoma, neuroblastoma, and advanced embryonal rhabdomyosarcoma, have been identified as important leukemogens. Pui et al. demonstrated that the risk of secondary acute myelogenous leukemia (AML) in patients treated for acute lymphoblastic leukemia was related to the administration of epipodophyllotoxins, with the cumulative frequency of AML being approximately 12% among those treated twice weekly or weekly, compared to approximately 2% among those treated with the drug less frequently or not at all (102). The risk of secondary AML depends upon the cumulative dose of drug administered, as well as the schedule of administration, with the frequency reported to be 0% among germ cell tumor patients treated with less than 2000 mg/m^2, compared to approximately 11% among those receiving more than 2000 mg/m^2 (103). Hawkins reported an increasing risk of secondary leukemia with increasing cumulative dose of epipodophyllotoxin, but did not find that the risk of secondary leukemia was zero for cumulative doses below 2000 mg/m^2 (104).

The carcinogenic potential of the anthracycline doxorubicin was suggested by the results of a case-control study of risk factors for leukemia as an SMN, in which increasing doxorubicin dose was associated with an increasing relative risk of leukemia as an SMN after adjustment for the AAD score (99). This finding is of interest as doxorubicin is now known to have as one of its targets topoisomerase II, the same target as that of the epipodophyllotoxins. A case-control study of risk factors for bone sarcoma as an SMN did not identify any effect of doxorubicin therapy on

TABLE 4-4. Second Malignant Tumors in Childhood Cancer Patients

Years Included	Number of Patients	Patient Selection	Surgery Only	Radiation Therapy	Chemotherapy
1946–1973 (91)	410*	5-year relapse-free survivors	N/A	69%	84%
1945–1979 (92)	9170	2-year survivors	N/A	N/A	N/A
1962–1979 (93) (1940–1979)***	9285**	3-year survivors	16%	58%	37%
1942–1969 (94)	634****	5-year survivors	9%	83%	49%
1960–1990 (95)	1406	All newly diagnosed patients	6%	58%	85%

*Of patients treated with chemotherapy, 40% (137/346) received dactinomycin as a single agent.

**Excludes retinoblastoma; no treatment details available for 18% of the patients.

***Additional patients included from selected institutions with patient rosters.

****Solid tumor patients only; 47% (250/528) of the irradiated patients were treated with orthovoltage radiation therapy.

the risk of developing such SMNs (96). A recent analysis of risk factors for any SMN in a large cohort of childhood cancer patients demonstrated that treatment with doxorubicin was the only factor identified, in addition to treatment with BCNU, which increased the risk of an SMN (95), a finding apparently extending the earlier suggestion that doxorubicin was leukemogenic, and supported by the identification of doxorubicin therapy as the only important factor modifying the risk of an SMN in irradiated survivors of Wilms tumor (105).

Although most studies of the carcinogenicity of chemotherapeutic agents have focused on the development of leukemia following treatment, it is clear that solid tumor induction is also possible following exposure to one or more chemotherapeutic agents. The best example of this is the occurrence of solid SMNs in genetically predisposed retinoblastoma patients who were treated with cyclophosphamide only following enucleation (106).

Increasingly the data suggest that, although specific exposures, whether to a particular chemotherapeutic agent or to ionizing radiation, may be linked to the occurrence of a new malignancy, the most important factor in the pathogenesis of many SMNs, previously suspected but until recently poorly documented, may be the genetic susceptibility of the patient. As our ability to identify genetically predisposed patients improves, our understanding of the apparent anomaly of solid tumor induction following systemic exposure to a carcinogenic agent will increase.

Patients known to be at greater risk for the occurrence of a second malignant tumor include those with hereditary retinoblastoma. Future research may identify other groups, such as those with germ line *p53* gene mutations (107), as having an increased risk of developing a second malignant tumor. The interaction between genetic predisposition, female sex (108,109), and treatment is not defined at present. These groups should be followed closely for the development of a new cancer.

SUMMARY

The improvement in the survival rates of children and adolescents with cancer is the result several factors, including the conduct of therapeutic trials by the national pediatric cancer clinical trials groups (Pediatric Oncology Group, Children's Cancer Study Group, National Wilms Tumor Study Group, and Intergroup Rhabdomyosarcoma Study Group), treatment in a referral center by trained specialists in childhood cancer who utilize modern multimodality therapeutic programs and increased awareness of physicians of the signs and symptoms of childhood cancer.

Although the success of therapy is frequently evaluated using endpoints such as 5 year disease-free or 5 year overall survival, additional endpoints such as employment rates, marriage rates, fertility rates, and survival percentages at 15 and more years after diagnosis must be evaluated to adequately assess the success or failure of a treatment approach. This goal requires the continued interest of the pediatric oncologist, as well as the concern of the obstetrician/gynecologist, internist, and medical oncologist to whom former pediatric cancer patients turn frequently for routine health evaluations or the diagnosis and management of a late complication, such as a second malignant tumor. Primary care physicians are an important source of information for the childhood cancer survivor, some of whom may not be aware that they were treated for cancer during childhood (110). It is important that, as the number of survivors increases, these caregivers be aware of the problems that may be encountered to facilitate early intervention. One possible intervention would be smoking cessation among long-term survivors, approximately 30% of whom are current smokers (111).

Additional research is required to define the effects of diagnosis, age at diagnosis, family history, and treatment on a variety of endpoints of interest. The large number of variables that must be analyzed generally precludes the conduct of such studies by a single institution due to the inability of such studies to provide statistically powerful analyses. Thus, as has been the case for therapeutic research in child hood cancer, research on survivors of childhood cancer will require the development of multi-institutional collaborative studies.

REFERENCES

1. Young JL Jr, Ries LG, Silverberg E, Horm JW, Miller RW. Cancer incidence, survival and mortality for children younger than 15 years of age. Cancer 1986;58:598–602.
2. Ries LAG, Miller BA, Hankey BF, Kosary CL, Harras A, Edwards BK, eds. SEER Cancer Statistics Review: 1973–1991. National Cancer Institute, NIH Publ No 94-2789. Bethesda, 1994.
3. Bleyer WA. The impact of childhood cancer on the United States and the world. CA 1990;40(6):355–367.
4. Sullivan MP, Chen T, Dyment PG, Hvizdala E, Steuber CP. Equivalence of intrathecal chemotherapy and radiotherapy as central nervous system prophylaxis in children with acute lymphatic leukemia: A Pediatric Oncology Group Study. Blood 1982;60:948–958.
5. Ochs JJ, Berger P, Brecher ML, Sinks LF, Kinkel W, Freeman AI. Computed tomography brain scans in children with acute lymphocytic leukemia receiving methotrexate alone as central nervous system prophylaxis. Cancer 1980;45:2274–2278.
6. Brouwers P, Moss H, Poplack D. Retrospective and prospective studies of the effect of preventive central nervous system therapy on neuro-psychological functioning in longterm survivors of childhood cancer. In: Last BF, van Veldhuizen AMH, eds. Developments in paediatric psychosocial oncology. Lisse: Swets and Zeitlinger, 1991.
7. Mulhern RK, Wasserman AL, Fairclough D, Ochs J. Memory function in disease-free survivors of childhood acute lymphocytic leukemia given CNS prophylaxis with or without 1,800 cGy cranial irradiation. J Clin Oncol 1988;6:315–320.
8. Ochs J, Mulhern R, Fairclough D, et al. Comparison of neuropsychologic functioning and clinical indicators of neurotoxicity in long-term survivors of childhood leukemia given cranial radiation or parenteral methotrexate: A prospective study. J Clin Oncol 1991;9:145–151.
9. Kelaghan J, Myers MH, Mulvihill JJ, et al. Educational achievement of long-term survivors of childhood and adolescent cancer. Med Pediatr Oncol 1988;16:320–326.
10. Meadows AT, McKee L, Kazak AE. Psychosocial status of young adult survivors of childhood cancer: A survey. Med Pediatr Oncol 1989;17:466–470.
11. Von Hoff DD, Layard MW, Basa P, et al. Risk factors for doxorubicin-induced congestive heart failure. Ann Intern Med 1979;91:710–717.
12. Pratt CB, Ransom JL, Evans WE. Age-related cardiotoxicity in children. Cancer Treat Rep 1978;62:1381–1385.
13. Smith PJ, Ekert H, Waters KD, Matthews RN. High incidence of cardiomyopathy in children treated with adriamycin and DTIC in combination chemotherapy [letter]. Cancer Treat Rep 1977;61:1736–1738.
14. Prout MN, Richards MJS, Chung KJ, Joo P, Davis HL Jr. Adriamycin cardiotoxicity in children. Cancer 1977;39:62–65.
15. Bhanot P, Cushing B, Phillipart A, Das L, Farooki Z. Hepatic irradiation and adriamycin cardiotoxicity. J Pediatr 1979;95:561–563.
16. Pinkel D, Camitta B, Kun L, Howarth C, Tang T. Doxorubicin cardiomyopathy in children with left-sided Wilms' tumor. Med Pediatr Oncol 1982;10:483–488.
17. Mefferd JM, Donaldson SS, Link MP. Pediatric Hodgkin's's disease: Pulmonary, cardiac and thyroid function following combined modality therapy. Int J Radiat Oncol Biol Phys 1989;16:679–685.

18. Bristow MR, Mason JW, Billingham ME, Daniels JR. Doxorubicin cardiomyopathy: Evaluation by phonocardiography, endomyocardial biopsy and cardiac catheterization. Ann Intern Med 1978;88:168–175.
19. Lipshultz SE, Colan SD, Gelber RD, Perez-Aatayde AR, Sallan SE, Sanders SP. Late cardiac effects of doxorubicin therapy for acute lymphoblastic leukemia in childhood. N Engl J Med 1991;324:808–815.
20. Goorin AM, Chauvenet AR, Perez-Atayde AR, Cruz J, McKone R, Lipshultz SE. Initial congestive heart failure six to ten years after doxorubicin chemotherapy for childhood cancer. J Pediatr 1990;116:144–147.
21. Green DM, Breslow NE, Moksness J, D'Angio GJ. Congestive heart failure following initial therapy for Wilms tumor. A report from the National Wilms Tumor Study. Pediatr Res 1994;35:161A. [Abstr.]
22. Steinherz LJ, Steinherz PG, Tan C. Cardiac failure and dysrhythmias 6–19 years after anthracycline therapy: A series of 15 patients. Med Pediatr Oncol 1995;24:352–361.
23. Davis LE, Brown CEL. Peripartum heart failure in a patient treated previously with doxorubicin. Obstet Gynecol 1988;71:506–507.
24. Steinherz LJ, Steinherz PG, Tan CTC, Heller G, Murphy ML. Cardiac toxicity 4 to 20 years after completing anthracycline therapy. JAMA 1991;266:1672–1677.
25. Lipshultz SE, Lipsitz SR, Mone SM, et al. Female sex and higher drug dose as risk factors for late cardiotoxic effects of doxorubicin therapy for childhood cancer. N Engl J Med 1995;332:1738–1743.
26. Silber JH, Jakacki RI, Larsen RL, Goldwein JW, Barber G. Increased risk of cardiac dysfunction after anthracyclines in girls. Med Pediatr Oncol 1993;21:477–479.
27. Aronin PA, Mahaley MS Jr, Rudnick SA, et al. Prediction of BCNU pulmonary toxicity in patients with malignant gliomas. N Engl J Med 1980;303:183–188.
28. O'Driscoll BR, Haselton PS, Taylor PM, Poulter LW, Gattamaneni HR, Woodcock AA. Active lung fibrosis up to 17 years after chemotherapy with carmustine (BCNU) in childhood. N Engl J Med 1990;323:378–382.
29. Balikian JP, Jochelson MS, Bauer KA, et al. Pulmonary complications of chemotherapy regimens containing bleomycin. Am J Roentgenol 1982;139:455–461.
30. Blum RH, Carter SK, Agre K. A clinical review of bleomycin–A new antineoplastic agent. Cancer 1973;31:903–914.
31. Goldiner PL, Schwiezer O. The hazards of anesthesia and surgery in bleomycin treated patients. Semin Oncol 1979;6:121–124.
32. Goldiner PL, Carlon GC, Cvitkovic E, Schweizer O, Howland WS. Factors influencing postoperative morbidity and mortality in patients treated with bleomycin. Br Med J 1978;1:1664–1667.
33. Meijer S, Sleijfer DT, Mulder NH, et al. Some effects of combination chemotherapy with cis-platinum on renal function in patients with nonseminomatous testicular carcinoma. Cancer 1983;51:2035–2040.
34. Boyer M, Raghavan D, Harris PJ, et al. Lack of late toxicity in patients treated with cisplatin-containing combination chemotherapy for metastatic testicular cancer. J Clin Oncol 1990;8:21–26.
35. Dentino M, Luft FC, Yum MN, Williams SD, Einhorn LH. Long term effect of cis-diamminedichloride platinum (CDPP) on renal function and structure in man. Cancer 1978;41:1274–1281.
36. Osanta S, Bukman A, Van Hoek F, Sterk PJ, De Laat JAPM, Hermans J. Long-term effects of chemotherapy in patients with testicular cancer. J Clin Oncol 1992;10:574–579.
37. Hutchison FN, Perez EA, Gandara DR, Lawrence HG, Kaysen GA. Renal salt wasting in patients treated with cisplatin. Ann Intern Med 1988;108:21–25.
38. Schacht RG, Feiner HD, Gallo GR, Lieberman A, Baldwin DS. Nephrotoxicity of nitrosoureas. Cancer 1981;48:1328–1334.
39. Harmon WE, Cohen HJ, Schneeberger EE, Grupe WE. Chronic renal failure in children treated with methyl CCNU. N Engl J Med 1979;300:1200–1203.
40. Goren MP, Wright RK, Pratt CB, et al. Potentiation of ifosfamide neurotoxicity, hematotoxicity and tubular nephrotoxicity by prior cis-diamminedichloroplatinum (II) therapy. Cancer Res 1987;47:1457–1460.
41. Pratt CB, Horowitz ME, Meyer WH, et al. Phase II trial of ifosfamide in children with malignant solid tumors. Cancer Treat Rep 1987;71:131–135.
42. Skinner R, Pearson ADJ, Price L, Coulthard MG, Craft AW. Nephrotoxicity after ifosfamide. Arch Dis Child 1990;65:732–738.
43. Pratt CB, Meyer WH, Jenkins JJ, et al. Ifosfamide, Fanconi's syndrome and rickets. J Clin Oncol 1991;9:1495–1499.
44. Suarez A, McDowell H, Niaudet P, Comoy E, Flamant F. Long-term follow-up of ifosfamide renal toxicity in children treated for malignant mesenchymal tumors: An International Society of Pediatric Oncology report. J Clin Oncol 1991;9:2177–2182.

45. Jayalakshmamma B, Pinkel D. Urinary-bladder toxicity following pelvic irradiation and simultaneous cyclophosphamide therapy. Cancer 1976;38:701–707.
46. Lawrence HJ, Simone J, Aur RJA. Cyclophosphamide-induced hemorrhagic cystitis in children with leukemia. Cancer 1975;36:1572–1576.
47. Gellman E, Kissane J, Frech R, Vietti T, McAlister W. Cyclophosphamide cystitis. J Can Assoc Radiol 1969;20:99–101.
48. Johnson WW, Meadows DC. Urinary-bladder fibrosis and telangiectasia associated with long-term cyclophosphamide therapy. N Engl J Med 1971;284:290–294.
49. Brock N, Stekar J, Pohl J, Neimeyer U, Scheffler G. Acrolein, the causative factor of urotoxic side-effects of cyclophosphamide, ifosfamide, trofosfamide and sufosfamide. Arzneimittel Forschung/Drug Research 1979;29:659–661.
50. Green DM. Long term complications of treatment for cancer during childhood and adolescence. Baltimore: Johns Hopkins University Press, 1989.
51. Chapman RM, Sutcliffe SB, Malpas JS. Cytotoxic-induced ovarian failure in women with Hodgkin's's disease. I. Hormone function. JAMA 1979;242:1877–1881.
52. Schilsky RL, Sherins RJ, Hubbard SM, Wesley MN, Young RC, DeVita VT. Long-term follow-up of ovarian function in women treated with MOPP chemotherapy for Hodgkin's's disease. Am J Med 1981;71:552–556.
53. Andrieu JM, Ochoa-Molina ME. Menstrual cycle, pregnancies and offspring before and after MOPP therapy for Hodgkin's's disease. Cancer 1983;52:435–438.
54. Whitehead E, Shalet SM, Blackledge G, Todd I, Crowther D, Beardwell CG. The effect of combination chemotherapy on ovarian function in women treated for Hodgkin's's disease. Cancer 1983;52:988–993.
55. King DJ, Ratcliffe MA, Dawson AA, Bennett F, MacGregor JE, Klopper AI. Fertility in young men and women after treatment for lymphoma: A study of a population. J Clin Pathol 1985;38:1247–1251.
56. Byrne J, Fears TR, Gail MH, et al. Early menopause in long-term survivors of cancer during adolescence. Am J Obstet Gynecol 1992;166:788–793.
57. Chapman RM, Sutcliffe SB, Malpas JS. Cytotoxic-induced ovarian failure in Hodgkin's's disease. II. Effects on sexual function. JAMA 1979;242:1882–1884.
58. Waxman JHX, Terry YA, Wrigley PFM, et al. Gonadal function in Hodgkin's's disease: Long-term follow-up of chemotherapy. Br Med J 1982;285:1612–1613.
59. Chapman RM, Sutcliffe SB. Protection of ovarian function by oral contraceptives in women receiving chemotherapy for Hodgkin's's disease. Blood 1981;58:849–851.
60. Green DM, Yakar D, Brecher ML, Lindsay AN, Voorhess ML, MacGillivray MH. Ovarian function in adolescent women following successful treatment for non-Hodgkin's's lymphoma. Am J Pediatr Hematol/Oncol 1983;5:27–31.
61. Siris ES, Leventhal BG, Vaitukaitis JL. Effects of childhood leukemia and chemotherapy on puberty and reproductive function in girls. N Engl J Med 1976;294:1143–1146.
62. DeVita VT, Arseneau JC, Sherins RJ, Canellos GP, Young RC. Intensive chemotherapy for Hodgkin's's disease: Long-term complications. Natl Cancer Inst Mono 1973;36:447–454.
63. Asbjornsen G, Molne K, Klepp O, Aakvaag A. Testicular function after combination chemotherapy for Hodgkin's's disease. Scand J Haematol 1976;16:66–69.
64. Sherins RJ, Olweny CLM, Ziegler JL. Gynecomastia and gonadal dysfunction in adolescent boys treated with combination chemotherapy for Hodgkin's's disease. N Engl J Med 1978;299:12–16.
65. Chapman RM, Rees LH, Sutcliffe SB, Edwards CRW, Malpas JS. Cyclical combination chemotherapy and gonadal function. Lancet 1979;1:285–289.
66. Chapman RM, Sutcliffe SB, Malpas JS. Male gonadal dysfunction in Hodgkin's's disease. JAMA 1981;245:1323–1328.
67. da Cunha MF, Meistrich ML, Fuller LM, et al. Recovery of spermatogenesis after treatment for Hodgkin's's disease: Limiting dose of MOPP chemotherapy. J Clin Oncol 1984;2:571–577.
68. Charak BS, Gupta R, Mandrekar P, et al. Testicular dysfunction after cyclophosphamide-vincristine-procarbazine-prednisolone chemotherapy for advanced Hodgkin's's disease. A long-term follow-up study. Cancer 1990;65:1903–1906.
69. Clark ST, Radford JA, Crowther D, Swindell R, Shalet SM. Gonadal function following chemotherapy for Hodgkin's's disease: A comparative study of MVPP and a seven-drug hybrid regimen. J Clin Oncol 1995;13:134–139.
70. Viviani S, Santoro A, Ragni G, Bonfante V, Bestetti O, Bonadonna G. Gonadal toxicity after combination chemotherapy for Hodgkin's's disease. Comparative results of MOPP vs ABVD. Eur J Cancer Clin Oncol 1985;21:601–605.
71. Roeser HP, Stocks AE, Smith AJ. Testicular damage due to cytotoxic drugs and recovery after cessation of therapy. Aust NZ J Med 1978;8:250–254.

72. Green DM, Brecher ML, Lindsay AN, et al. Gonadal function in pediatric patients following treatment for Hodgkin's's disease. Med Pediatr Oncol 1981;9:235–244.
73. Whitehead E, Shalet SM, Morris-Jones PH, Beardwell CG, Deakin DP. Gonadal function after combination chemotherapy for Hodgkin's's disease in childhood. Arch Dis Child 1982;47:287–291.
74. Shafford EA, Kingston JE, Malpas JS, et al. Testicular function following the treatment of Hodgkin's's disease in childhood. Br J Cancer 1993;68:1199–1204.
75. Clark ST, Radford JA, Crowther D, Swindell R, Shalet SM. Gonadal function following chemotherapy for Hodgkin's's disease: A comparative study of MVPP and a seven-drug hybrid regimen. J Clin Oncol 1995;13:134–139.
76. Shalet SM, Hann IM, Lendon M, Morris-Jones PH, Beardwell CG. Testicular function after combination chemotherapy for acute lymphoblastic leukemia. Arch Dis Child 1981;56:275–278.
77. Lendon M, Palmer MK, Morris-Jones PH, Hann IM, Shalet SM. Testicular histology after combination chemotherapy in childhood for acute lymphoblastic leukaemia. Lancet 1978;2: 439–441.
78. Blatt J, Poplack DG, Sherins RJ. Testicular function in boys after chemotherapy for acute lymphoblastic leukemia. N Engl J Med 1981;304:1121–1124.
79. Li FP, Fine W, Jaffe N, Holmes GE, Holmes FF. Offspring of patients treated for cancer in childhood. J Natl Cancer Inst 1979;62:1193–1197.
80. Hawkins MM, Smith RA, Curtice LJ. Childhood cancer survivors and their offspring studied through a postal survey of general practitioners: Preliminary results. J Royal Coll Gen Pract 1988;38:102–105.
81. Mulvihill JJ, Byrne J, Steinhorn SA, et al. Genetic disease in offspring of survivors of cancer in the young. Am J Hum Genet 1986;39:A7a. [Abstr.]
82. Green DM, Fine WE, Li FP. Offspring of patients treated for unilateral Wilms' tumor in childhood. Cancer 1982;49:2285–2288.
83. Byrne J, Mulvihill JJ, Connelly RR, et al. Reproductive problems and birth defects in survivors of Wilms' tumor and their relatives. Med Pediatr Oncol 1988;16:233–240.
84. Li FP, Gimbrere K, Gelber RD, et al. Outcome of pregnancy in survivors of Wilms' tumor. JAMA 1987;257:216–219.
85. Hawkins MM, Smith RA. Pregnancy outcomes in childhood cancer survivors: Probable effects of abdominal irradiation. Int J Cancer 1989;43:399–402.
86. Hawkins MM. Is there evidence of a therapy-related increase in germ cell mutation among childhood cancer survivors? J Natl Cancer Inst 1991;83:1643–1650.
87. Green DM, Zevon MA, Lowrie G, Siegelstein N, Hall B. Pregnancy outcome following treatment with chemotherapy for cancer in childhood and adolescence. N Engl J Med 1991;325:141–146
88. Mulvihill JJ, Myers MH, Connelly RR, et al. Cancer in offspring of long-term survivors of childhood and adolescent cancer. Lancet 1987;2:813–817.
89. Hawkins JJ, Draper GJ, Smith RA. Cancer among 1,348 offspring of survivors of childhood cancer. Intl J Cancer 1989;43:975–978.
90. Li FP. Second malignant tumors after cancer in childhood. Cancer 1977;40:1899–1902.
91. Li FP, Cassady JR, Jaffe N. Risk of second tumors in survivors of childhood cancer. Cancer 1975;35:1230–1235.
92. Tucker MA, Meadows AT, Boice JD Jr, Hoover RN, Fraumeni JF Jr. Cancer risk following treatment of childhood cancer. In: Boice JD Jr, Fraumeni JF Jr, eds. Radiation carcinogenesis, epidemiology and biological significance. New York: Raven Press, 1984, pp 211–224.
93. Hawkins MM, Draper GJ, Kingston JE. Incidence of second primary tumors among childhood cancer survivors. Br J Cancer 1987;56:339–347.
94. de Vathaire F, Schweisguth O, Rodary C, et al. Long-term risk of a second malignant neoplasm after a cancer in childhood. Br J Cancer 1989;59:448–452.
95. Green DM, Zevon MA, Reese PA, et al. Second malignant tumors following treatment during childhood and adolescence for cancer. Med Pediatr Oncol 1994;22:1–10.
96. Tucker MA, D'Angio GJ, Boice JD, et al. Bone sarcoma linked to radiotherapy and chemotherapy in children. N Engl J Med 1987;317:588–593.
97. Ron E, Modan B, Boice JD Jr, et al. Tumors of the brain and nervous system after radiotherapy in childhood. N Engl J Med 1988;319:1033–1039.
98. Tucker MA, Morris-Jones PH, Boice JD Jr, et al. Therapeutic radiation at a young age is linked to secondary thyroid cancer. Cancer Res 1991;51:2885–2888.
99. Tucker MA, Meadows AT, Boice JD Jr, et al. Leukemia after therapy with alkylating agents for childhood cancer. J Natl Cancer Inst 1987;78:459–464.
100. Heyn R, Haeberlen V, Newton WA, et al. Second malignant neoplasms in children treated for rhabdomyosarcoma. J Clin Oncol 1993;11:262–270.

101. Travis LB, Curtis RE, Glimelius B, et al. Bladder and kidney cancer following cyclophosphamide therapy for non-Hodgkin's's lymphoma. J Natl Cancer Inst 1995;87:524–530.
102. Pui C-H, Ribaeiro RC, Hancock ML, et al. Acute myeloid leukemia in children treated with epipodophyllotoxins for acute lymphoblastic leukemia. N Engl J Med 1991;325:1682–1687.
103. Pedersen-Bjergaard J, Daugaard G, Hansen SW, Philip P, Olsen-Larsen S, Rorth M. Increased risk of myelodysplasia and leukaemia after etoposide, cisplatin, and bleomycin for germ cell tumours. Lancet 1991;338:359–363.
104. Hawkins MM, Kinnier Wilson LM, Stovall MA, et al. Epipodophyllotoxins, alkylating agents and radiation and risk of secondary leukaemia after childhood cancer. Br Med J 1992;304:951–958.
105. Breslow NE, Takashima JR, Whitton JA, Moksness J, D'Angio GJ, Green DM. Second malignant neoplasms following treatment for Wilms tumor: A report from the National Wilms Tumor Study Group J Clin Oncol 1995;13:1851–1859.
106. Draper GJ, Sanders BM, Kingston JE. Second primary neoplasms in patients with retinoblastoma. Br J Cancer 1986,53:661–671.
107. Malkin D, Jolly KW, Barbier N, et al. Germ line mutations of the *p53* tumor-suppressor gene in children and young adults with second malignant neoplasms. N Engl J Med 1992;326:1309–1315.
108. Beaty O III, Hudson MM, Greenwald C, et al. Subsequent malignancies in children and adolescents after treatment for Hodgkin's's disease. J Clin Oncol 1995;13:603–609.
109. Tarbell NJ, Gelber RD, Weinstein HJ, Mauch P. Sex differences in risk of second malignant tumours after Hodgkin's's disease in childhood. Lancet 1993;341:1428–1432.
110. Byrne J, Lewis S, Halamek L, Connelly RR, Mulvihill JJ. Childhood cancer survivors; knowledge of their diagnosis and treatment. Ann Intern Med 1989;110:400–403.
111. Haupt R, Byrne J, Connelly RR, et al. Smoking habits in survivors of childhood and adolescent cancer. Med Pediatr Oncol 1992;20:301–306.

Adjuvant Therapy of Cancer VIII, edited by Sydney E. Salmon. Lippincott–Raven Publishers, Philadelphia © 1997.

5
Use and Coverage of Novel Cancer Agents in Managed Care

Joseph S. Bailes

Managed care plans currently insure a growing minority of individuals in the United States. Enrollment in managed care plans is likely to increase regardless of legislative action on health care reform. As more than 1 million Americans are diagnosed with cancer each year (1), it is critical for such plans to ensure access to effective cancer treatment.

Cancer is unique in that its routine management depends on novel therapies to a greater extent than other diseases, with the possible exception of acquired immunodeficiency syndrome, an analogous disease. Novel therapies are those that have been recently approved by the Food and Drug Administration (FDA) but are not yet in widespread use, are not yet FDA-approved for a particular indication (i.e., off-label use), or are still under investigation. Patients with life-threatening illnesses do not have the luxury of waiting for drug approval. Novel therapy is often the only therapeutic alternative for the cancer patient who has exhausted standard treatment options (2).

Resistance to providing coverage for novel therapies is a source of tension between managed care plans and oncologists. Such restrictions are misguided for several reasons. Reflex denial of novel therapy coverage does not necessarily save money. Some novel therapies cost no more than conventional therapy, and the prospect for successful outcome may be better with the novel therapy. Furthermore, such restrictions may jeopardize the plan's competitive edge because a managed care plan must offer the same type of therapy as other organizations to be considered competitive. This will become increasingly important when anticipated outcome data demonstrate the benefit of novel therapies.

In addition, plans my be liable if they fail to provide access to novel therapy. For example, a woman who did not receive an autologous bone marrow transplant for breast cancer successfully sued a large managed care plan in Southern California (3). The issue was not whether she should have received the transplant, which is controversial; the problem arose from the managed care plan's refusal to honor and cover the patient's request for a second opinion from someone outside the organization.

The purpose of this paper is to identify some of the potential problems for cancer patients enrolled in managed care plans and to offer solutions.

Originally published in *Seminars in Oncology*, Supplement 14, Vol. 21, No. 6, 1994.

PROBLEMS WITH ACCESS TO NOVEL CANCER THERAPIES IN MANAGED CARE

The need for universal access to health care is a driving force behind health care reform. Paradoxically, cancer patients enrolled in managed care plans often experience problems with access to health care (Table 5-1).

As a threshold matter, state-of-the-art care depends on access to physicians and facilities that specialize in cancer treatment. Oncologists are more familiar with treatment options available to patients with cancer than nonspecialists. The National Cancer Institute has an extensive research and treatment network, both in the community and in specially designated facilities, and patients without access to this network are less likely to receive state-of-the-art care. This is true particularly in the case of childhood cancer because these cancers are biologically distinct from adult cancers. The likelihood of successful outcome is increased if care is provided by pediatric cancer specialists within referral cancer centers compared with community physicians (4). Unfortunately, some managed care plans do not have pediatric oncologists on their panels.

Financial incentives may interfere with appropriate treatment. In the gatekeeper approach, primary care physicians determine the need for referral to specialists. The primary care physician also may be financially responsible for the drugs and procedures ordered by the specialist.

Another problem in managed care plans is limited access to comprehensive drug therapy due to closed drug formularies. This concept, which attempts to reduce drug costs by controlling inventory size, is rapidly gaining acceptance. In 1993, the percentage of health maintenance organization formularies that were closed increased to 35%, from 25% in 1992 (5). Closed formularies create barriers for physicians who prescribe nonformulary drugs. Some organizations are slow to add new drugs to their formularies.

Another popular cost-control measure is restricting off-label drug uses or services. This approach, in essence, allows appropriate drug therapy to be determined by the FDA and not necessarily by clinical trials. FDA approval is often delayed because research outpaces the drug approval process and because pharmaceutical companies may not wish to incur the expense of applying for supplemental indications. This can be a major point of contention between oncologists and managed

Table 5–1. Barriers to Access to Novel Therapy Encountered by Patients Enrolled in Managed Care Plans

Restrictions on patient access to oncology specialists and specialized facilities
Limited use of new agents
Closed drug formularies
Delays in adding new FDA-approved agents to list of reimbursable treatments
Restrictions on off-label uses
Denial of coverage for patient care costs incurred during clinical trials

care plans because many indications supported by major medical compendia are considered state-of-the-art care but are nonetheless off label (2,6). For example, paclitaxel did not have approval for breast cancer until recently and, consequently, may not have been available to many women enrolled in managed care plans.

Cancer patients enrolled in managed care plans encounter problems in gaining access to clinical trials. Protocol treatment often offers the best chance of survival, particularly for patients whose cancer does not respond to standard therapy. Restriction of experimental or investigational therapies was originally intended to protect patients from therapies that may be harmful or that lack therapeutic value. However, this policy has increasingly been used to reflexively deny coverage for state-of-the-art care associated with clinical trials (7).

Coverage of patient care costs associated with clinical trials is often disputed. For example, an organization may cover the cost of a third- or fourth-line therapy such as mitomycin for colon cancer; however, the same organization may deny health care coverage for an individual enrolled in a clinical trial whose therapy is provided by the sponsor.

SOLUTIONS

One of the first solutions is to develop criteria to ensure that novel cancer therapies are used appropriately and rationally. But before considering specific criteria that managed care plans should develop, it is useful to review federal and state trends regarding coverage of off-label uses of cancer therapies.

Federal regulations stipulate that both Medicare and Medicaid programs must cover off-label uses of an FDA-approved drug if that use is referenced in one of the three major compendia (i.e., *American Medical Association Drug Evaluations*, *American Hospital Formulary Service Drug Information*, and *United States Pharmacopoeia Drug Information*) or peer-reviewed medical literature (8). The Health Care Financing Administration, which oversees the federal Medicaid and Medicare programs, has remained silent as to whether biologic substances should be included in these provisions. It is unlikely that the Health Care Financing Administration will render an opinion on this issue, but the law clearly indicates that biologic substances are included.

States are actively considering legislation to require managed care plans to cover off-label indications for cancer drugs. Several states have enacted such laws, and bills are pending in additional states.

The major gap in coverage of off-indications for cancer drugs is created by the Employer Retirement Income Security Act (ERISA). Under ERISA, self-insured corporate benefit plans are immune from state regulation. When this act was passed in 1974, it was intended for company pension plans, not health insurance; however, it has since been applied to health plans. This has widespread implications because most insurance mandates in this country are a result of state legislation; the majority of working Americans are covered under potential ERISA plans. Consequently, recent state initiatives do not improve coverage for cancer patients covered by ERISA plans.

Developing Coverage Criteria

Regardless of federal and state trends, managed care plans should develop specific coverage criteria. The first is to ensure access to physicians and facilities that specialize in cancer to the extent that is considered medically appropriate. All oncologic specialties should be included. Oncologists should contribute to quality assurance and utilization review standards. One often overlooked method of accomplishing this is through the basic contract, which can be used to negotiate involvement.

Solving the problem of access to specialized practitioners and facilities will require comprehensive health care reform. The reform package must include a standard benefit package that also applies to or eliminates ERISA plans. Ideally, the cancer specialist, not the primary care physician, should be the gatekeeper who determines access to tertiary care facilities, handles follow-up, and monitors orders for tests and therapies.

Access to comprehensive drug therapy can be improved by adding new drugs to open formularies immediately after FDA approval. If the plan has a closed formulary, an oncologist should be involved in the formulary committee to prevent delays. Off-label use of approved cancer drugs should be covered if the indication is supported by one of the major medical compendia or by peer-reviewed literature. The off-label issue must be addressed at the federal level because of the ERISA loophole for plans that do not want to cover off-label uses of FDA-approved drugs despite state mandates.

Managed care plans should cover clinical treatment protocols, including the costs of hospital, physician, and other health care services, as well as approved agents for labeled or unlabeled uses. The American Society of Clinical Oncology has developed specific criteria that address these issues (Table 5-2) (7).

The first criterion is therapeutic intent to improve patient outcome as measured by survival or quality of life. The protocol should be approved by a research entity and by the institution's own research board. The facility and personnel providing the treatment must be capable of doing so by virtue of their experience or training.

Table 5–2. American Society of Clinical Oncology Criteria for Determining Reimbursement Eligibility for Clinical Treatment Protocols

Therapeutic Intent
Approval by National Cancer Institute, National Cancer Institute-designated center or program, FDA, Veterans Administration, or qualified nongovernmental research entity
Approval by institutional review board
Qualified personnel and facility
No clearly superior noninvestigational treatment
Protocol therapy equal to or better than standard therapy

There should be no clearly superior noninvestigational or standard treatment. If all these criteria are met, the managed care plan should provide reimbursement.

CONCLUSION

Managed care organizations and oncologists share the goal of providing comprehensive, state-of-the-art care for cancer patients. Managed care organizations and oncologists must work together to achieve this goal. Managed care organizations should take the steps required to ensure state-of-the-art care for their cancer patients. Cancer specialists should take the time to become involved by participating in utilization review, quality assurance, and formulary committees.

REFERENCES

1. American Cancer Society. Cancer facts & figures—1993. Atlanta, GA: American Cancer Society; 1993.
2. National Committee to Review Current Procedures for Approval of New Drugs for Cancer and AIDS. Final report. Bethesda, MD: National Cancer Institute, August 15, 1990.
3. News Services. Family awarded $89.1 million from HMO in cancer death. The Washington Post, December 30, 1993. p A12.
4. Shah NR. The community physician's involvement in clinical trials and home treatment. Cancer 1986;58(Suppl):504–507.
5. F-D-C Reports. PCS manages 21% of retail dispensed prescriptions—Walsh American data: Out-of-pocket scripts dip below 50% of market, HMO formulary compliance nears 90%. The Pink Sheet. Chevy Chase, MD: F-D-C Reports, Inc., March 14, 1994. pp 11–12.
6. Tennenbaum D. Testimony before the National Committee to Review Current Procedures for Approval of New Drugs for Cancer and AIDS, October 25, 1989.
7. American Society of Clinical Oncology. Reimbursement and coverage implications of clinical trials in treatment of cancer. Am Soc Clin Oncol Press Release, February 19, 1993.
8. Plocher D. Statement of the Health Insurance Association of America (HIAA) on coverage for unapproved drugs and drug-related costs. Presented before the National Committee to Review Current Procedures for Approval of New Drugs for Cancer and AIDS, October 25, 1989.

II

Airway Tumors

Adjuvant Therapy of Cancer VIII, edited by Sydney E. Salmon. Lippincott–Raven Publishers, Philadelphia © 1997.

6

Advances in the Biological Study, Prevention, and Therapy of Head and Neck Cancer

E. H. Bernicker, F. R. Khuri, S. M. Lippman, and W. K. Hong

Head and neck cancer represents a major international health problem, with more than 500,000 cases a year world wide and more than 40,000 cases annually in the United States (1). Despite intensive investigation in the areas of prevention and therapy, long-term survival rates have not improved in the past 30 years and survival rates for African Americans have actually declined (2). Many neoadjuvant trials have demonstrated that head and neck cancer is a chemosensitive disease but, frustratingly, high chemotherapy response rates have not translated into consistent survival advantages in phase III studies (3). The importance of the anatomic structures involved and the significant morbidity from radical surgery for locally advanced disease continues to drive the integration of primary chemotherapy into organ preservation strategies.

The majority (>90%) of head and neck cancers are squamous cell carcinomas (2,4). The most important risk factors are tobacco and alcohol (2,4). Dietary factors are also postulated to play a role (5). Tumors of the salivary glands and the nasopharynx have different risk factors than the other head and neck sites. Nasopharyngeal carcinogenesis is tightly linked to Epstein-Barr virus; viral DNA can be isolated from premalignant and malignant nasopharyngeal lesions (6).

Standard therapy for early stage cancer continues to be radiation therapy or surgery. Surgery can give slightly better local control in some sites but surgical salvage of radiation failures is often excellent, leading to equivalent survival rates (2). Unfortunately, only approximately one third of patients present with early stage disease. The majority present with either advanced local and/or regional disease, for which surgery followed by radiotherapy remain standard therapy but with poor results—fewer than 30% of patients will be cured (2,4). The two major patterns of failure after primary therapy of head and neck squamous cell carcinoma are primary disease recurrence (local, regional or distant), or the development of a second primary tumor.

BIOLOGY

Carcinogenesis of the upper aerodigestive tract is believed to occur through a multistep process characterized by the accumulation of genetic damage and morphologic progression through a series of distinct stages ranging from hyperplasia to increasing degrees of dysplasia to invasive cancer. The rapid development and application of molecular techniques to the study of head and neck carcinogenesis has begun to illuminate many of the genetic changes that preceed the development of cancer and should provide new and exciting advances in the early detection, prevention and therapy for head and neck cancer.

It has long been recognized that patients with head and neck cancer are at risk for the development of second primary tumors. This fact has been ascribed to the upper aerodigestive tract's common and repeated exposure to particular carcinogens, such as tobacco and alcohol. This concept was originally proposed by Slaughter et al. (7) who observed diffuse histopathologic changes (hyperplasia, dysplasia and in-situ and invasive cancer) in tissue surrounding head and neck cancer resection specimens. Recent study of *p53* has provided strong molecular genetic evidence for this concept. Brennan et al. (8) sequenced exons 5-9 of the *p53* gene in 102 patients with newly diagnosed head and neck cancer and 27 patients with recurrent cancer. The results revealed that the highest incidence and spectrum of mutations occurred in patients who both smoked and consumed alcohol. Additionally, it was discovered that 100% of the *p53* mutations in nonsmokers and nondrinkers occurred at endogenous hot spots containing cytidine phosphate guanosine dinucleotides, whereas only 23% of the *p53* mutations in smokers occurred in such areas. This evidence suggests that tobacco exposure causes *p53* mutations at non-endogenous sites in the genome and provides a molecular corollary to the observed epidemiology of tobacco-related cancers.

Further work on *p53* has led to new, critical insights on the nature of carcinogenesis in head and neck cancer and strengthened the field carcinogenesis concept. Chung et al. (9) extracted DNA from primary head and neck cancers and the associated second primary tumors from 31 patients. The DNA from exons 5–8 of the *p53* gene was analyzed. Twenty-one of 31 patients had *p53* mutations in the primary or second primary tumor. In all 21 cases there was discordance of the genetic changes, indicating that the development of second primary tumors occurs as an independent clonal event.

Gene *p53* mutations have been examined for prognostic information. Brennan et al. (10) studied 25 patients with *p53* positive (mutated) primary head and neck tumors after complete resections with negative surgical margins by conventional histopathology. Thirteen patients had *p53* mutations in the surgical margins, five of whom later had local recurrence as compared with no local recurrences in the 12 patients with margins negative for *p53*. An on-going multi-institutional trial has been launched to analyze the impact of molecular analysis of surgical margins and lymph nodes in head and neck cancer.

Alterations of *p53* in the tumor specimen itself, rather than the histopathologically negative margins or lymph nodes, also have been evaluated for prognostic significance. Shin et al. (11) performed immunohistochemical staining with a *p53*-specific monoclonal antibody in 69 tumor samples from patients who received definitive local treatment for head and neck cancer. The patients whose tumors had *p53* protein accumulation had a significantly shorter time to recurrence, time to development of a second primary tumor, and overall survival. Other genetic markers may identify subsets of patients with poor outcomes, such as cyclin D1 amplification (12).

Recently, preneoplastic lung cancer lesions were shown through loss of heterozygosity (LOH) studies to have allele-specific loss of chromosome 3p and 9p, the sites of putative tumor suppressor genes (13,14). Studies have confirmed similar deletions in head and neck cancer. Van der Riet et al. (15) using a PCR-based microsatellite analysis, found a high rate of LOH at 9p21 and 3p12 in dysplasias and carcinoma *in situ* lesions, similar to deletions noted in invasive carcinoma. Mao et al. (16) evaluated oral leukoplakia samples and also found LOH, using microsatellite markers for 9p21 and 3p14, in 51% of premalignant lesions. Thirty-seven percent of patients with LOH have subsequently developed squamous cell carcinoma compared with only 1 of the 18 patients without LOH. These studies suggest that clonal genetic alterations are present early in premalignant lesions and may provide intermediate biomarkers of lesion risk and chemopreventive drug activity.

CHEMOTHERAPY

Recurrent Disease

Chemotherapy has demonstrated activity against squamous cell carcinoma of the head and neck. The most active agents are cisplatin, carboplatin, methotrexate, bleomycin, and 5FU, which have produced 15–30% response rates in recurrent disease. To date, despite higher response rates to combination chemotherapy, single agents provide equivalent survival times (17,18). New agents under investigation include the taxanes, paclitaxel and docotaxel; ifosfamide; topotecan; and gemcitabine. Taxol, in particular, appears promising in phase II single agent studies (19,20). Single agent methotrexate remains the drug of choice in the palliative (recurrent disease) setting, due to its activity, low cost and favorable toxicity profile. The best-studied regimen in this setting is the combination of cisplatin with infusional 5-FU which produces an overall response rate of 70–80%, 20–30% complete (20). Similiar results have been achieved with other cisplatin-based regimens (2,4,20). Modifications of 5-FU with leucovorin may provide higher complete response rates but with increased toxicities (21).

Locally Advanced Disease

In the neoadjuvant setting, combinations that provide a higher response rate are sought in order to improve both local and distant control and ultimately improve survival. There are approximately 45 phase III trials of neoadjuvant and/or adjuvant therapy in the treatment of head and neck cancer (20). The small number of patients and heterogeneous patient populations in most studies, however, have made analysis of the data difficult. Indeed, many of the trials were too small to have the power to detect a clinically important survival advantage (20,22). Eight studies have assessed true adjuvant therapy (20)—therapy given after definitive treatment to eradicate presumed micrometastatic disease. Most of the phase III trials of primary chemotherapy have assessed neoadjuvant and/or adjuvant therapy. The rationale for employing primary chemotherapy prior to definitive radiotherapy or surgery relates to better patient tolerance, ability to assess clinical and histologic response, early eradication of micrometastatic disease, and improved drug delivery due to intact vasculature.

The first large phase III trial to assess neoadjuvant and adjuvant chemotherapy was the NCI-sponsored Head and Neck Contracts Program, which randomized 462 patients between (a) induction chemotherapy consisting of a single course of cisplatin and bleomycin followed by standard therapy with surgery and postoperative radiation, (b) induction chemotherapy followed by standard treatment and then maintenance chemotherapy with six cycles of monthly cisplatin, and finally (c) standard therapy alone (23). There was no survival difference between the three arms but the maintenance group had a reduced incidence of distant relapse. Subgroup analysis revealed that patients with oral cavity cancer who were on the maintenance arm had a significantly improved 3 year survival (67% versus 49% on the standard arm and 44% on the induction arm) and that patients with N2 disease also had a statistically significant survival advantage on maintenance (24).

The Southwest Oncology Group (SWOG) randomized patients with locally advanced head and neck cancers to standard surgery and radiation versus combination chemotherapy with cisplatin, methotrexate, bleomycin, and vincristine prior to surgery and then radiation therapy (25). The complete response rate to chemotherapy was 19% with an overall response rate of 70% but there was no survival advantage to preoperative chemotherapy. However, the trial did show that there was no increase in surgical complications in the group that received neoadjuvant therapy and that the induction group had a reduction in the development of distant metastases—28% versus 49%.

Laramore et al. (26) reported on a study of 442 patients with fully resected head and neck cancer who were randomized to either radiotherapy alone or three cycles of cisplatin at 100 mg/m^2 and 5-FU at 1000 mg/m^2/day for 5 days followed by radiotherapy. There were no statistically significant differences in disease free survival or local/regional failure rate, but there was a measurable difference in the development of distant metastases favoring the combined therapy arm, 23% versus 13%. Studies such as this one continue to indicate that adjuvant chemotherapy can decrease the rate of distant metastases, but does not improve in overall survival in squamous cell carcinoma of the head and neck.

Neoadjuvant chemotherapy has also been studied in three phase III trials in the treatment of nasopharyngeal carcinoma. Chan et al. (27) randomized patients with locally advanced nasopharyngeal carcinoma to either definitive radiotherapy or induction cisplatin and 5-FU immediately prior to definitive radiotherapy followed by four cycles of postradiotherapy chemotherapy. The complete response rate to the chemoradiotherapy was 100% and there were no treatment related deaths. There were no statistically significant differences between the two arms in regards to 2 year overall survival, local-regional relapse rate, distant metastatic rate or median time to relapse. The lack of detectable chemotherapy benefit in this study may be due to the inclusion of a large percentage of relatively early stage patients who are effectively treated with primary radiotherapy alone. The excellent 2 year survival rates of approximately 80% in each arm are consistent with this possibility. A potential impact of primary therapy in this disease may be more apparent in patients with more advanced local-regional disease, such as those with extensive cervical adenopathy. This possibility is supported by recent findings from the other two trials.

Eschwege et al. (28) compared neoadjuvant cisplatin, epirubicin, and bleomycin (3 cycles) to primary radiation therapy in 339 patients with N2-3 disease. The 4 year disease-free survival was significantly increased in the chemoradiotherapy (42%) arm compared with the radiotherapy (29%) arm ($P = 0.0006$).

Al-Sarraf et al. randomized patients with stage III or IV nasopharyngeal carcinoma to radiation therapy alone versus radiation and concurrent cisplatin followed by three courses of cisplatin with 5-flurouracil. The study was halted prematurely because of a statistically significant difference in disease free and overall survival favoring the chemotherapy arm (Al-Sarraf, personal communication).

The morbidity associated with total larygectomy (29) and the demonstration that cisplatin-based chemotherapy could produce high response rates in locally advanced disease led the Department of Veterans Affairs Laryngeal Cancer Study Group to design a trial of organ preservation utilizing neoadjuvant chemotherapy followed by definitive radiation therapy (30). Patients with locally advanced (stage III or IV) squamous cell carcinoma of the larynx were randomized to either standard therapy with surgery and radiation therapy versus neoadjuvant chemotherapy with cisplatinum 100 mg/m^2 and 5-FU 1000 mg/m^2 day for 5 days by continuous infusion followed by radiation therapy. If the patients showed either a CR or PR to the chemotherapy after two cycles they received a third; if there was less than a PR or progression, they underwent salvage laryngectomy. Eight patients died during treatment, five in the chemotherapy group and three in the standard treatment group. Thirty-one percent of the patients receiving chemotherapy obtained a CR following two cycles and 54% had a PR for an overall response rate of 85%. There was no difference in overall survival between the two groups and the larynx was preserved in 62% of the patients assigned to chemotherapy. Salvage laryngectomy was more likely to be required in the stage IV patients than the stage III. Smaller tumor size, increased DNA content and infiltrating histology correlated with response to chemotherapy (31). The results of the trial have recently been updated—the two arms continue to have an similar 8 year survival rate of approximately 35% (G. T. Wolf, personal communication).

While the overall survival is poor and suggests the need to develop better strategies, larynx sparing therapy is well tolerated and does not sacrifice a survival advantage compared with total laryngectomy. The criticism of the study centers around the fact that there was not a group randomized to radiotherapy alone, which has led to the current RTOG protocol randomizing patients to radiotherapy alone, concomitant radiotherapy and cisplatin, and neoadjuvant cisplatin and 5-fluorouracil followed by radiotherapy.

Investigators have attempted organ preservation trials at other sites in the head and neck. The EORTC randomized untreated patients with squamous cell carcinoma of the hypopharynx to either extensive standard surgery (total laryngectomy with partial pharyngectomy and radical neck dissection) and postoperative radiotherapy or induction chemotherapy followed by radiation therapy for the complete clinical responders. The chemotherapy utilized was 5-FU and cisplatin; patients with less than complete response went to salvage surgery. Preliminary evaluation of the data revealed an equivalence in survival between the two arms and, after 3 years, the group treated with chemotherapy and radiation had 28% of patients without evidence of disease and with preservation of their hypopharynx (32). This study suggests that even in poor prognostic sites, such as the hypopharynx, organ preservation is a feasible strategy.

Other strategies of alternating chemotherapy with radiotherapy or giving chemotherapy concurrently with radiation are ongoing. In general, concurrent therapy can give higher response rates but with the expense of increased toxicity (mucositis). The rationale behind using concurrent radiotherapy and chemotherapy consists of spatial cooperation, chemotherapy inhibition of sublethal radiation repair, and decreased tumor bulk with improved blood supply, leading to increased radio and chemosensitivity (2,4). Single agent synchronous chemoradiotherapy has been compared with radiotherapy alone in over 20 phase III trials including 9 with bleomycin, 4 of 5-FU and 2 of cisplatin. Most have shown nonsignificant trends towards improved survival in the chemoradiotherapy arm (20).

In an early phase III study, Fu et al. (33) randomized 104 patients with stage III or IV head and neck cancer to either radiotherapy alone or radiotherapy with concommitant chemotherapy consisting of bleomycin, followed by bleomycin and methotrexate after completion of radiation. While the overall survival curves were not significantly different, the concommitant group had a higher complete response rate (45% versus 67%) and 2 year control rate, as well as a decreased incidence of distant metastases.

5-FU has provided promising survival results in this setting. In the most recent study, Browman et al. (34) gave 5-FU along with radiotherapy versus a placebo infusion and increased the complete response rate (68% versus 56%). The concurrent group experienced more toxicity but the delivery of the radiotherapy was not compromised.

Bachaud et al. (35) gave weekly adjuvant cisplatin at 50 mg/m^2 concurrently with radiation to patients with stage III or IV head and neck cancer with extracapsular spread of tumor in the lymph node metastases. The combined modality arm had a higher incidence of toxicity but showed a significant disease free survival at 2 years (65% versus 41%). The only phase III study of synchronous cisplatin-radiotherapy in locally advanced disease, however, was negative (2,4,20).

Concomittant multiagent chemoradiotherapy has been compared to radiotherapy alone in five phase III trials and to sequential chemoradiotherapy in seven (20). This approach is associated with much greater toxicity than single agent programs and, therefore, has generally required suboptimal radiotherapy schedules (e.g., alternating or interrupted radiotherapy).

The most important chemoradiotherapy trial published to date compared alternating chemotherapy and radiation to radiation alone. Merlano et al. (36) took previously untreated stage III or IV patients and randomly assigned them to receive either radiation therapy alone (up to 70 Gy) or four cycles of cisplatin 20 mg/m^2/day and 5-FU at 200 mg/m^2/day for 5 days alternating with radiotherapy in three two week courses (20 Gy per course). The CR rate in the alternating group was 42% as compared to 22% in the radiotherapy group; the 3 year survival was 41% in the alternating group and 23% in the radiotherapy group ($P < 0.05$). The toxicity was comparable between the two arms. The study was stopped prior to accruing the planned study sample size due to the difference in survival between the two arms; however, the study has subsequently been criticized owing to the fact that the survival in the radiotherapy only arm was worse than that of historical controls.

Taylor et al. (37) reported a phase III trial of sequential versus concomitant therapy in 214 patients with untreated stage III and IV disease. The CR rate was similar in both groups (50% and 52%) but there were more PRs in the concomitant group and more stable disease or progression in the sequential group. The rate of distant metastases were low and identical in the two groups but the rate of regional recurrences were lower in the concomitant arm. While death from cancer was lower in the concomitant arm, there were more deaths from other causes and thus there was no survival advantage

Chemoradiotherapy is now being studied in patients who have failed prior local therapy. Vokes et al. (38) gave 39 inoperable patients daily radiotherapy with concurrent 5 FU at 800 mg/m^2/day with escalating doses of hydroxyurea. Fourteen of 15 evaluable patients previously treated with local therapy responded, six with a CR. Seventeen patients who had not had prior therapy all responded, 12 with a CR. At a dose of hydroxyurea less than 2000 mg/day there was mild to moderate myelosuppression that still permitted greater than 80% of the 5 FU dose to be administered All patients developed mucositis. Further studies looking at innovative combinations of chemotherapy and radiotherapy are warranted.

CHEMOPREVENTION

Patients who survive their head and neck cancer are at high long-term risk for the development of second primary tumors, which occurs at a rate of 5–7% per year (2,3). Therefore, interventions able to decrease the rate of second primary tumors in these patients could produce significant advances in the long-term survival of head and neck cancer patients.

Few areas have generated as much exciting research in oncology in the past decade as the evolving work on retinoids (39,40). The success of retinoids to reverse premalignant lesions has led to intensive investigation to elucidate their mechanism of actions. Retinoids, which are vitamin A analogues, have demonstrated the ability to modulate proliferation, differentiation and apoptosis. They appear to act by binding to specific nuclear receptors, either retinoic acid receptors (RAR) or retinoid X receptors (RXR), which subsequently bind to specific nuclear sites and function as transcription factors. The first study of these receptors in premalignancy and chemoprevention was recently reported by Lotan et al. (41). In this study, 52 patients had their oral premalignant lesions studied for mRNA expression of retinoic acid receptors (RARs) and retinoid X receptors (RXRs) prior to and after therapy with 13-*cis*-retinoic acid. These samples were compared to seven normal controls (nonsmoking volunteers). All of the normal specimens expressed RAR-β mRNA, but only 40% of the premalignant lesions had detectable RAR-β mRNA. After retinoid therapy, 31 of the 39 studied specimens expressed RAR-β. These data indicate that RAR-β is selectively downregulated in oral premalignant lesions and that treatment with high-dose 13-*cis*-retinoic acid can upregulate it, along with effecting a clinical response. Further studies are needed to clarify the mechanism of RAR-β suppression in oral premalignancy and its association with carcinogenic progression. Very recent data suggest that RAR-β expression is linked to intracellular retinoic acid levels (42). Other translations studied in the retinoid-oral premalignant lesion system are focused on the specific genetic events preceding neoplasia (43,44).

Retinoids, in particular 13-*cis*-retinoic acid, have been shown to be effective in reversing oral premalignant lesions (40). The first randomized trial, reported by Hong et al. (45), included 44 patients with the premalignant lesion oral leukoplakia randomized to receive either placebo or 13-*cis*-retinoic acid at 1–2 mg/kg/day for 3 mo. There were major decreases in the sizes of the lesions in 67% of the patients given the drug and in 10% of the placebo group; dysplasia was reversed in 54% of the retinoid group and in 10% of the placebo. Toxicity consisted of cheilitis, skin peeling and facial erythema. Nine of 16 patients relapsed within 3 months of discontinuing the drug.

Because of the high toxicity and relapse rate, a subsequent study was designed to assess maintenance therapy with low dose 13-*cis*-retinoic acid at 0.5 mg/kg/day or β carotene after a 3 month high-dose 13-*cis*-retinoic acid induction (46). The rate of response of leukoplakia to the high dose therapy was 55%. Of the group that responded and went on to maintenance, 92% of the retinoid arm continued to have stable (or further responding) lesions as compared with 45% of the β carotene arm.

Three other randomized studies have evaluated the benefits of retinoids in reversing oral leukoplakia (40). Stich et al. (47) gave tobacco-betel nut chewers in India with leukoplakia either vitamin A (200,000 units/week) versus placebo and found a remission rate of 57% versus 3%. In addition, 21% of the placebo treated patients developed new lesions versus none of the vitamin A patients. Chiesa et al. (48) gave patients no treatment versus 4-HPR following surgically resected oral leukoplakia and found a recurrence rate of 3 in the treated patients and 12 in the control.

The documented efficacy of retinoids to reverse premalignant lesions of the upper aerodigestive tract led to its study in patients with treated head and neck cancer who were at risk for both recurrence and second primary tumors (SPTs) (49). One hundred three patients disease free after primary treatment for squamous cell cancers of the head and neck were randomized to either placebo or 13-*cis*-retinoic acid at 50 to 100 mg/m^2 a day for 1 year. There was no difference between the two groups in regards to local, regional or metastatic recurrences of their primary tumors but there was a marked difference in the rate of formation of SPTs between the two groups (4% versus 24%). A recent update of the data continues to show that retinoid treated patients have fewer primary tumors overall (14% versus 31%) and within the aerodigestive tract (7% versus 33%, $P = 0.008$) (50). The success of that trial has led to further trials with other retinoids, as well as two ongoing trials of low dose 13-*cis*-retinoic acid versus placebo in early head and neck cancer and non-small cell lung cancer. Large intergroup trials are currently underway in the United States, Europe, and Australia, and the results should be available in late 1999 or 2000.

Another randomized study has assessed retinoid effects on SPTs. Bolla et al. (51) gave etretinate to patients following treatment for squamous cell carcinoma of the oral cavity or oral pharynx. Patients were randomized to etretinate at 50 mg/day for 1 month followed by 25 mg/day for 2 years versus placebo. There was no reduction noted in second primary tumors between the two arms, but the trial did confirm the high rate of second primary tumors following treatment for early stage head and neck cancer: one quarter of the patients developed a second primary, 79% within the upper aerodigestive tract.

CONCLUSION

Despite intensive efforts in the prevention and therapy of head and neck cancer, survival rates have not improved, and this disease remains a major worldwide cause of morbidity and mortality. Nevertheless, head and neck carcinogenesis research has advanced in many areas.

Biological study advances include important new insights into the understanding of field and multistep carcinogenesis. Studies of *p53* provide the first molecular-genetic evidence of field carcinogenesis. Microsatellite studies of oral premalignant lesions have shown that loss of heterozygosity frequently occurs at chromosome 9p21 and 3p14. This is the first evidence of clonal expansion in these lesions. That biological study is important to the clinical control of head and neck carcinogenesis is illustrated by recent data showing that *p53* gene mutations and *p53* protein accumulation may be useful predictors of treatment failure after definitive local therapy.

Several recent major advances also have occurred in chemotherapy of head and neck cancer. Now in development, taxanes show promise as a new active class of agents in this disease. Although not significantly improving survival, neoadjuvant chemotherapy for organ preservation has emerged as an important control of morbidity in the head and neck. The VA laryngeal preservation study established sequential cisplatin-based chemotherapy followed by radiation as an equivalent alternative to total laryngectomy and radiation for treating resectable locally advanced laryngeal cancer. A recent long-term update of this seminal study indicates that the chemotherapy and surgery arms both have 8 year survival rates of 35%. A recent positive phase III study in hypopharyngeal cancer provides further support for organ preservation strategies in the head and neck. Two of the three recent phase III neoadjuvant trials in nasopharyngeal cancer, which has a very different biology and sensitivity to chemotherapy and radiation than typical head and neck squamous cell cancers, have had success with primary cisplatin-based chemotherapy in advanced local-regional disease. Concomitant chemo-radiotherapy is the most promising primary treatment approach in head and neck cancer. The primary goals of this aggressive approach are to develop ways to reduce the severe mucositis it causes and to determine optimal radiation programs and chemotherapy drugs, doses and schedules.

All randomized head and neck chemoprevention studies have involved retinoids. Five of these trials were in oral premalignant lesions, and all showed significant activity. The other two randomized retinoid trials were conducted to prevent second primary tumors. One was positive, one was negative. The primary goals of head and neck chemoprevention are to develop new agents, including receptor-selective retinoids and retinamides, and to pursue translational studies that will add to our understanding of premalignant-lesion biology and mechanisms of drug activity.

REFERENCES

1. Parker SL, Tong T, Colden S, et al. Cancer statistics. 1996;CA46:5–27.
2. Wolf GT, Lippman SM, Laramore GE, Hong WK. Head and neck cancer. In: Holland JF, et al., eds. Cancer medicine, 3rd ed. Philadelphia: Lea and Febiger, 1993. p 1211.
3. Vokes EE, Mick R, Lester EP, Panje WR, Weichselbaum RR. Cisplatin and fluorouracil chemotherapy does not yield long term benefit in locally advanced head and neck cancer: Results from a single institution. J Clin Oncol 1991;9:1376.
4. Vokes EE, Weichselbaum RR, Lippman SM, Hong WK. Head and neck cancer. N Engl J Med 1993;328:184.
5. McLaughlin JK, Gridley G, Block G, Winn DM, Preston-Martin S, Schoenberg JB. Dietary factors in oral and pharyngeal cancer. J Natl Cancer Inst 1988;80:1237.
6. Pathmanathan R, Prasad U, Sadler R, Flynn K, Raab-Traub N. Clonal proliferations of cells infected with Epstein-Barr virus in preinvasive lesions related to nasopharyngeal carcinoma. N Engl J Med 1995;333:693.
7. Slaughter DP, Southwick HW, Smejkal W. "Field cancerization" in oral stratification squamous epithelium: Clinical implications of mutocentric origin. Cancer 1953:6:963.
8. Brennan JA, Boyle JO, Koch WM, Goodman SN, Hruban RH, Eby YJ, et al. Association between cigarette smoking and mutation of the p53 gene in squamous-cell carcinoma of the head and neck. N Engl J Med 1995;332:712.
9. Chung KY, Mukhopadhyay T, Kim J, Casson A, Ro JY, Goepfert H, et al. Discordant p53 gene mutations in primary head and neck cancers and corresponding second primary cancers of the upper aerodigestive tract. Cancer Res 1993;53:1676.
10. Brennan JA, Mao L, Hruban RH, Boyle JO, Eby YJ, Koch WM, et al. Molecular assessment of histopathological staging in squamous cell carcinoma of the head and neck. N Engl J Med 1995;332:429.
11. Shin DM, Lee JS, Lippman SM, Lee JJ, Tu ZN, Choi G, et al. p53 expression: Predicting recurrence and second primary tumors in head and neck squamous cell carcinoma. J Natl Cancer Inst. 1996;88(8):519–529.
12. Callender T, El-Naggar AK, Lee MS, Frankenthaler R, Luna MA, Batsakis JG. Prad-1 (CCND1)/cyclin D1 oncogene amplification in primary head and neck squamous cell carcinoma. Cancer 1994;74:152.
13. Hung J, Kishimoto U, Sugio S, Virami A, Mcintire DD, Minna JD, et al. Allele-specific chromosome 3p deletions occur at an early stage in the pathogenesis of lung carcinoma. JAMA 1995;273:1908.
14. Kishimoto Y, Sugio K, Hung JY, Virami AK, Mcintire DD, Minna JD, et al. Allele-specific loss in chromosome 9p loci in preneoplastic lesions accompanying non-small cell lung cancers. J Natl Cancer Inst 1995;87:1224.
15. Van der Riet P, Califano J, Westra W, Sidransky D. Loss of heterozygosity on chromosome 3p12 and 9p21 in preinvasive head and neck tumors: Toward a progression model for head and neck squamous cell carcinoma. Proc Am Assoc Cancer Res 1995;36:A3264.
16. Mao L, Lee JS, Fan YH, Ro JY, Batsakis JG, Lippman S, et al. Frequent microsatellite alterations at chromosomes 9p21 and 3p14 in oral premalignant lesions and their value in cancer risk assessment. Nature Med 2 1996;682–685.
17. Hong WK and Bromer R. Chemotherapy in head and neck cancer: Current concepts. N Engl J Med 1983;308:75.
18. Jacobs C, Lyman G, Velez-Garcia E, et al. A phase III randomized study comparing cisplatin and fluorouracil as single agents and in combination for advanced squamous cell carcinoma of the head and neck. J Clin Oncol 1992;10:257.
19. Forastiere AA, Neuberg D, Taylor SG IV, DeConti R, Adams G. Phase II evaluation of taxol in advanced head and neck cancer: An Eastern Cooperative Oncology Group trial. Proc Am Soc Clin Oncol 1993;12:277. [Abstr.]

20. Lippman SM, Hong WK. Chemotherapy and chemoprevention. In: Myers E, Suen JY, eds. Cancer of the head and neck, 3rd ed. W. B. Saunders Co., 1996.
21. Dreyfuss AI, Clark JR, Wright JE, et al. Continuous infusion high-dose leucovorin with 5-fluorouracil and cisplatin for untreated stage IV carcinoma of the head and neck. Ann Intern Med 1990;112:167.
22. El-Sayed S, Nelson N. Adjuvant and adjunctive chemotherapy in the management of squamous cell carcinoma of the head and neck region: A meta-analysis of prospective and randomized trials. J Clin Oncol 1996;14(3):838.
23. Head and Neck Contracts Program. Adjuvant chemotherapy for advanced head and neck squamous carcinoma. Final report of the Head and Neck Contracts Program. Cancer 1987;60:301.
24. Jacobs C, Makuch R. Efficacy of adjuvant chemotherapy for patients with resectable head and neck cancer: A subset analaysis of the head and neck contracts program. J Clin Oncol 1990;8:838.
25. Schuller DE, Metch B, Stein DW, Mattox D, McCracken JD. Preoperative chemotherapy in advanced resectable head and neck cancer: Final report of the Southwest Oncology Group. Laryngoscope 1988;98:1205.
26. Laramore GE, Scott CB, Al-Sarraf M, Haselow RE, Ervin TJ, Wheeler R, et al. Adjuvant chemotherapy for resectable squamous cell carcinomas of the head and neck: Report on Intergroup Study 0034. Int J Radiat Oncol Biol Phys 1992;23:705.
27. Chan ATC, Teo PML, Leung TWT, Leung SF, Lee WY, Yeo W, et al. A prospective randomized study of chemotherapy adjunctive to definitive radiotherapy in advanced nasopharyngeal carcinoma. Int J Radiat Oncol Biol Phys 1995;33:569.
28. Eschwege F, et al. Randomized phase III trial of neoadjuvant chemotherapy (NACT) with bleomycin (B), epirubicin (E), cisplatin (C) followed by radiotherapy versus radiotherapy alone in undifferentiated carcinoma of nasopharyngeal type (UCNT): Preliminary results. Radiat Oncol Biol Phys 1995;32(Suppl 1):192.
29. McNeil BJ, Weichselbaum R, Pauker SG. Speech and survival: Trade-offs between quality and quantity of life in laryngeal cancer. N Engl J Med 1981;305:982.
30. The Department of Veterans Affairs Laryngeal Cancer Study Group. Induction chemotherapy plus radiation compared with surgery plus radiation in patients with advanced laryngeal cancer. N Engl J Med 1991;324:1685.
31. Spaulding MB, Fisher SG, Wolf GT. Tumor response, toxicity, and survival after neoadjuvant organ preserving chemotherapy in advanced laryngeal cancer. J Clin Oncol 1994;12:1592.
32. Lefebvre JL and Sahmoud T. Larynx preservation in hypopharynx squamous cell carcinoma: Preliminary results of a randomized study (EORTC 24891). Proc Annu Meet Am Soc Clin Oncol 1994;13:A912. [Abstr.]
33. Fu KK, Phillips TL, Silverberg IJ, Jacobs C, Goffinet DR, Chun C, et al. Combined radiotherapy and chemotherapy with bleomycin and methotrexate for advanced inoperable head and neck cancer: Update of a Northern California Oncology Group randomized trial. J Clin Oncol 1987;5:1410.
34. Bowman GP, Cripps C, Hodson DI, Eapen L, Sathya J, Levine MN. Placebo-controlled randomized trial of infusional fluorouracil during standard radiotherapy in locally advanced head and neck cancer. J Clin Oncol 1994;12:2648.
35. Bachaud JM, David JM, Boussin G, Daly N. Combined postoperative radiotherapy and weekly cisplatin infusion for locally advanced squamous cell carcinoma of the head and neck: Preliminary report of a randomized trial. Int J Radiat Oncol Biol Phys 1991;20:243.
36. Merlano M, Vitale V, Rosso R, Benasso M, Corvo R, Cavallari M, et al. Treatment of advanced squamous cell carcinoma of the head and neck with alternating chemotherapy and radiotherapy. N Engl J Med 1992;327:1115.
37. Taylor IV SG, Murthy AK, Vannetzel JM, Colin P, Dray M, Caldarelli DD, et al. Randomized comparison of neoadjuvant cisplatin and flurouracil infusion followed by radiation versus concomitant treatment in advanced head and neck cancer. J Clin Oncol 1994;12:385.
38. Vokes EE, Panje WR, Schilsky RL, Mick R, Awan AM, Moran WJ, et al. Hydroxyurea, flurouracil, and concomitant radiotherapy in poor prognosis head and neck cancer: A phase I–II study. J Clin Oncol 1989;7:761.
39. Smith MA, Parkinson DR, Cheson BD, et al. Retinoids in cancer therapy. J Clin Oncol 1992;10:839.
40. Lippman SM, Benner SE, Hong WK. Cancer chemoprevention. J Clin Oncol 1994;12:851.
41. Lotan R, Xu XC, Lippman SM, Ro JY, Lee JS, Lee JJ. Suppression of retinoic acid receptor beta in premalignant oral lesions and its up-regulation by isotretinoin. N Engl J Med 1995;332:1405.
42. Xu XC, Zile MH, Lippman SM, Lee JS, Lee JJ, Hong WK, Lotan R. Anti-retinoic acid (RA) antibody binding to human premalignant oral lesions, which occurs less frequently than binding to normal tissue, increases after 13-*cis*-RA treatment *in vivo* and is related to RA receptor beta expression. Cancer Res 1995;55:5507.

43. Lippman SM, Shin DM, Lee JJ, Batsakis JG, Lotan R, Tainsky MA, Hittelman WN, Hong WK: p53 and retinoid chemoprevention of oral carcinogenesis. Cancer Res 1995;55:16.
44. Hong WK, Lippman SM, Hittelman WN, et al. Retinoid chemoprevention of aerodigestive cancer from basic research to the clinic. Clin Cancer Res 1995;1:677.
45. Hong WK, Endicott J, Itri LM, Doos W, Batsakis JG, Bell R, et al. 13-*cis*-Retinoic acid in the treatment of oral leukoplakia. N Engl J Med 1986;315:1501.
46. Lippman SM, Batsakis JG, Toth BB, Weber RS, Lee JJ, Martin JW, et al. Comparison of low-dose isotretintoin with beta carotene to prevent oral carcinogensis. N Engl J Med 1993;328:15.
47. Stich HF, Hornby AP, Matthew B, Sankeranarayanan R, Nair MK. Response of oral leukoplakia to the administration of vitamin A. Cancer Letters 1988;40:93.
48. Chiesa F, Tradati N, Marazzo M, Rossi N, Boracchi P, Mariani L, et al. Prevention of local relapses and new localization of oral leukoplakias with the synthetic retinoid fenretinide 4-HPR. Preliminary results. Eur J Cancer 1992;28:95.
49. Hong WK, Lippman SM, Itri LM, Karp DD, Lee JS, Byers RM, et al. Prevention of second primary tumors with isotretinoin in squamous-cell carcinoma of the head and neck. N Engl J Med 1990;323:795.
50. Benner SE, Pajak TF, Stetz J, Lippman SM, Hong WK, Schantz SP. Prevention of second primary tumors with isotretinoin in patients with squamous cell carcinoma of the head and neck: Long term follow-up. J Natl Cancer Inst 1994;86:140.
51. Bolla M, Lefur R, Ton Van J, Domenge C, Badet JM, Koskas Y, et al. Prevention of second primary tumours with etretinate in squamous cell carcinoma of the oral cavity and oropharynx. Results of a multicentric double-blind randomised study. Eur J Cancer 1994;6:767.

Sydney E. Salmon, Ed. *Adjuvant Therapy of Cancer VIII.*

7
Adjuvant Chemotherapy of Non–Small-Cell Lung Cancer

Olivier Rixe and Thierry Le Chevalier

The main curative treatment of early stage NSCLC is surgery. Nevertheless, after surgical resection, more than 50% of patients with clinical stage I or II will die of tumor progression. In 70% of cases, recurrence will occur outside the chest and the development of effective adjuvant treatments remain one of the most important goals for the therapeutic strategy of lung cancer.

Postoperative treatments have been widely evaluated during the last decades. Thoracic radiotherapy preceding or following surgical resection does not appear to have any impact on survival and this may be due to an improved quality of mediastinal dissection by thoracic surgeons.

Adjuvant chemotherapy has also been widely tested after local treatment in NSCLC. Two trials (1,2) have shown encouraging results with chemotherapy given after surgical resection of NSCLC. However, because of the limited number of patients enrolled in these trials, the role of adjuvant chemotherapy cannot be clearly established in early stage NSCLC. For this reason, the Medical Research Council and Institut Gustave-Roussy decided to perform a large meta-analysis using updated individual data (3). In the group comparing surgery alone to surgery followed by adjuvant chemotherapy, 14 trials have been registered including 4357 patients (of whom 2574 died). The results for the five trials using long-term alkylating agents showed a 15% increase in the risk of death translating to an absolute detriment of chemotherapy of 5% at 5 years. In the seven trials using a cisplatin-based regimen, a 13% reduction in the risk of death was observed, suggesting an absolute benefit from adjuvant chemotherapy of 5% at 5 years. Chemotherapy was randomly added to surgery and radiotherapy in a total of 807 patients and a 6% reduction in the risk of death was observed, suggesting a 2% absolute benefit at 5 years. Neither gender nor performance status, age, or histological subtype had any impact on this effect. This constitutes a rationale for large scale trials and several adjuvant studies have already been initiated worldwide. Among these, the IALT (International Adjuvant Lung Cancer Trial) protocol was started in February 1995 and 3300 patients have to be included in this study to demonstrate a survival benefit of 5% according to the hypothesis emerging from the meta-analysis.

Another approach in operable patients is to propose neoadjuvant chemotherapy and numerous phase II studies have reported promising results in terms of response and resectability. In stage IIIA, two important randomized trials have recently been published comparing surgery alone or neoadjuvant chemotherapy prior surgery. The first, reported by Rosell et al. (4) used three courses of cisplatin, ifosfamide and mitomycin and was stopped early due to significant improvement of survival in the neoadjuvant arm (median survival: 26 months) compared to the control arm (median survival: 8 months). Both arms received post operative radiation therapy in this study. In the M. D. Anderson Study (5), six cycles of neoadjuvant cyclophosphamide, etoposide and cisplatin were compared to surgery alone. Radiation therapy was not a part of either treatment regimen. Sixty patients were randomized and the median survival was 64 months in the neoadjuvant arm compared to 11 months in the control group. These two trials have shown encouraging results but the groups were small and the populations heterogeneous. It is still unclear whether neoadjuvant chemotherapy can provide a significant survival advantage in resectable NSCLC. An ongoing multicenter french trial (6) has already included more than 300 patients with early stage NSCLC. In this trial, two cycles of MIP (mitomycin, ifosfamide, cisplatin) are given before and after radical surgery in the investigational group and patients in the control group have surgery alone. This study should clarify the role of preoperative chemotherapy in this setting.

The role of chemotherapy has also been evaluated in patients with locally advanced NSCLC. The standard treatment of such patients is radiotherapy but this therapeutic option does not give more than 5% survivors at 5 years. The meta-analysis performed by the MRC and Institut Gustave-Roussy pooled the results of 22 trials having included a total of 3033 patients. Five trials used long-term alkylating agents, 6 used other non-cisplatin regimens, and 11 used cisplatin based regimens. A 13% reduction in the risk of death was observed, suggesting an absolute benefit from adjuvant therapy of 4% at 2 years and 2% at 5 years. Again in this category of patients, none of the classical prognostic factors (age, sex, performance status, histological subtype) influenced this impact of chemotherapy on survival. More recent drug combinations, radiotherapy timing and fractionation and combined chemoradiotherapy modalities should improve these results.

The optimal systemic chemotherapy for NSCLC is still controversal. The most effective and commonly used regimens are cisplatin combined with etoposide or vinca alcaloids (vinorelbine, vinblastine, vindesine). We reported the superiority of cisplatin and vinorelbine over cisplatin and vindesine and vinorelbine alone in a randomized trial including 612 patients (7). This regimen appears to be one of the most active protocols using "conventional" chemotherapeutic agents. Furthermore, the emergence of several drugs active in advanced disease (taxoids, topoisomerase I inhibitors, and gemcitabine) could increase the benefit of adjuvant chemotherapy preceding or following local treatment in case of limited disease.

REFERENCES

1. Holmes EC, Gail M, for The Lung Cancer Study Group. Surgical adjuvant therapy for stage II and stage III adenocarcinoma and large-cell undifferentiated carcinoma. J Clin Oncol 1986;4:710–715.
2. Niiranen A, Niitamo-Korhonen S, Kouri M, et al. Adjuvant chemotherapy after radical surgery for non-small-cell lung cancer: A randomized study. J Clin Oncol 1992;10:1927–1932.
3. Non Small Cell Lung Cancer Collaborative Group. Chemotherapy in non-small cell lung cancer: A meta-analysis using updated data on individual patients from 52 randomized clinical trials. Br Med J 1995;311:899–909.

4. Rosell R, Gomez-Codina J, Comps C, et al. A randomized trial comparing preoperative chemotherapy plus surgery with surgery alone in patients with non-small cell lung cancer. N Engl J Med 1994;330:153–158.
5. Roth JA, Fossella F, Kamoski R, et al. A randomized trial comparing perioperative chemotherapy and surgery with surgery alone in resectable stage IIIa non-small cell lung cancer. J Natl Cancer Inst 1994;86:673–680.
6. Depierre A, Milleron B, Chastang C, et al. Phase III randomized study of neo-adjuvant chemotherapy-surgery in non-small cell lung cancer: Preliminary results. Cancer treatment: An update. Paris: Springer-Verlag, 1994.
7. Le Chevalier T, Brisgand D, Douillard JY, et al. Randomized study of vinorelbine cisplatin versus vindesine and cisplatin versus vinorelbine alone in advanced non-small cell lung cancer: Results of a European multi-center trial including 612 patients. J Clin Oncol 1994;12:360–367.

III

Breast Cancer

Large-Scale Adjuvant Trials

Adjuvant Therapy of Cancer VIII, edited by Sydney E. Salmon. Lippincott–Raven Publishers, Philadelphia © 1997.

8

Update of the Milan Cancer Institute Studies in Operable Breast Cancer

Gianni Bonadonna, Pinuccia Valagussa, Angela Moliterni, Milvia Zambetti, Monica Terenziani, Laura Ferrari, and Cristina Brambilla

Over the past quarter of this century, adjuvant systemic treatment of high-risk operable breast cancer has become widely used in clinical practice after seminal biological concepts were corroborated by clinical results (1,2). This paper will review and update the most relevant findings achieved through multidisciplinary approaches by the Milan Cancer Institute.

FIRST GENERATION OF ADJUVANT TRIALS

In June 1973, we started the first prospective randomized study with combination chemotherapy as an adjuvant to surgical treatment. The case series included premenopausal and postmenopausal women who had histologically positive lymph nodes after radical mastectomy; a combination of 12 monthly cycles of CMF (cyclophosphamide, methotrexate, and fluorouracil) was administered to women allocated to receive adjuvant therapy after surgery (3). The long-term analysis of this trial demonstrates a significant advantage of CMF adjuvant chemotherapy that persists for at least 20 years after surgery (Table 8-1). Treatment with CMF result-

TABLE 8-1. First CMF Study: Essential Results at 20 Years

	Control Group (%) (179 Patients)	CMF Group (%) (207 Patients)	Relative Risk (95% CI)
Relapse-free survival	25	32	0.65 (0.51–0.83) $P < 0.001$
Total 1st relapses	73	64	
Locoregional	15	13	
Distant	54	44	
Contralateral breast	4	7	
Total survival	23	34	0.76 (0.60–0.97) $P = 0.03$

ed in the suppression, albeit moderate, of micrometastases regardless of their anatomical sites. Overall, the benefit translated into a 34% reduction in the relative risk of relapse and in a 26% reduction in the relative risk of death, although the magnitude of the changes differed among various subgroups of patients (4). Our results after 20 years of follow-up confirmed our initial observation underlying the importance of avoiding reduced doses of chemotherapy if maximal benefit is to be achieved (4,5). This finding has also been supported by recent data from a prospective randomized study carried out by investigators of the Cancer and Leukemia Group B (6).

The second Milan study with adjuvant standard CMF randomly tested 12 versus 6 monthly cycles and was started in September 1975. Here too the long term results (18 years; Table 8-2) confirmed the early observations showing similarity in treatment outcome between the two treatment groups (7). This finding should be interpreted as an indirect sign of resistant cell lines.

The last study with adjuvant CMF was activated in December 1980 in node-negative and estrogen receptor-negative breast cancer patients (8). To avoid arbitrary dose reductions in the administration of oral cyclophosphamide, we designed a new regimen where all the three drugs were given intravenously every 3 weeks for a total of 12 courses (i.e., for approximately 9 months). The 12-year results confirmed that full dose intravenous CMF significantly improved relapse-free (71% versus 48%, $P = 0.008$) and total survival rates (80% versus 50%, $p = 0.03$) compared to locoregional treatment alone. Despite the limited number of patients we could enroll in this study, the benefit from adjuvant chemotherapy was evident in all patient subsets.

SECOND GENERATION OF ADJUVANT TRIALS

In the attempt to circumvent the phenomenon of primary drug resistance, early in the 1980s we designed new adjuvant trials testing sequential non-cross resistant agents (1). In patients presenting with 1 to 3 positive nodes (9), the administration of four cycles of Adriamycin (75 mg/m^2 every 3 weeks) after 8 courses of intravenous CMF failed to improve treatment outcome compared to the delivery of 12 intravenous courses of CMF alone (Table 8-3).

TABLE 8-2. Second CMF Study: 18-Year Results

	CMF 12 Cycles (%) (243 Patients)	CMF 6 Cycles (%) (216 Patients)
Relapse-free survival	35	38
Total 1st relapses	63	59
Locoregional	12	10
Distant	45	42
Contralateral breast	6	7
Total survival	38	45

TABLE 8-3. Sequential CMF and Adriamycin (DOX) in Patients with 1 to 3 Positive Nodes. Ten-Year Results

	CMF IV (%) (275 Patients)	CMF→DOX (%) (277 Patients)
Relapse-free survival	59	57
Total 1st relapse	37	39
Locoregional	10	8
Distant	23	27
Contralateral breast	4	4
Total survival	75	75

In patients presenting with >3 positive nodes we tested a sequential approach with 4 cycles of Adriamycin given before CMF versus the alternating administration of CMF and Adriamycin (1). The recently published results (1) confirming the superiority of sequential chemotherapy over alternating chemotherapy held up to the 10-year analysis (10). The essential results are reported in Table 8-4. Both adjuvant regimens included the same drugs, doses and treatment duration and the received dose intensity for all drugs was comparable in the two treatment groups. With the only variation being drug sequence, the median duration of relapse-free was almost doubled after the sequential (86 months) compared with the alternating (47 months) regimen. This observation confirmed that the scheduling of drugs is important for treatment improvement.

Another important prospective non-randomized trial involved the sequential administration of high-dose (HDS) non-cross resistant agents. The aim of the HDS regimen, combined with hematopoietic growth factor and autografting of cryopreserved peripheral blood progenitor cell support, was to assess its efficacy, toxicity and applicability as adjuvant therapy for patients with ≥10 positive nodes (11). At

TABLE 8-4. Sequential Adriamycin (DOX) and CMF vs Alternating CMF and DOX in Patients with > 3 Positive Nodes. Ten-year results

	DOX →CMF (%) (201 Patients)	CMF/DOX (%) (202 Patients)	Relative Risk (%) (95% CI)
Relapse-free survival	42	28	1.53 (1.19-2.01) $P = 0.001$
Total 1st relapses	53	66	
Locoregional	15	21	
Distant	34	45	
Contralateral breast	4	1	
Total survival	58	44	1.66 (1.23–2.56) $P < 0.001$

5 years, treatment outcome was significantly superior for the 67 women treated with HDS compared to a similar patient subgroup given sequential Adriamycin and CMF, the relapse-free total survival rates being 57% and 70%, respectively, after HDS. Overall, this novel regimen was of a short duration (median 70 days), subjectively well tolerated and required limited transfusional support.

TRIALS WITH PRIMARY CHEMOTHERAPY

Having established that the outcome of primary treatment is not related to the extent of surgery (2) and that systemic adjuvant therapy significantly reduces the annual odds of recurrence and death (1,12), the use of primary (neoadjuvant) chemotherapy has become one of the next attractive approaches to explore, particularly in women whose tumor characteristics are at high risk of harboring distant micrometastases.

Primary chemotherapy for breast cancer was first introduced in 1973 as part of the multidisciplinary approach that the Milan Cancer Institute had designed for locally advanced inoperable breast cancer (1). The review of the 10-year results showed that the benefit of treatment was inversely related to the tumor mass and significantly influenced by adjuvant chemotherapy delivered after the locoregional modality (13).

Based on the above-mentioned observations, in January 1988 we started clinical studies with primary chemotherapy in women who were otherwise candidates for modified radical mastectomy (15). The first trial included 227 women presenting with a breast tumor of 3 cm or more in largest diameter. Five different drug regimens (CMF, anthracycline- or mitoxantrone-containing combinations, Adriamycin alone) were tested as primary chemotherapy. The second study was started in October 1990 in patients with tumors measuring more than 2.5 cm in widest diameter (15,16). Initially, 210 women were given 3 cycles of primary Adriamycin (75 mg/m^2 every 3 weeks); subsequently, epidoxorubicin was delivered (at the dose of 90–120 mg/m^2) in the remaining 99 patients. Overall, treatment results were superimposable between the two studies: complete remission on clinical grounds was documented in 16% of the total 536 patients and tumor shrinkage >50% in 321 women (60%) for a total objective response rate of 76%. Tumor progression while on primary chemotherapy was documented in only 3% of the entire case series. Table 8-5 summarizes the most relevant findings at surgery. Detailed histopathologic findings on the first 424 women have been recently reported (15).

Following primary chemotherapy, conservative surgery plus breast irradiation was performed in 87% of the patients. Adjuvant chemotherapy was delivered in all women presenting with histologically positive nodal involvement as well as in high-risk node-negative breast cancers (namely negative estrogen receptors, undifferentiated and/or highly proliferating tumors).

After a median follow-up of 44 months, the 4-year results of the two studies with primary chemotherapy are reported in Table 8-6. Briefly, considering that the vast majority of patients (>85%) presented with breast cancer at high-risk of disease relapse, present results compare favorably with our long-term experience with adjuvant chemotherapy. In women undergoing breast-saving procedures, the 4-year cumulative risk of local relapse was 4.7%.

TABLE 8-5. Essential Results with Primary Chemotherapy in Two Successive Studies at the Milan Cancer Institute

Initial Tumor Diameter	Number Subjected to Surgery	Pathological CR Gross (%)	Pathological CR Micro (%)	Tumor 0.1–2 cm at Surgery (%)	Conservative Surgery (%)
≤ 4.0 c m	283	5	3	55	93
4.1–5.0 cm	156	10	3	47	87
> 5.0 cm	81	12	1	25	64
Total	520	8	3	48	87

CONCLUSIONS

After 20 years of successive clinical trials, the results achieved at the Milan Cancer Institute have helped to establish the effectiveness of adjuvant combination chemotherapy in high-risk women with resectable breast cancer and represent an important step in the contemporary evolution of breast cancer treatment. As far as primary chemotherapy is concerned, initial studies have confirmed that this novel approach can provide effective downstaging of the locoregional disease (15). However, the usefulness of this modality should not be limited to increasing the frequency of breast-sparing procedures. From our studies, the knowledge is clearly emerging that the degree of pathologic tumor regression (Table 8-6) appears to represent a

TABLE 8-6. Follow-up Results in Two Successive Studies of Primary Chemotherapy (Data are at 4 years from Surgery)

	%
Relapse-free survival	
Total	63
Pathologic response	
Complete	83
Good partial	67
Minor	49
Type of surgery	
Conservative	66
Mastectomy	46
Nodal status	
Negative	78
N^+ 1 to 3	61
N^+ >3	43
Local relapse after conservative surgery*	4.7

* As first event alone

marker of treatment outcome. As a consequence, the achievement of complete pathologic remission will become the major goal of properly intensified drug regimens to ensure a durable relapse-free survival rate. To further improve treatment outcome over current results, newer drug regimens of appropriate dose size and dose intensity should be conceived and tested in high-risk patients.

ACKNOWLEDGMENTS

These studies were supported in part by contracts N01-CM-33714 and N01-CM-07338 with the Division of Cancer Treatment, National Cancer Institute, National Institutes of Health, Bethesda, Maryland, and a grant from the Associazione Italiana per la Ricerca sul Cancro, Milano, Italy. We are indebted to the many clinical associates of the Milan Cancer Institute for their cooperation in these studies.

REFERENCES

1. Bonadonna G. Evolving concepts in the systemic adjuvant treatment of breast cancer. Cancer Res 1992;52:2127.
2. Fisher B. The evolution of paradigms for the management of breast cancer: A personal perspective. Cancer Res 1992;52:2371.
3. Bonadonna G, Brusamolino E, Valagussa P, et al. Combination chemotherapy as an adjuvant treatment in operable breast cancer. N Engl J Med 1976;294:405.
4. Bonadonna G, Valagussa P, Moliterni A, Zambetti M, Brambilla C. Adjuvant cyclophosphamide, methotrexate, and fluorouracil in node-positive breast cancer. The results of 20 years of follow-up. N Engl J Med 1995;332:901.
5. Bonadonna G, Valagussa P. Dose-response effect of adjuvant chemotherapy in breast cancer. N Engl J Med 1982;304:10.
6. Wood WC, Budman DR, Korzun AH, et al. Dose and dose intensity of adjuvant chemotherapy for stage II, node-positive breast cancer. N Engl J Med 1994;330:1253.
7. Tancini G, Bonadonna G, Valagussa P, Marchini S, Veronesi U. Adjuvant CMF in breast cancer: Comparative 5-year results of 12 versus 6 cycles. J Clin Oncol 1983;1:2.
8. Zambetti M, Bonadonna G, Valagussa P, et al. CMF for node-negative and estrogen receptor-negative breast cancer. J Natl Cancer Inst Monogr 1992;11:79.
9. Moliterni A, Bonadonna G, Valagussa P, Ferrari L, Zambetti M. Cyclophosphamide, methotrexate, and fluorouracil with and without doxorubicin in the adjuvant treatment of resectable breast cancer with one to three positive axillary nodes. J Clin Oncol 119;9:1124.
10. Bonadonna G, Zambetti M, Valagussa P. Sequential or alternating doxorubicin and CMF regimens in breast cancer with more than three positive axillary nodes: Ten-year results. JAMA 1995;273:542.
11. Gianni AM, Siena S, Bregni M, et al. Efficacy, toxicity and applicability of high-dose sequential chemotherapy as adjuvant treatment in operable breast cancer with 10 or more axillary nodes involved. J Clin Oncol 1996. In press.
12. Early Breast Cancer Trialists' Collaborative Group. Systemic treatment of early breast cancer by hormonal, cytotoxic, or immune therapy: 133 randomised trials involving 31000 recurrences and 24000 deaths among 75000 women. Lancet 1992;399:1 (Part I) and 71 (Part II).
13. Valagussa P, Zambetti M, Bonadonna G, Zucali R, Mezzanotte G, Veronesi U. Prognostic factors in locally advanced noninflammatory breast cancer: Long-term results following primary chemotherapy. Breast Cancer Res Treat 1990;15:137.
14. Bonadonna G, Veronesi U, Brambilla C, et al. Primary chemotherapy to avoid mastectomy in tumors with diameters of three centimeters or more. J Natl Cancer Inst 1990;82:1539.
15. Bonadonna G, Valagussa P, Zucali R, Salvadori B. Primary chemotherapy in surgically resectable breast cancer. CA Cancer J Clin 1995;45:227.
16. Bonadonna G, Valagussa P. Primary chemotherapy in operable breast cancer. Semin Oncol 1996. In press.

Adjuvant Therapy of Cancer VIII, edited by Sydney E. Salmon. Lippincott–Raven Publishers, Philadelphia © 1997.

9

Recent Findings from Three NSABP Clinical Trials Evaluating Systemic Adjuvant Therapy in Patients with Primary Breast Cancer and Negative Axillary Nodes

Bernard Fisher and James Dignam

Since 1958 approximately 50,000 women who either had primary breast cancer or who were at high risk for the disease participated in 26 clinical trials conducted by the National Surgical Adjuvant Breast and Bowel Project (NSABP). Information obtained from those trials has been presented at each of the seven international conferences on the adjuvant therapy of cancer by one of the authors (B.F.), who has been closely associated with the hypothesis generation, design, and conduct of those studies. This report provides an overview of some of the recent findings from three NSABP trials evaluating systemic adjuvant therapy for node-negative breast cancer.

SEQUENTIAL METHOTREXATE AND 5-FLUOROURACIL (M→F) FOR THE TREATMENT OF NODE-NEGATIVE BREAST CANCER PATIENTS WITH ESTROGEN-RECEPTOR (ER)-NEGATIVE TUMORS

In 1981, the NSABP began a randomized trial (B-13) to determine the worth of M→F therapy in node-negative breast cancer patients with ER-negative tumors (<10 fmol). Initial findings, reported in 1989 (1) after 4 years of follow-up, indicated a significant improvement in disease-free survival (DFS) for women treated with M→F compared to those receiving no systemic therapy. The advantage from M→F was observed in women aged ≤49 years as well as in those aged ≥50 years. No significant survival benefit was observed.

Because cyclophosphamide, methotrexate, and 5-fluorouracil (CMF) had been shown to demonstrate a benefit in patients similar to those in B-13, in October 1988, the NSABP implemented another clinical trial, B-19, to compare the worth of M→F with conventional CMF. Findings from B-13 were recently reported through 8 years of follow-up and those from B-19, through 5 years of follow-up (2).

There was a significant benefit in DFS from M→F therapy given for 12 cycles in B-13 at 4 years; this benefit persisted through 8 years of follow-up (74% vs. 59%; $P < 0.001$) (Figure 9-1). The overall survival advantage was of borderline significance ($P = 0.06$). The DFS benefit was present in women aged ≤49 years (69% vs. 56%; $P = 0.006$) as well as in those aged ≥50 years (81% vs. 63%; $P = 0.002$) (Figure 9-2). A survival advantage was evident only in the older patients (89% vs. 80%; $P = 0.03$)

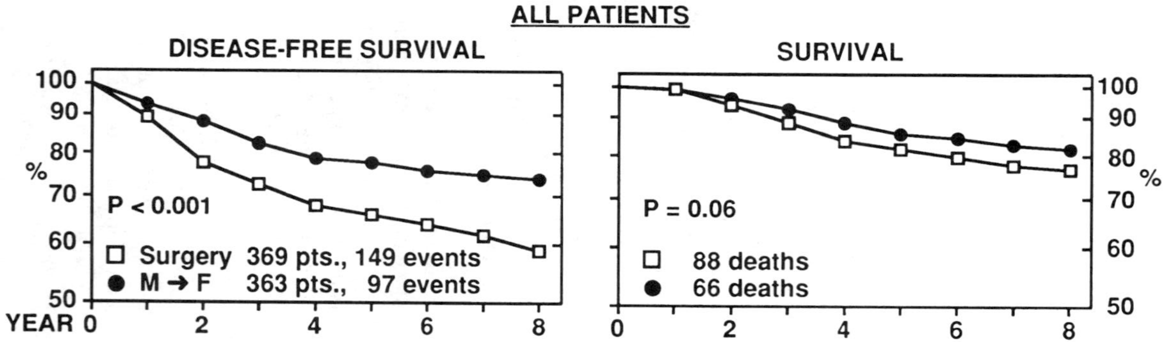

Figure 9-1. Disease-free survival and survival, through 8 years of follow-up, all patients: NSABP B-13.

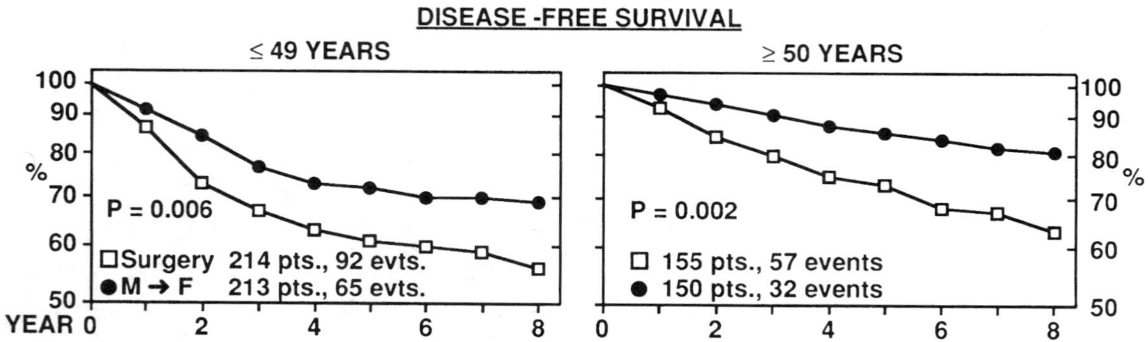

Figure 9-2. Disease-free survival, through 8 years of follow-up, according to age: NSABP B-13.

(Figure 9-3). The findings from B-13 indicated that the benefit was achieved without the use of an alkylating agent.

In B-19, there was an overall DFS advantage (82% vs. 73%; $P < 0.001$) and a borderline survival advantage (88% vs. 85%; $P = 0.06$) following CMF, when compared with M→F given for 6 cycles (Figure 9-4). The DFS (84% vs. 72%; $P < 0.001$) in women aged ≤49 years was clearly better following CMF (Figure 9-5). In patients aged ≥50 years, the DFS findings with regard to the relative worth of M→F and CMF were less clear ($P = 0.13$) (Figure 9-5). When survival outcome was evaluated within age groups, 89% of CMF-treated patients ≤49 years of age were alive at 5 years, compared with 84% of such women who received M→F ($P = 0.04$). In patients ≥50 years of age, 88% of patients treated with CMF and 86% of patients who received M→F were alive at 5 years ($P = 0.64$) (data not shown).

Findings regarding dose reduction and toxicity in B-19 patients failed to indicate that those parameters had any bearing on the response to CMF in either older or younger women. Findings indicated that the absence of a clear benefit from CMF in patients aged ≥50 years was not related to the amount of drug received.

We concluded that both M→F and CMF are effective for node-negative patients with ER-negative tumors. The incidence of local-regional and distant metastases and of ipsilateral breast tumor recurrence (IBTR) following lumpectomy and breast irradiation decreased after either therapy was employed. Although the benefit from either therapy was evident in all patients regardless of age, the advantage was found to be greater from CMF, particularly in younger women. Because of its lesser toxicity, M→F may be of value in treating patients with associated medical problems that would prohibit their receiving CMF. For a more in-depth discussion of these findings and of the possible mechanisms responsible for them, the reader is referred to the recent publication (2).

TAMOXIFEN FOR THE TREATMENT OF NODE-NEGATIVE BREAST CANCER PATIENTS WITH ESTROGEN-RECEPTOR (ER)-POSITIVE TUMORS

In 1982 the NSABP initiated a randomized clinical trial (B-14) to assess the worth of adjuvant tamoxifen therapy (20 mg/day) in patients with histologically negative nodes and ER-positive tumors (≥10 fmol). Previous reports of findings from that study indicated a highly significant prolongation of DFS through 5 years of follow-up in patients of all ages (3,4). There was a decreased rate of treatment failure at local and distant sites and a decrease in both the incidence of IBTR after lumpectomy and breast irradiation and in the occurrence of second primary cancers in the contralateral breast. Moreover, the advantages were achieved in all subgroups with an acceptable incidence of toxicity. Findings have recently been obtained relative to the outcome, through 10 years of follow-up, of over 2800 patients initially randomized to receive either tamoxifen or placebo. In addition, the outcome of patients who received more than 5 years of tamoxifen therapy has been compared with that of those who discontinued tamoxifen after 5 years. Findings have also been obtained with regard to the adverse effects of prolonged tamoxifen therapy. The updated

Text continues on page 88

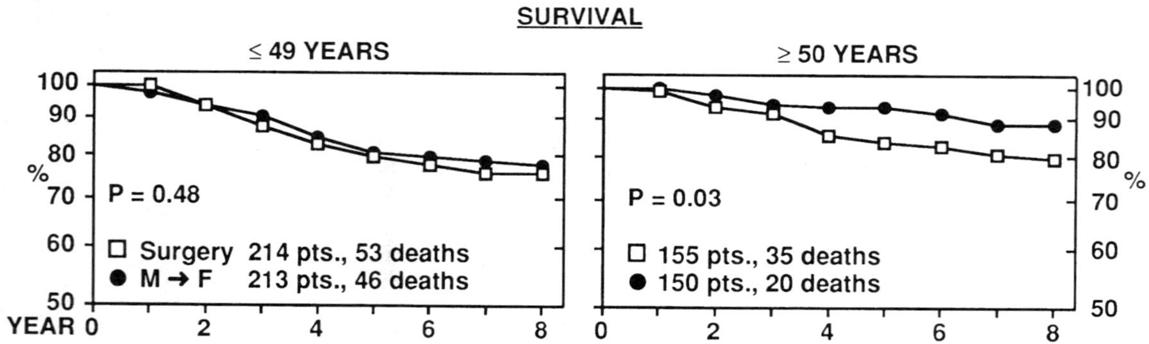

Figure 9-3. Survival, through 8 years of follow-up, according to age: NSABP B-13.

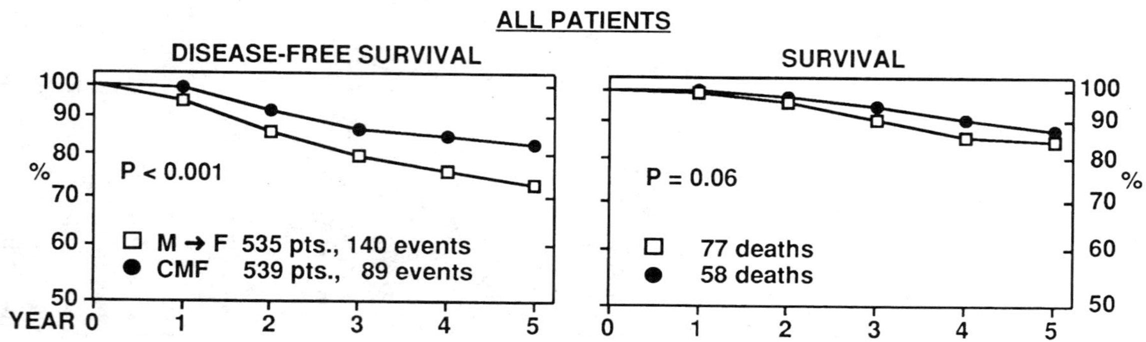

Figure 9-4. Disease-free survival and survival, through 5 years of follow-up, all patients: NSABP B-19.

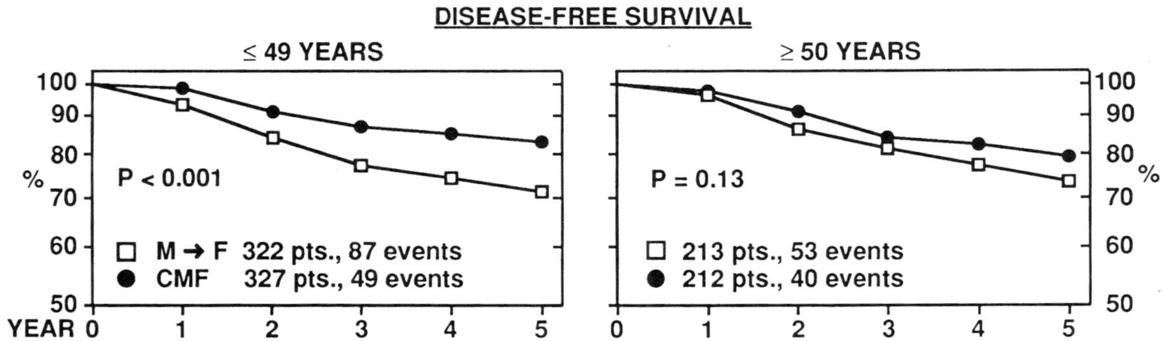

Figure 9-5. Disease-free survival, through 5 years of follow-up, according to age: NSABP B-19.

findings from B-14 were considered in light of some of prevailing biologic concepts regarding tamoxifen's mechanism of action. For a more comprehensive account of the design and results of this study, which are beyond the scope of this presentation, the reader is referred to the recent publication (5).

The findings from B-14 indicate that the magnitude of the benefit from tamoxifen first reported after 4 years of follow-up remains undiminished through 10 years. A significant DFS advantage was observed (69% vs. 57% at 10 years [$P < 0.0001$]; relative risk 0.66 [95% CI 0.58-0.74]) (Figure 9-6). The benefit from tamoxifen was observed in those aged ≤49 years ($P < 0.0001$) as well as in those ≥50 years of age ($P < 0.0001$) (Figure 9-6). There was also a significant advantage from tamoxifen in distant disease-free survival ($P < 0.0001$; Figure 9-7) and in survival (80% vs. 76% at 10 years; $P = 0.02$) (Figure 9-7). Tamoxifen significantly reduced both the rate of treatment failure at local, regional, and distant sites and the incidence of IBTR after lumpectomy and breast irradiation. The reduction in the incidence of contralateral breast cancer was of particular significance (31%; $P = 0.005$) (not shown).

To determine the length of tamoxifen administration necessary to maintain a maximum benefit, tamoxifen-treated patients who remained disease-free after 5 years were randomized to either continue therapy after 5 years or to discontinue tamoxifen and receive placebo. Through 4 years after the second randomization, there was a DFS advantage (92% vs. 86%; $P = 0.003$) for those who discontinued tamoxifen (Figure 9-8). In both age groups, the findings favored those who discontinued tamoxifen therapy. Continuing tamoxifen therapy beyond 5 years failed to result in a reduction in events at distant disease sites, as was observed at 5 years. Survival through 4 years was 96% for those who discontinued tamoxifen and 94% for those who continued it ($P = 0.08$) (Figure 9-8).

The counterintuitive findings of a better outcome from discontinuing tamoxifen were considered in light of prevailing biological concepts regarding tamoxifen resistance and tamoxifen dependence. It is possible that, after withdrawal of the drug, tumor foci dependent on tamoxifen for their growth became indolent, resulting in a decrease in the rate of treatment failure. Whatever the mechanism of action, there was no evidence to indicate that additional benefit was obtained from the administration of tamoxifen beyond 5 years. It is important to point out that, because of the nature of the study design, it was not possible to determine whether patients who received more than 5 years of tamoxifen therapy might have experienced some benefit or harm compared with patients who *never* received tamoxifen.

It is also important to emphasize that the precise time for discontinuing tamoxifen in all patients is arbitrary. Whether stopping the drug at 4 years or at 6 years in any particular patient would have provided similar results is conjectural. Moreover, in view of our findings, it seems more prudent to recommend discontinuing tamoxifen after 5 years for node-positive patients until data are available to indicate otherwise.

The incidence of non-life-threatening side effects from tamoxifen was, in most instances, similar to that in placebo patients. The incidence of thromboembolic events increased in the tamoxifen-treated patients (1.8%) over that in the placebo

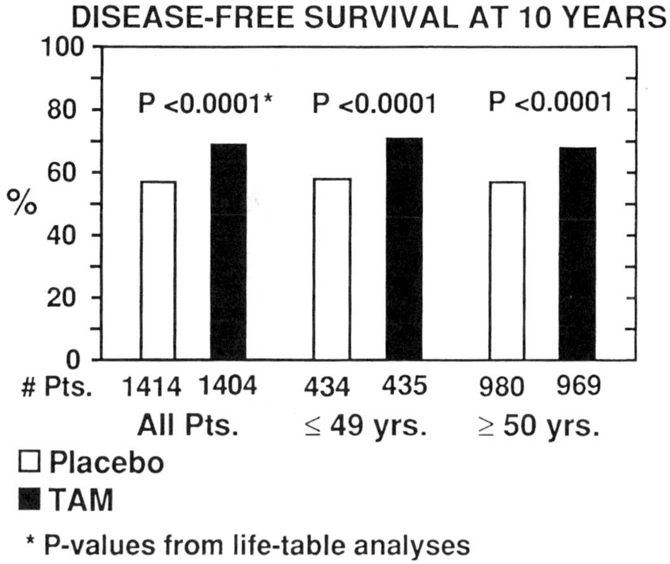

Figure 9-6. Disease-free survival of all patients and disease-free survival according to age through 10 years after first randomization: NSABP B-14.

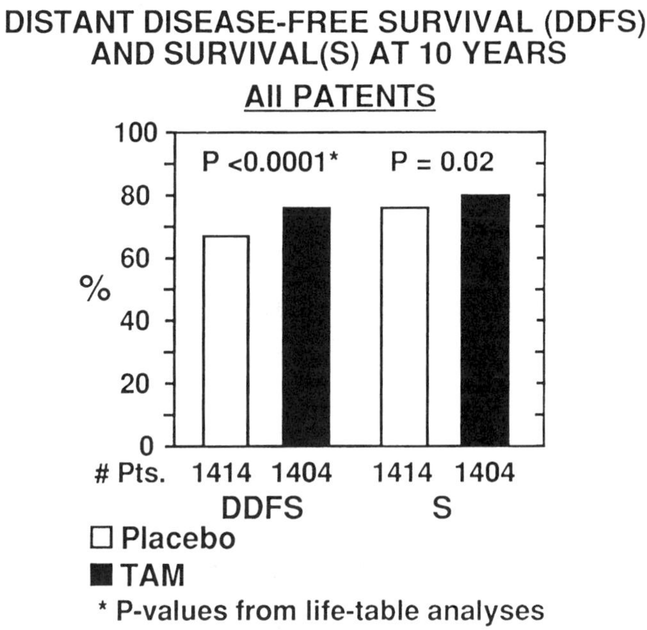

Figure 9-7. Distant disease-free survival and survival through 10 years after first randomization, all patients: NSABP B-14.

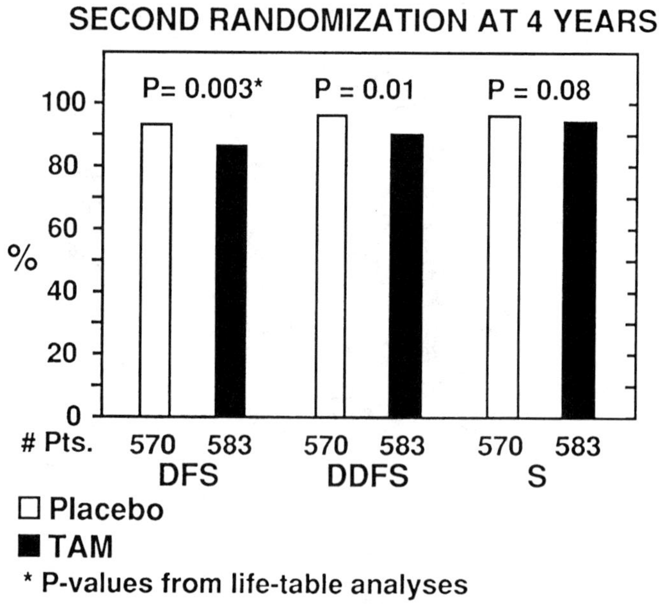

Figure 9-8. Disease-free survival, distant disease-free survival, and survival through 4 years after second randomization, all patients: NSABP B-14.

group (0.6%); more than 60% of the events occurred in tamoxifen-treated patients ≥60 years of age. Except for endometrial cancer, the incidence of second primary tumors did not increase in the tamoxifen group. The incidence of endometrial cancer was 1.6% in the tamoxifen group and 0.4% in the placebo group. The estimated annual incidence rate of endometrial cancer in tamoxifen-treated women was 1.9 cases/1000 patients, a rate similar to that previously reported (6).

We concluded that, when compared to placebo, the benefits from 5 years of tamoxifen, including a significant survival advantage, persisted through 10 years of follow-up and that no additional advantage was obtained from continuing tamoxifen therapy for longer than 5 years. Finally, we found that the side effects from tamoxifen failed to preclude its use for the treatment of breast cancer. Moreover, in view of the benefits from tamoxifen, the findings with regard to the drug's undesirable side effects did not justify the recent political and media attack that created confusion in the minds of all women regarding the appropriateness of its use.

ACKNOWLEDGMENTS

This investigation was supported by Public Health Service grants from the National Cancer Institute (NCI-U10-CA-12027, NCI-U10-CA-37377, and NCI-U10-CA-39086) and by a grant from the American Cancer Society (ACS-R-13).

REFERENCES

1. Fisher B, Redmond C, Dimitrov NV, et al. A randomized clinical trial evaluating sequential methotrexate and fluorouracil in the treatment of patients with node-negative breast cancer who have estrogen-receptor-negative tumors. N Engl J Med 1989;320:473.
2. Fisher B, Dignam J, Mamounas EP, et al. Sequential methotrexate and fluorouracil for the treatment of node-negative breast cancer patients with estrogen receptor-negative tumors: Eight-year results from National Surgical Adjuvant Breast and Bowel Project (NSABP) B-13 and first report of findings from NSABP B-19 comparing methotrexate and fluorouracil with conventional cyclophosphamide, methotrexate, and fluorouracil. J Clin Oncol 1996;14:1982.
3. Fisher B, Costantino J, Redmond C, et al. A randomized clinical trial evaluating tamoxifen in the treatment of patients with node-negative breast cancer who have estrogen-receptor-positive tumors. N Engl J Med 1989;320:479.
4. Fisher B, Redmond C. Systemic therapy in node-negative patients: Updated findings from NSABP clinical trials. J Natl Cancer Inst Monogr 1992;11:105.
5. Fisher B, Dignam J, Bryant J, et al. Five versus more than five years of tamoxifen therapy for breast cancer patients with negative lymph nodes and estrogen receptor-positive tumors. J Natl Cancer Inst. In press.
6. Fisher B, Costantino JP, Redmond CK, et al. Endometrial cancer in tamoxifen-treated breast cancer patients: Findings from the National Surgical Adjuvant Breast and Bowel Project (NSABP) B-14. J Natl Cancer Inst 1994;86:527.

Adjuvant Therapy of Cancer VIII, edited
by Sydney E. Salmon. Lippincott–Raven
Publishers, Philadelphia © 1997.

10

Impact of FAC-Adjuvant Therapy on Mortality of Early Breast Cancer: Long-Term Results of the M. D. Anderson Cancer Center Studies

Aman U. Buzdar, Gabriel N. Hortobagyi, S. Eva Singletary, Frankie A. Holmes, Richard Theriault, Ronald Walters, Kapil Dhingra, Daniel Booser, Angela Morris, Lina Asmar, Vance Wright-Browne, Eleni Diamandidou, Maria A. Witjaksono, Eric Strom, Marsha McNeese, and Frederick Ames

Between 1974 and 1986, four prospective adjuvant chemotherapy studies were carried out at the M. D. Anderson Cancer Center. In these trials, 1107 patients were treated. Earlier findings of these trials have been published (1–4). The updated results of these studies, including the efficacy of doxorubicin-containing combinations (FAC) and the long-term safety profile of this drug regimen, are presented in this chapter.

PATIENTS AND METHODS

A total of 1107 patients with either stage II or III disease were treated in four prospective studies following definitive breast surgery. The details of pretreatment characteristics and the chemotherapy programs have been published earlier (1–4). The number of patients in each study, including those who remain alive, those who have died from causes other than breast cancer, and the median follow-up of living patients are shown in Table 10-1. The disease-free and overall survival of these FAC-treated patients were compared to a consecutive series of 186 historical control patients. The details of the historical control group have been published earlier (1). These patients had similar stages of disease, but were treated with only regional therapy and received no systemic adjuvant therapy. Follow-up data of the historical control group is also shown in Table 10-1. Information on all patients was updated through September 1995. The cause of death for each patient was evaluated. The risks of developing a second primary breast cancer, non-breast malignancies and cardiac dysfunction, were also updated.

The Kaplan-Meier technique and Gehan's test were used to estimate survival rates, and statistical differences between outcomes were measured by two-tailed p-values. Survival was calculated from the start of chemotherapy. All deaths due to any cause (including causes other than breast cancer) were counted as deaths in computing survival curves.

TABLE 10-1. Survival and Follow-up Data of Four Studies

Study Number	Total Patients	# Alive (%)	Dead (Without Recurrence of Cancer)	Median Follow-up Living Patients (months)
1	222	90 (41)	34 (15)	204
2	238	103 (43)	22 (9)	189
3	336	190 (43)	16 (5)	155
4	311	181 (58)	18 (6)	123
Historical Controls	186	28 (15)	29 (16)	221

RESULTS

At this update, 564 patients were alive and the median follow-up of living patients in the combined FAC studies was 12.4 years. The 10-year estimated survival rates by stage, age, and nodal status are shown by individual study in Table 10-2. Approximately 72% of the patients with 1–3 positive nodes, 55% of those with 4–10 positive nodes, and 36% of the patients with >10 positive nodes were alive at 10 years. Overall, there were no significant differences in the survival between the studies, but there was a trend (non-significant) for improved survival of patients treated in the last two studies, compared to the earlier two studies. The estimated reduction in mortality at 15 years compared with the historical control group was approximately 50% (53% vs. 27% in FAC and Controls were alive) and 30% (31% vs. 17% in FAC and Controls were alive) for patients with stage II and III disease, respectively. Patients <50 years of age had a 57% (61% vs. 20% in FAC and controls were alive) reduction in mortality, and those ≥50 years of age had a 44% (42% vs. 20% in FAC and controls were alive) reduction in the risk of death. Patients with stage II disease and with 1–3 positive nodes had a 62% (63% vs. 29% in FAC and controls were alive); 4–10 positive nodes a 47% (48% vs. 30% in FAC and controls were alive); and those with >10 positive nodes had a 24% (27% vs. 13% in FAC and controls were alive) reduction in mortality in comparison with historical controls. The disease-free survival of combined patients in four studies treated with adjuvant FAC chemotherapy is shown in Figure 10-1 by stage of disease. Most recurrences were observed in the first 6–7 years, and very few late recurrences have been observed with longer follow-up. The disease-free and overall survival data of all patients with stage II treated with FAC compared with historical controls are illustrated in Figure 10-2. With additional follow-up the differences in survival have persisted.

The survival of all FAC treated patients who were ≥50 years of age was evaluated by cause-specific mortality. As would be expected, with longer follow-up a significant number of patients have died from causes other than cancer (Figure 10-3).

TABLE 10-2. Percent Disease Free and Overall Survival at 10 Years by Individual Study

	Percent Disease Free					Percent Survival				
	Study 1	**Study 2**	**Study 3**	**Study 4**	***P***	**Study 1**	**Study 2**	**Study 3**	**Study 4**	***P***
Stage II	58	53	58	57	.82	61	55	67	60	.25
Nodal Involvement										
1–3	64	73	66	65	.80	73	64	72	72	.79
4–10	55	49	56	51	.66	55	53	68	53	.44
>10	36	28	22	33	.80	37	33	32	38	.99
Stage III	32	31	37	43	.41	37	33	45	46	.36
All Pts.	49	45	54	55	.07	53	46	62	58	<.01

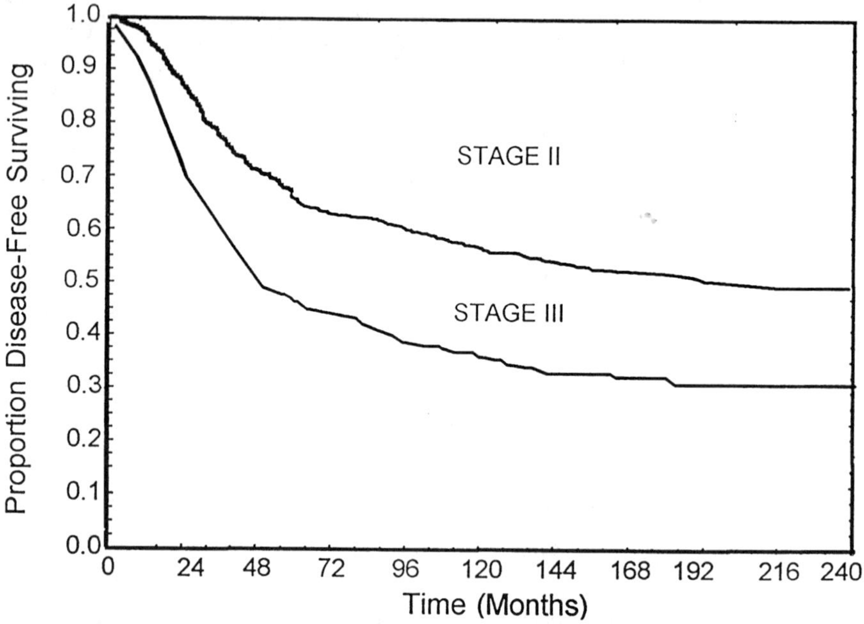

Figure 10-1. Disease-free survival of combined patients in four studies by stage of disease, treated with FAC-Combination Chemotherapy.

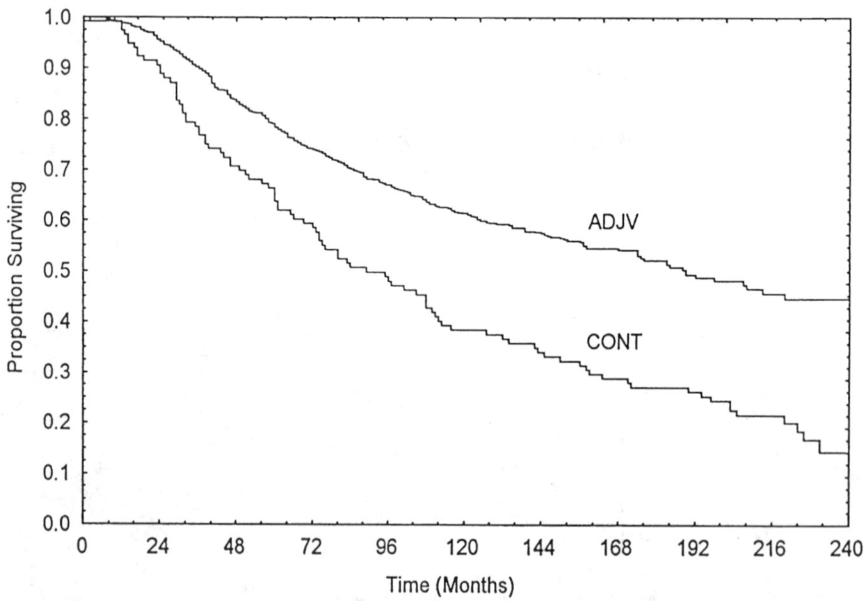

Figure 10-2. Disease-free survival of stage II treated with FAC-Combination, and the historical control group (ADJV = FAC; CONT = historical control group)

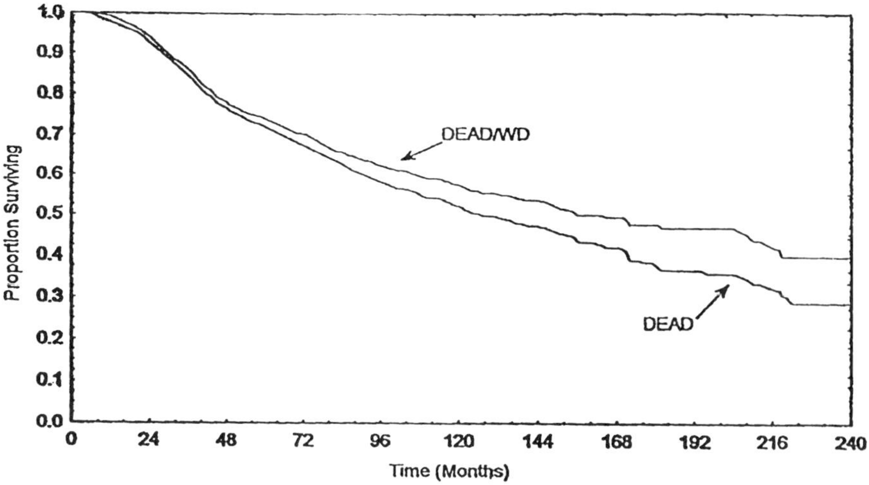

Figure 10-3. Survival of FAC patients ≥ 50 years of age (stage II), mortality from cancer and all causes (DEAD/WD = death with disease; DEAD = death from any cause)

In our third study, we evaluated the role of an alternate, potentially non-cross resistant chemotherapy regimen. Patients whose tumors were either estrogen receptor-positive, or unknown, were randomized to receive either tamoxifen alone for 6 months, or tamoxifen with methotrexate and vinblastine after completion of FAC. The 13-year estimated disease-free survival rates for patients who had estrogen receptor-positive tumors were 64% and 55%, for patients treated with tamoxifen alone and with additional chemotherapy, respectively. The disease-free survival rate of patients with estrogen receptor-negative tumors was 51%, and these patients received treatment with methotrexate and vinblastine.

The incidence of cardiotoxicity was 1% for patients treated in the initial two studies; and these patients had a maximum dose of 300 mg/m^2 of doxorubicin administered by bolus. Most episodes of cardiac dysfunction occurred within a few months of the last dose of doxorubicin. With longer follow-up, no delayed cardiac toxicity has been observed. In the fourth study doxorubicin was given as a 72-hr continuous infusion, and total cumulative dose delivered was 430 mg/m^2. In this group, one patient with preexisting heart disease developed heart failure. Several additional patients later developed cardiac dysfunction, but these had recurrent disease and required additional treatment with cardiotoxic drugs (Table 10-3). The hazard rate for cardiac failure from the last dose of doxorubicin is shown graphically in Figure 10-4, by the method of drug administration. Patients treated with continuous infusion doxorubicin had a 30% higher cumulative dose of the drug, and yet had lower risk of cardiac dysfunction ($P = 0.06$).

The risk of leukemia was also evaluated in these patients; those who received radiation therapy in addition to FAC chemotherapy had a somewhat higher risk of leukemia (2.5%; 95% confidence intervals 1.0–5.1%) compared to the patients who

TABLE 10-3. Cardiotoxicity Data of FAC Studies

Study	Cumulative Doxorubicin (mg/m²)	Doxorubicin-related Congestive Heart Failure	Congestive Heart Failure (Other Causes)
1	300	2 (1%)	7 (4.1%)
2	300	2 (1%)	1 (<1%)
4*	430	1 (<1%)	5 (2%)

* Study #3 complete data were not available at this review

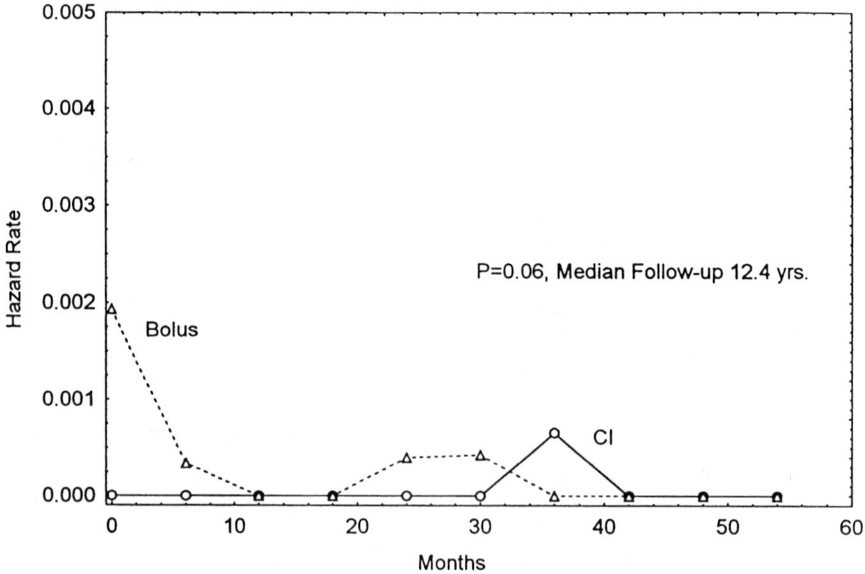

Figure 10-4. Hazard rates for congestive heart failure from last dose of doxorubicin by schedules of administration of the drug ($P = 0.06$).

received only FAC (0.6%; 95% confidence intervals 0.1–2.4%) (5). Thirty-four cases of second primary breast cancer were diagnosed. Of those, 24 patients were in the subgroup ($n = 512$) of patients who received irradiation and chemotherapy. The risk of developing contralateral primary breast cancer was somewhat higher in patients treated with chemotherapy and irradiation (6).

DISCUSSION

The long-term data of four prospective studies compared with historical controls showed that FAC chemotherapy is effective in reducing the risk of death from

TABLE 10-4. Percent Disease free at 10 Years in Milan and FAC Studies

Groups	A-CMF	CMF-A	FAC
4–10 Nodes	47	29	55
10 + Nodes	29	21	36

breast cancer. The reduction in mortality for patients under 50 years of age was a striking 57%. A 25–30% reduction was observed for patients with either stage III disease, or those with stage II disease and >10 positive nodes. Our results compare favorably to a recently reported study of doxorubicin as a single agent followed by CMF therapy 7, and these are shown in Table 10-4. In comparable prognostic subgroups of patients, the FAC combination resulted in a higher fraction of patients remaining alive and free of disease at 10 years, compared with doxorubicin followed by CMF 7.

Long-term follow-up of these studies showed that the incidence of cardiac failure with bolus doxorubicin was roughly 1%, and it was markedly reduced when the drug was administered by a 72-hour continuous infusion schedule. The role of the newly available cardioprotective agent, desrazoxane needs to be evaluated in the adjuvant setting, since doxorubicin-containing therapies are becoming the standard of care. Patients treated with FAC chemotherapy had a small but definite excess risk of developing leukemia or second primary breast cancer. This risk was somewhat higher in patients who received radiation therapy in addition to chemotherapy.

The role of additional treatment with potentially non-cross resistant drugs was evaluated in one of our studies, and the data do suggest an additional reduction in recurrence with this approach. However, the sample size was too small to detect differences with statistical significance. Recently we completed accrual in another prospective randomized study to evaluate this hypothesis. Newer cytotoxic drugs, including paclitaxel and vinorelbine, with significant activity against doxorubicin-resistant tumors have recently become available. These drugs need to be evaluated as potentially non-cross resistant alternate therapies with FAC, to further reduce the risk of death. The role of some of these drugs is being evaluated in current studies.

REFERENCES

1. Buzdar AU, Blumenschein GR, Gutterman JU, Tashima CK, Hortobagyi GN, Smith TL, Campos LT, Wheeler WL, Hersh EM, Freireich EJ, Gehan EA. Postoperative adjuvant chemotherapy with 5-fluorouracil, doxorubicin, cyclophosphamide, and BCG vaccine: A follow-up report. JAMA 1979;242:1509–1513.
2. Buzdar AU, Blumenschein GR, Smith TL, Powell KC, Hortobagyi GN, Yap HY, Schell FC, Barnes BC, Ames FC, Martin RG, Hersh EM. Adjuvant chemotherapy with fluorouracil, doxorubicin, and cyclophosphamide (FAC) with or without BCG and with or without irradiation in operable breast cancer: A prospective randomized trial. Cancer 1984;53:384–389.
3. Buzdar AU, Hortobagyi GN, Kau SW, Smith TL, Fraschini G, Holmes FA, Gutterman JU, Hug VM, Singletary SE, Ames FC, McNeese MD. Adjuvant therapy with escalating doses of doxorubicin and cyclophosphamide with or without leukocyte α-interferon for stage II or III breast cancer. J Clin Oncol 1992;10:1540–1546.

4. Buzdar AU, Hortobagyi GN, Kau S, Smith TL, Fraschini G, Holmes FA, Hug V, Gutterman JU, McNeese MD, Singletary SE, Ames F. Doxorubicin-containing adjuvant therapy for patients with stage II breast cancer: MD Anderson Cancer Center experience. In: Salmon SE, ed. Adjuvant therapy of cancer VI. W. B. Saunders Co., 1990, pp 210–215.
5. Diamandidou E, Buzdar A, Smith T, Frye D, Witjaksono M, Hortobagyi G. Treatment-related leukemia in breast cancer patients treated with FAC chemotherapy. Breast Cancer Res Treatment 1996;37(Suppl):36. [Abstr.]
6. Wright-Browne V, Buzdar AU, Smith TL, McNeese M, Strom E, Dye C, Hortobagyi GN. The incidence of second primary breast cancer (SPBC) in women treated with chemotherapy alone versus women treated with doxorubicin-containing chemotherapy (FAC) and radiotherapy (XRT). Breast Cancer Res Treatment 1996;37(Suppl):36. [Abstr.]
7. Bonadonna G, Zambetti M, Valagussa P. Sequential or alternating doxorubicin and CMF regimens in breast cancer with more than three positive nodes. JAMA 1995;273:542–547.

Adjuvant Therapy of Cancer VIII, edited
by Sydney E. Salmon. Lippincott–Raven
Publishers, Philadelphia © 1997.

11

CMF Versus Tamoxifen Plus Goserelin as Adjuvant Treatment of ER-Positive Pre-Perimenopausal Breast Cancer Patients: Preliminary Results of an Ongoing Italian Breast Cancer Adjuvant Study Group (GROCTA) Trial

F. Boccardo, A. Rubagotti, D. Amoroso, M. Liquori, M. Mesiti, O. Geraci, P. Delia, E. Villa, D. Aldrighetti, F. Genta, C. De Sanctis, L. Irtelli, D. Donati, P. Pacini, A. Farris, T. Scotto, G. Schieppati, and other participants in the GROCTA, National Institute for Cancer Research, Genoa, Italy

Chemotherapy still represents the standard treatment for premenopausal women at risk of relapse following mastectomy (1). However, we had previously showed that in women with ER positive tumors prolonged treatment with tamoxifen can achieve equivalent if not better results than chemotherapy with less acute side effects (2,3). Because these results came out from subgroup analysis, we initiated a confirmatory trial, the preliminary results of which are the subject of the present report.

PATIENTS AND METHODS

Patient Eligibility

Since January 1989, 237 premenopausal or perimenopausal women (i.e., those women without regular menses for a maximum of 12 months at the time of mastectomy) with surgically removed breast cancer were entered into this trial provided they met the following criteria: age above 35; modified radical mastectomy or quadrantectomy with axillary clearance for women with a tumor of 2 cm or less in diameter (in these patients radiotherapy of the residual breast through two opposing irradiating fields for a total dose of 50 Gy plus 10 Gy on the tumor bed was mandatory); positive axillary lymph nodes or negative lymph nodes in the presence of a high TLI (>2.8%) or a high S phase (>8%); positive ER assay (>10 fmol/mg of protein); adequate bone marrow reserve (WBC ≥4000; platelets ≥120,000); creatinine and bilirubin less than 1.5 N; no co-morbid diseases or geographic reasons that might alter patients compliance to the planned treatment or to follow-up examinations.

Allocated Treatments

Within 4 weeks since mastectomy (or quadrantectomy) patients were randomly allocated to receive either six cycles of CMF (cyclophosphamide: 100 mg/m^2 per os days 1–14; methotrexate: 40 mg/m^2 IV days 1 and 8; 5-fluorouracil: 600 mg/m^2 IV days 1 and 8; every 4 weeks) or tamoxifen (30 mg daily) for a total of 5 years. In patients allocated to CMF, who had been previously treated with quadrantectomy, radiotherapy was usually administered during chemotherapy. Patients allocated to tamoxifen treatment were given also the depot formulation of goserelin (one injection subcutaneously every 4 weeks) for the first 2 years. A few patients were treated with ovarian irradiation.

Follow-Up Studies

Patients were clinically examined every 3 months for the first 3 years, then every 4 months until the fifth year. A clinical check-up every 6 months was planned thereafter for 5 more years. During the first 5 years, blood counts were repeated every 3 months, chest x-ray every 6 months, and bone scan yearly. Chest tomography, bone survey and/or tomography, liver scan and/or ultrasonography, and all other investigations were done whenever deemed necessary by the patient's physician. The vital status of any patient failing to present for examination was checked by phone.

Statistical Analysis

The events used as end points for assessment of disease-free survival included first local recurrence of disease, regional and distant metastases, recurrent disease in the ipsilateral breast, controlateral breast cancer, second malignancy, and death due to whatever cause. The last event was used for the analysis of overall survival. Times were measured from the date of randomization. Survival and disease-free survival were estimated by the Kaplan-Meier method (4). The log-rank procedure was used to assess the statistical significance of treatment differences in events distribution (5). The disease-free survival of patients with drug-induced amenorrhea was compared to the disease-free survival of patients still regularly menstruating during chemotherapy using the method first described by Mantel and Byar (6) in which subjects are compared according to their status (amenorrhea yes or not) at each time of the follow-up. All p values were derived from a two-sided test for significance.

Sample Size Assessment

In the previous study (3) a trend of about 10% favored tamoxifen with respect to chemotherapy in premenopausal women. However, the difference was not significant, due to the small number of patients left by subgroup analysis. Considering that the reported 5-year relapse-free survival for the premenopausal women treated with 6 cycles of standard CMF, i.e., the same regimen we used in the present study, in the Milan studies was about 55% (7) and that even better results might be expected by the combination of tamoxifen with ovarian ablation in ER positive patients, it was thought that 300 patients, recruited in 3 years, could be enough to allow us to detect a difference between 10 and 15% in the 5-year relapse-free survival in favor of the patients allocated to endocrine therapy assuming an error equal to 0.05 and a power of 80%.

RESULTS

The main characteristics of study patients are summarized in Table 11-1. Patients in the two arms are well balanced with respect to age, menopausal status, tumor size, tumor grade, number of involved nodes and treatment of primary. At a median follow-up time of 36 months (range: 1–81 months) 4 patients (1.7%) were lost to follow-up, 62 progressed, and 22 died. There was no difference so far between the two treatment arms either in terms of disease free survival (Figure 11-1) or in terms of overall survival (Figure 11-2). Results were equivalent also after stratifying patients on the basis of tumor grade (grade 1–2 vs. grade 3 vs. grade unknown) or number of involved nodes (nodes = 0 vs. nodes = 1–3 vs. nodes ≥ 4) (data not shown). First

TABLE 11-1. Main Characteristics of Study Patients

	CMF (%)	**TMX + GOS (%)**
No. patients	116	121
Median age in years (range)	45 (32-58)	46 (30–57)
Menopausal status		
Premenopause	104 (89.7)	106 (87.6)
Perimenopause	2 (10.3)	15 (12.4)
Tumor grade		
G1–2	77 (66.4)	88 (72.7)
G3	14 (12.0)	8 (6.6)
Gx	25 (21.6)	25 (20.7)
Tumor size		
≤2 cm	62 (53.4)	55 (45.4)
>2 cm	54 (46.6)	66 (54.6)
No. of involved nodes		
0*	17 (14.7)	17 (14.0)
1–3	73 (62.9)	72 (59.5)
≥4	26 (22.4)	32 (26.5)
Treatment of primary		
Mastectomy	61 (52.6)	69 (57.0)
Quart	55 (47.4)	52 (43.0)

*Includes only high TLI or S phase Tumors

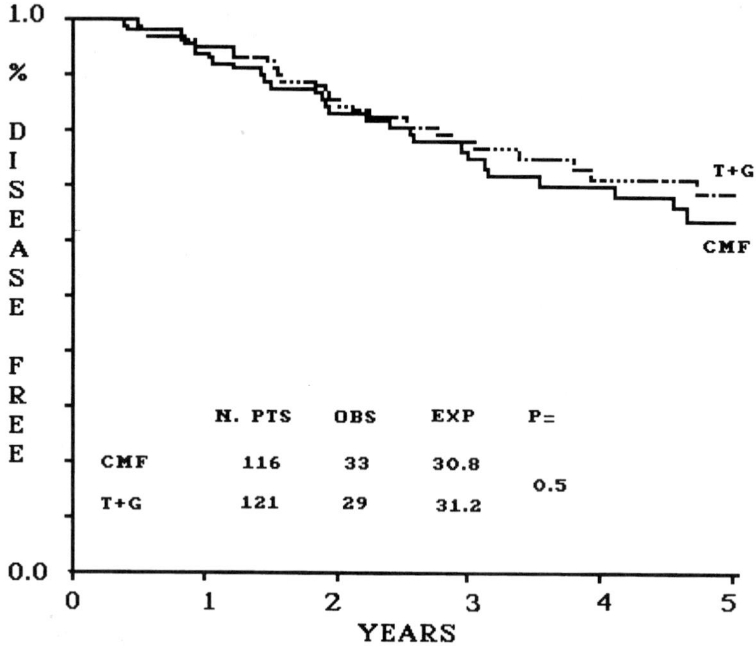

Figure 11-1. Comparative 5-year disease-free survival for all patients.

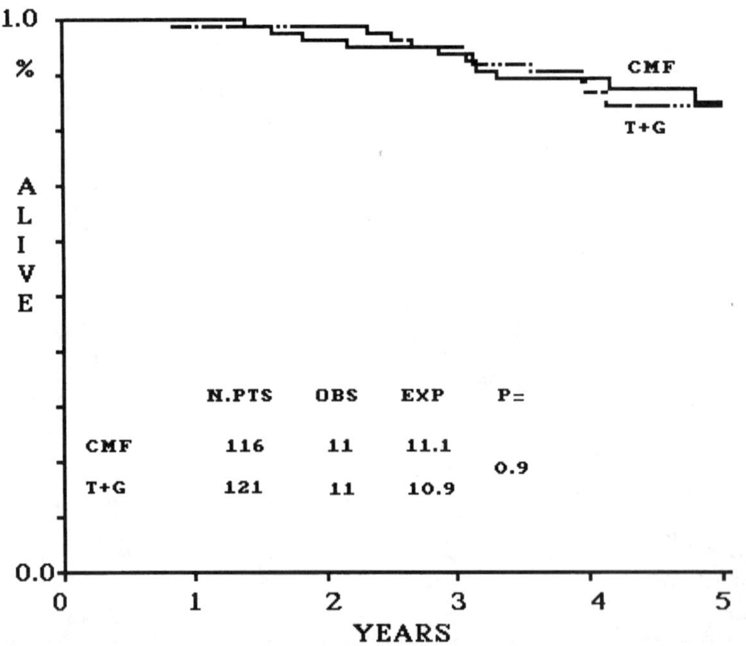

Figure 11-2. Comparative 5-year survival for all patients.

site of disease progression was also comparable (Table 11-2). In the CMF group there was a significant trend ($P = 0.04$) in favor of the patients achieving drug-induced amenorrhea in course of treatment. Moreover, the 5-year disease-free survival of these patients was comparable to that of women treated with tamoxifen plus goserelin (Figure 11-3). Treatment toxicity is summarized in Table 11-3. Leukopenia, nausea and vomiting, stomatitis, diarrhea, and alopecia were significantly more com-

TABLE 11-2. First Site of Disease Progression

Site	CMF (n = 33)	TMX + GOS (n = 29)
Local-regional		
Chest wall + axilla	3	2
Ipsilateral breast	2	—
Distant		
Skin/nodes	4	4
Bone	10	11
Viscera	3	6
Multiple sites	4	2
Local-regional plus distant	5	2
New primaries	2	2

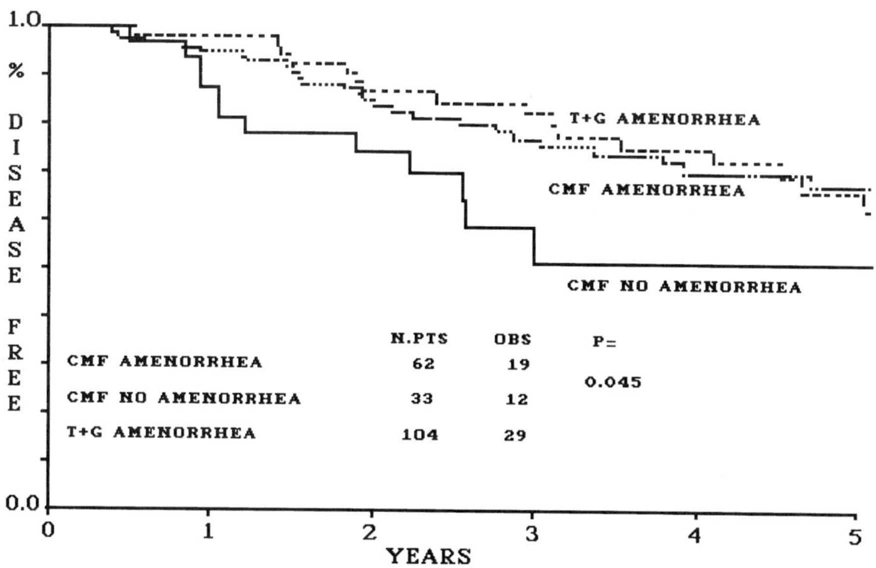

Figure 11-3. Comparative 5-year disease-free survival for patients in the tamoxifen (TMX) group and for patients in the CMF group according to drug-induced amenorrhea.

TABLE 11-3. Main Differences in Side Effects (any degree)

	CMF (n = 116)	TMX + GOS (n = 121)	P
Leukopenia	46.0%	7.4%	0.000
Thrombocitopenia	8.5%	2.4%	N.S.
Nausea	64.0%	5.7%	0.000
Vomiting	50.0%	0.8%	0.000
Stomatitis	13.0%	—	0.000
Diarrhea	8.0%	0.8%	0.02
Alopecia	30.3%	1.6%	0.000
Hot flushes	4.3%	37.0%	0.000
Spotting	—	11.0%	0.000

mon in patients allocated to CMF, while hot flushes and vaginal spotting were significantly more common in patients allocated to tamoxifen plus goserelin.

DISCUSSION

When this trial was initiated, an accrual of about 100 patients per year for a total of 3 years was expected. This projection appeared to be reasonable in view of the recruitment rate achieved in the previous study (2,3). However, after 6 years only 237 patients had been recruited. Therefore, an interim analysis was performed to decide whether recruitment should continue. At the time of this analysis the study is still unpowered, having a power of about 60% to detect a difference of 10% or more in disease-free survival between the two groups on study. However, it seems to us that it provides preliminary information that deserve some interest, although they should be considered with caution. In fact, it confirms that endocrine therapy represents a safe alternative to chemotherapy in premenopausal women with ER positive tumors. These results are particularly relevant if it is considered that a full dose chemotherapy was used by us in the present trial, as it is demonstrated by the high median dose-intensity of each of the drugs employed. In fact, the median ratio between the actually delivered and the planned dose was 0.83 for cyclophophamide, 0.85 for methotrexate and 0.84 for 5-fluorouracil.

Present results confirm on a prospective basis our previous findings and are in keeping with the results of a recent Scottish trial showing the superiority of oophorectomy over CMF treatment in the premenopausal women bearing ER positive tumors (8). Indeed, in our study no clear-cut superiority of endocrine therapy over CMF emerged so far. However, median follow-up time is still short. Moreover, the CMF-based chemotherapy we used was more prolonged and more intense than the chemotherapy employed by the Scottish investigators, who in addition used a higher cutoff to define their patients as ER positive ones. Our study confirms also that in premenopausal women adjuvant chemotherapy works at least in part through the endocrine effects it induces, even when it is administered with an adequate intensity. Moreover, the absolute comparability of the results achieved by chemotherapy in women developing persistent amenorrhea and of those achieved by tamoxifen plus goserelin, provides a rationale for the use of LH-RH analogs in those women who do not achieve castration in course of chemotherapy. Finally, the present trial confirms that chemotherapy causes significantly more side effects than endocrine therapy, although the long-term effects on quality life of symptoms like hot flushes and vaginal spotting and of the other symptoms related to estrogen deprivation must deserve further concern. However, these symptoms are likely to develop also in women who are castrated by chemotherapy, who represented the great majority of those allocated to receive this treatment modality also in the present study.

In conclusion, our study clearly shows that prolonged tamoxifen treatment, with the concurrent use of goserelin, is equivalent to six cycles of CMF in premenopausal women with ER positive tumor, even in those subgroups at higher risk of relapse such as women with four or more involved nodes. However, because median follow-up time is still relatively short, we cannot rule out that the postulated superiority of endocrine therapy might come out in the long run, when all patients will have been treated with tamoxifen for 5 years and the events are numerous enough to ensure the expected statistical power of 80%. This will probably occur in the next 2 years, when about 50% of the patients will have relapsed.

APPENDIX—PARTICIPATING CENTERS (INVESTIGATORS)

Arcispedale S. Anna, Ferrara	D. Donati, P.Malacarne
Policlinico Careggi, Firenze	P. Pacini, M. Cappellini
Istituto Nazionale per la Ricerca sul Cancro, Genova	D. Amoroso, F. Boccardo
Ospedale Civile, Merate	S. Banducci
Istituto Scientifico S. Raffaele, Milano	D. Aldrighetti, A. Bolognesi, E. Villa
Ospedale Oncologico "M. Ascoli", Palermo	A. Traina, L. Castagnetta
Ospedale Spallanzani, Reggio Emilia	M. Sassi
Ospedale S.Giacomo, Roma	A. Beni
Ospedale Civile, Saronno	G. Schieppati
Cattedra di Oncologia Clinica, Università di Sassari	T. Scotto, A. Farris
Ospedale SS. Annunziata, Savigliano	L. Galletto
Cattedra di Ginecologia Oncologica, Università di Torino	C. De Sanctis, F. Genta, P. Sismondi
Centro Oncologico "M. Lovenati", Trieste	G. Mustacchi
Ospedali Galliera, Genova	C. Caroti, L. Gallo
Istituto di Clinica Oncologica, Università di Messina	P. Delia, O. Geraci, M. Mesiti
Cattedra di Oncologia Medica, Università "G. D'Annunzio" di Chieti	S. Iacobelli, L. Irtelli

ACKNOWLEDGMENTS

The study was partially supported by the Italian National Research Council, Project ACRO grant 93.02275.PF39. The helpful contribution by Mrs. G. De Stefano in data management and the skillful secretarial assistance by Miss A. Fossati are also acknowledged.

REFERENCES

1. Breast Cancer Chemotherapy Consensus Conference. JAMA 1985;254:3461.
2. Boccardo F, Rubagotti A, Bruzzi P, et al. Chemotherapy versus tamoxifen versus chemotherapy plus tamoxifen in node-positive, estrogen receptor-positive breast cancer patients: Results of a multicentric Italian study. J Clin Oncol 1990;8:1310.
3. Boccardo F, Rubagotti A, Amoroso D, et al. Chemotherapy versus tamoxifen versus chemotherapy plus tamoxifen in node-positive, oestrogen-receptor positive breast cancer patients. An update at 7 years of the 1st GROCTA (Breast Cancer Adjuvant Chemo-Hormone Therapy Cooperative Group) trial. Eur J Cancer 1992;28:673.
4. Kaplan ER, Meier P. Nonparametric estimation from incomplete observation. J Am Stat Assoc 1958;53:457.
5. Peto R, Pike MC, Armitage P, et al. Design and analysis of randomized clinical trials requiring prolonged observation of each patient. Part II, Analysis and examples. Br J Cancer 1977;35:1.
6. Mantel N, Byar DP. Evaluation of response-time data involving transient states: An illustration using heart transplant data. J Am Stat Assoc 1974;69:81.
7. Bonadonna G, Valagussa P, Rossi A, et al. Ten-year experience with CMF based adjuvant chemotherapy in resectable breast cancer. Breast Cancer Res Treat 1985;5:95.
8. Scottish Cancer Trials Breast Group and ICRF Breast Unit, Guy's Hospital, London. Adjuvant ovarian ablation versus CMF chemotherapy in premenopausal women with pathological stage II breast carcinoma: The Scottish trial. Lancet 1993;341:1293.

III

BREAST CANCER

HIGH-DOSE CHEMOTHERAPY

Adjuvant Therapy of Cancer VIII, edited by Sydney E. Salmon. Lippincott–Raven Publishers, Philadelphia © 1997.

12

High-Dose Chemotherapy with Stem Cell Protection: Tandem, Sequence, and Phenylalanine Mustard Studies

E. Frei III, J. Bitran, L. Ayash, A. Elias, D. Griswald, B. Teicher, P. Richardson, and C. Wheeler

High-dose chemotherapy with stem cell rescue (HD-SC) has increased the complete response (CR) rate, has probably improved survival, and has questionably produced a disease-free survival plateau (cure) rate of up to 20% in patients with early metastatic breast cancer. If a single HD-SC course is effective, two non-cross-resistant HD-SC courses might prove superior. This article presents preclinical and clinical data relating to double or tandom HD-SCs.

The three studies are indicated in Table 12-1. Induction with standard doxorubicin-based combinations was employed in all three studies. Study #1 involved a single HD-SC with CTCb (cyclophosphamide, thiotepa, carboplatin). Study #2 was similar save that HD-phenylalanine mustard (HD-P) was employed first, followed by CTCb. The third study involved the reverse sequence, i.e., HD-CT first followed by HD-P.The first two of these Phase II studies were conducted by the Dana-Farber Cancer Institute–Beth Israel Hospital; the third was undertaken at the University of Chicago. The demographics and prognostic factors for the three studies were similar.

The results in terms of CR induction are presented in Table 12-2. PRs are CRs for soft-tissue lesions in patients with bone metastases. Of note is the substantial jump in CR rate for Study #3 as a result of the second HD-SC in contrast to Study #2.

TABLE 12-1. The Three Clinical Trials (Studies)

			Intensification		
Study No.	**Induction**		**HD-SC#1**		**HD-SC#2**
I	D(MF) × 4	→	CTCb		
II	(D + CPA) × 6	→	P	→	CTCb
III	D(comb)a	→	CT	→	P

HD-SC = high dose chemotherapy with stem cell rescue.

D = doxorubicin; M = Methotrexate; F = fluorouracil; C = cyclophosphamide, T = thiotepa, Cb = carboplatin, P = PAM = phenylalinine mustard.

a = doxorubicin in various combinations.

TABLE 12-2. Frequency, Magnitude, and Timing of Tumor Response

Study	Induction	HD-SC #I	HD-SC#II
CR Following			
I	12 (19%)	18 (29%)	
II	17 (25%)	—	22 (33%)
III	4 (15%)	9 (33%)	15 (54%)
CR + PR* Following			
I	20 (32%)	27 (44%)	
II	26 (39%)	—	32 (48%)
III	4 (15%)	13 (51%)	18 (67%)

CR = complete response. PR* = CR for measured lesion but bone lesions present.

Failure-free survival (FFS) for the three studies is presented in Figure 12-1. For Study #1 relapses occurred during the first 2–3 years down to 20%, after which no further relapses occurred. The FFS for Study #2 was slightly inferior to Study #1. Thus, the addition of HD-P did not result in a superior initial response rate, failure free or overall survival.

For Study #3 the FFS at 2 and 3 years was 60% as compared to 20–30% for the other two studies. Since the difference between Study #2 and Study #3 is primarily

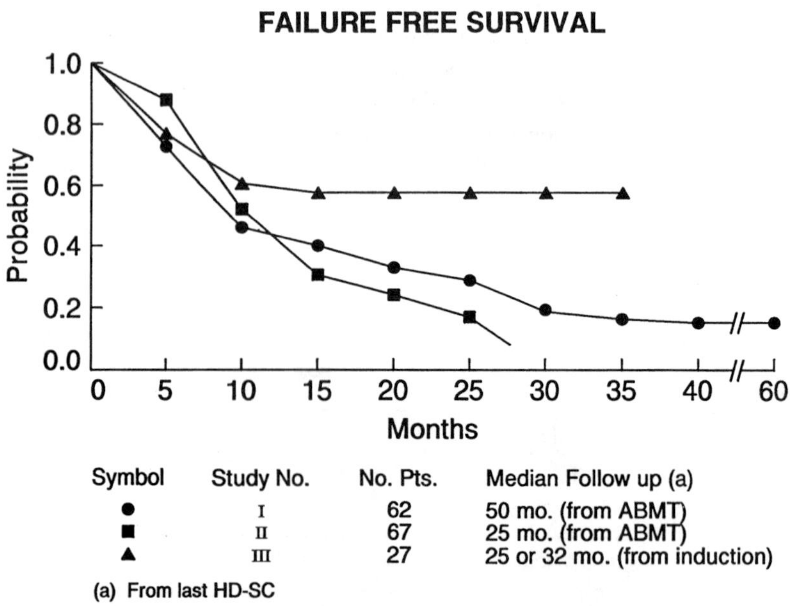

Figure 12-1. Failure-free survival for the three clinical studies.

related to the sequence of HD-SCs, we conducted laboratory studies of these relationships of alkylating agents.

We employed five human tumor cell lines, including the breast cancer line MCF7. Resistance was produced by selection pressure with increasing concentrations of the selecting agent. The resistant cell lines were then compared to their sensitive counterpart (parent line) for various properties, including cross-resistant and collateral sensitivity patterns (Table 12-3). For the PAM resistant cell lines there was a high rate (57%) of cross-resistance to the other alkylating agents as compared to CDDP, 4HC (cyclophosphamide), and HN2, where the frequency of cross-resistance was 5–17%. BCNU was intermediate. Interestingly, we found that when PAM was used as second-order treatment in cell lines resistant to other alkylating agents, collateral sensitivity was common.

Thus, in an alkylating agent sequence, PAM is the wrong drug to use first but the right drug to use as second-order treatment.

Similarly, in studies conducted at the Southern Research Institute, the p388 mouse leukemia made resistant to the various alkylating agents by serial passage in the presence of the agent *in vivo* were examined for cross-resistance (Table 12-4). In Table 12-4, S means sensitive and R means resistant; the numbers in the table mean log kill of tumor cells. Thus, a −7 indicates a 7 log kill with an LD_{10} dose. Cross resistance to PAM was common, occurring in 9 of 12 studies. In contrast, cross-resistance to the other alkylating agents occurred in only 4 of 26 (15%) of tests.

These preclinical studies are consistant with our clincial studies and will be discussed in terms of the biologic and clinical interpretations and implications.

What are the biochemical implications of these studies? The studies suggest that resistance to PAM may involve one or more mechanisms that are common to the alkylating agents and perhaps other agents as well. In contrast, resistance to some of the other alkylating agents may be specific. We and others have found multiple

TABLE 12-3. Summary of the Occurrence of Cross-Resistance in the Antitumor Alkylating Agent Resistant Cell Lines Grouped by Selecting Agent.

Resistant Cell Lines[a]	Number of Occurrences of Cross-Resistance				
	Major	Moderate	None or Minimal	Total	%
CDDP	0	3	21	3/24	13
4-HC	1	0	20	1/21	5
PAM	9	3	9	12/21	57
HN2	2	1	15	3/18	17
BCNU	8	0	13	8/21	38
TOTAL	20	7	78	27/105	25

[a]Total are five cell lines resistant to each AA.

TABLE 12-4. Cross-Resistance Among the Alkylating Agents in p388 Mouse Leukemia

	p388 Leukemia Sensitive (S) and Resistant (R) to							
	PAM		**CPA**		**cPlat**		**BCNU**	
	S	**R**	**S**	**R**	**S**	**R**	**S**	**R**
PAM	–7	0	–6	–7	–7	–7	–7	–7
CPA	–7	–7	–7	–1	–7	–7	–7	–7
cPlat	–7	+2	–3	–7	–6	+2	–3	–4
cPlat (repeat)	–7	+2	–5	–5	–6	+2	–7	–5
BCNU	–7	–8	–7	–7	–7	–8	–7	+2
Hepsulfama	–7	–1	–5	–6	–4	0	–4	–4
Spiromustine	–6	–2	–7	–5	–4	+1		
Tetraplat	–4	0			–4	–4		
Pyrizine-azo-OH	–7	–1		–6	–7			
X-resistant/total	*5/7*		*0/5*		*2/6*		*0/5*	
Resistance to non-alkylating Agents								
Doxorubicin	–7	–7	–5	–6	–7	–7		
Mitaxantrone	–6	–3			–3	–8		
AMSA	—	+2	–3	–6	–2	–7		
Merbarone	–7	–3			–5	–7		
Vincristine	–5	+1	–4	–4	–7	–7		
Penclomidine	–1	+2	–4	–1	–1	+1	–4	+1
X-resistant/total	*4/5*		*1/4*		*0/5*		*1/1*	

Number = log tumor cell kill per LD_{10} dose.

a = Busulfam analog; PAM = phenylalanine mustard; CPA = cyclophosphamide; cPlat = cisplain; BCNU = bis-chlorethyl nitrosourea; VCR = vincristine.

Spiromustine, tetraplatin, and pyizine diazo OH are nonclassical alkylating agents.

mechanisms for PAM resistant tumors, including decreased amino acid transport, and increased GSH and GST (glutathione transferase) activity. The protein sulfhydryl scavenger metallothionein may be increased. Finally, several DNA repair mechanisms capable of removing the alkylating agent cross-links have been shown to be elevated in PAM resistant cells. Of the above, only the transport mechanism would be specific for PAM.

Similarly, for the other alkylating agents both general and specific mechanisms for resistance exist and have been described. Specific mechanisms that could explain the resistance patterns and which have been described include increased expression of aldehyde dehydrogenase II for cyclophosphamide and the DNA O6 alkyl transferase DNA repair enzyme for BCNU and the DNA monitoring protein for cisplatin.

However, it has been difficult to correlate biologic resistance with biochemical events that could be responsible for the resistance. A major reason for this is that resistance is commonly multifactorial, involving three or more mechanisms.

Investigators generally report on one mechanism, the one in which they are interested. Even when that one is in fact involved in the resistance, dilution by other mechanisms makes correlation difficult. Such correlations will require examination for multiple mechanisms of resistance, a difficult task, particularly for alkylating agents and *in vivo*, particularly in patients.

Most of the studies of resistance involve tumor cells that have had long exposure to the selecting agent and are stably resistant. One might question whether mechanisms that apply here for development of stably resistant lines also are relevant after intensive short term exposure in the clinical setting. Such resistance is generally reversible. The above would suggest that with the long induction, stable resistance is genetic, whereas the labile resistance that occurs after intensive, short-term exposure is inductive. We are examining this question in model systems.

Another explanation for the broad pattern of cross-resistance to PAM may relate to mutagenicity. PAM, compared to the other alkylating agents, is more mutagenic at therapeutic doses. For example, in the adjuvant chemotherapy of breast cancer, secondary MDS and AML occurs much more commonly after PAM than after cyclophosphamide. To the extent that PAM is more mutagenic, it might be expected to produce more in the way of tumor heterogeneity and therefore greater numbers and variety of resistant daughter cells.

The major implications of these studies is that the antitumor alkylating agents differ substantially in terms of such critical issues as resistance, cross-resistance, collateral sensitivity, and reversibility of resistance, and that such factors may be critical to their optimal use in combination, sequence, high dose and other clinical trial variables.

REFERENCES

1. Ayash L, et al. J Clin Oncol 1994;12:37.
2. Bitran J, et al. Submitted.
3. Frei E III. Proc Natl Acad Sci USA 1985;82:2158.
4. Frei E III. Cancer Chemother Pharmacol 1993;13(2):113.

Adjuvant Therapy of Cancer VIII, edited
by Sydney E. Salmon. Lippincott–Raven
Publishers, Philadelphia © 1997.

13
High-Dose Chemotherapy for High-Risk Primary Breast Cancer

William P. Peters, Roger Dansey, Jared Klein, and D. Berry

Breast cancer is now the most common disease for which high-dose chemotherapy and autologous bone marrow transplantation is performed in the United States, surpassing non-Hodgkin's and Hodgkin's disease as indications. It is now estimated that over 4000 autotransplants have been done for breast cancer throughout the United States. Increasingly, the therapeutic modality is being used earlier in the disease, particularly in the high-risk adjuvant setting. This increased use reflects in part the general disappointment with available conventional dose approaches, particularly in the patients with primary breast cancer involving multiple axillary lymph nodes. The increased interest in the use of high-dose therapy also coincides with the rapidly decreasing toxicity associated with the use of the treatment modality. In experienced hands, with the use of colony stimulating factor primed peripheral blood progenitor cells (PBPC), the acute mortality of the treatment is less than 3–5% and in some centers, the procedure is largely performed as an outpatient, with average lengths of inpatient hospitalization as low as 5 days.

With some investigators emphasizing the importance of dose intensification in breast cancer (1–3), others have argued that the utilization of this therapeutic approach far exceeds its demonstrated value (4). Randomized, comparative trials have not yet been reported for treatment in the adjuvant setting, and although they are being conducted, results will not be available for another 3–4 years. Randomized trials of the use of high-dose chemotherapy with autologous cellular support in patients with metastatic breast cancer have recently been completed and reported indicating a statistically significant improvement in both disease-free and overall survival for patients treated with high-dose therapy and autologous cellular support (5,6). These data provide considerable encouragement to the conduct of the trials in primary breast cancer since many felt it unlikely that the magnitude of the benefit in metastatic disease would allow significant differences to be detected without very large trials. The study and widespread use of this treatment is complicated by medical insurance companies' concern about the potentially large and increasing total expenditures for this new therapeutic approach, despite the rapid decrease in the average overall charge for the treatment. Arbitrary and capricious denial of coverage for some patients (7) has resulted in litigation, sometimes with large punitive awards being subsequently given by juries.

Currently available data for patients with primary breast cancer examine single-institution studies with follow-up in excess of a median 5 years and a survey of the North American transplant centers (8,9). These data in combination provide a reasonable picture of the effectiveness of transplantation but do not provide the gold standard of comparative data, that is, results of prospective, randomized trials. Prospective randomized trials are underway in the United States and Europe, but the results of these trials are not likely to be available before near the turn of the century. The data reviewed here provide a view of the information available currently that can be used for guidance while waiting for the results of randomized trials in primary breast cancer.

MATERIALS AND METHODS

Single-Institution Data

Between 1987 and 1991, we treated 85 patients on a protocol prescribing induction chemotherapy with cyclophosphamide, doxorubicin, and fluorouracil (CAF) for four cycles followed by high-dose consolidation with cyclophosphamide, cisplatin, and carmustine with bone marrow and in two-thirds of the patients, peripheral blood progenitor cell support. The details of the patient selection and eligibility criteria as well as the treatment program have been described previously (10). The median follow-up for the study as presented is 6 years.

Survey of American Transplant Centers

In early 1994, we performed a survey of the American bone marrow transplant centers identified through the American Society of Blood and Marrow Transplantation. Results were obtained via electronic communication, compiled, and analyzed. Information on primary endpoints of disease-free survival and overall survival were considered the primary endpoints evaluated. Full details of the methodology are published elsewhere (8,9).

RESULTS

Single-Institution Data

Continued follow-up of patients treated and reported previously (11) provides information with a median follow-up of 6 years, a minimum follow-up of 4.5 years and a lead follow-up nearing 9 years. Figure 13-1 shows the event-free survival for the 85 patients treated with induction chemotherapy using cyclophosphamide, doxorubicin, and 5-fluorouracil (CAF) followed immediately by consolidation with high-dose cyclophosphamide, cisplatin, and carmustine with autologous cellular support. The data indicated that the event-free survival (including all relapses and therapy-related mortality) at 5 years is 64% (95% confidence interval: 53–74%). Figure 13-2 presents the overall survival for the patients in the study and at 5 years is estimated by Kaplan-Meier methodology to be 73% (95% CI: 63–83%). Table 13-1 presents the disease-free and overall survival data for patients treated as part of this high-dose intensification trial. In addition, data derived from comparable but non-randomized historical

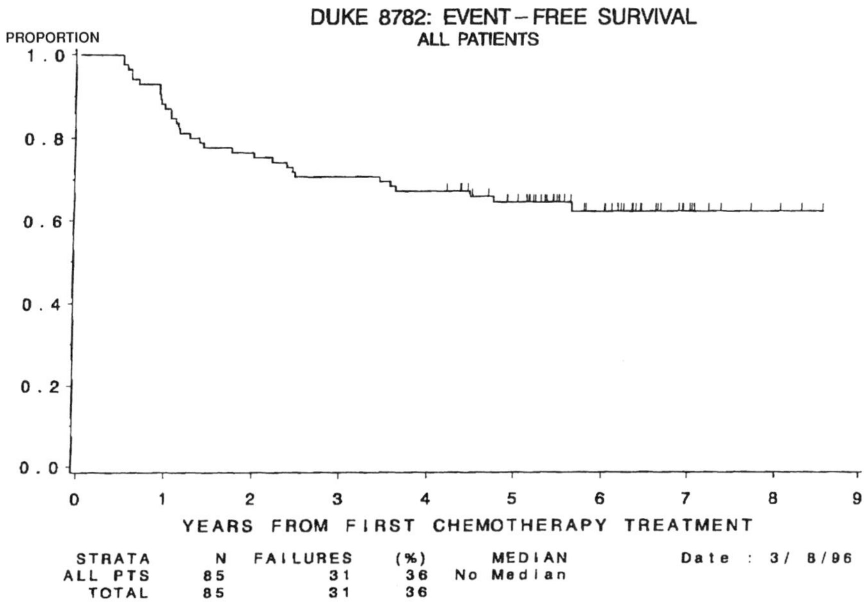

Figure 13-1. Event-free survival for 85 patients treated with four cycles of induction chemotherapy using CAF followed by high-dose consolidation with cyclophosphamide, cisplatin and carmustine (CPB) and autologous bone marrow and peripheral blood progenitor support. Details of the patient selection, eligibility, treatment and follow-up have been previously presented.

and contemporaneous control groups treated with conventional-dose chemotherapy are presented. These data compare favorably to the results seen from historical and contemporaneous control groups treated with conventional-dose chemotherapy and indicate an approximate 30% improvement in disease-free and overall survival for patients receiving high-dose consolidation.

SURVEY DATA

Results were obtained from 662 patients treated with high-dose chemotherapy and autologous cellular support for primary breast cancer. The vast majority of patients (78%) were found at initial diagnosis to have ten or more involved lymph nodes at the time of the initial surgery. Of interest in this survey, 15% of patients being treated with high-dose therapy for primary breast cancer had involvement of four to nine lymph nodes at the time of surgery. Table 13-2 shows the disease-free and overall survival for patients identified as part of this survey as treated with high-dose consolidation for primary breast cancer. These data are similar to those obtained from the single-institution trial presented above. In fact, the remarkable consistency of the treatment results across multiple regimens and multiple institutions provides some comfort in the validity of the data for this patient population.

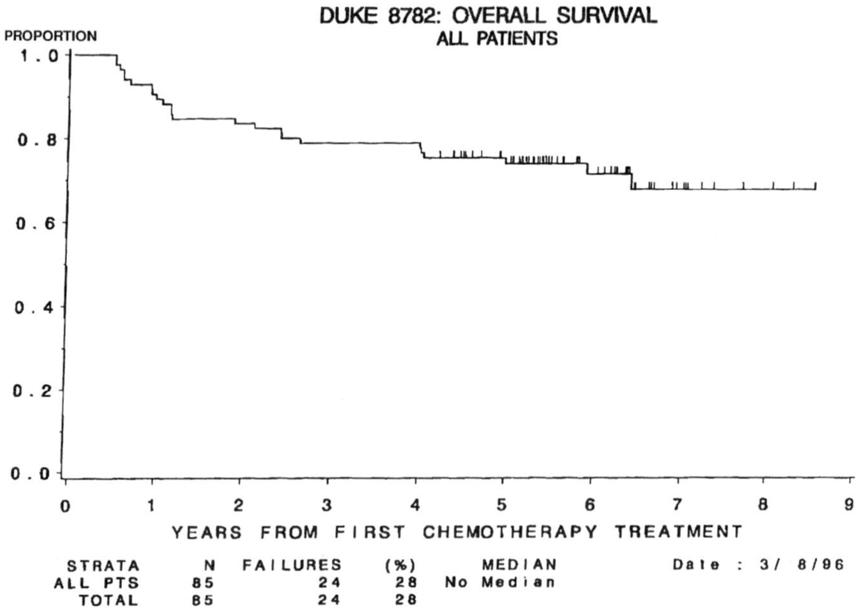

Figure 13-2. Overall survival for 85 patients treated with four cycles of induction chemotherapy using CAF followed by high-dose consolidation with cyclophosphamide, cisplatin and carmustine (CPB) and autologous bone marrow and peripheral blood progenitor support.

TABLE 13-1. Event-free and Overall Survival

Study		Number of Patients**	Event-free Survival#	Overall Survival#
Protocol 8782	CAF → HD CPB	85	64% (53–74%)	73% (63–83%)
CALGB 7581	CMFVP	111	30% (22–39%)	45% (36–54%)
CALGB 8082	CMFVP/VATH	120	30% (23–39%)	47% (38–55%)
CALGB 8541	CAF	58	35% (23–50%)	57% (43–70%)

*The details of the treatment programs have been previously reported. The updates on protocol 8782 represent an analysis to February, 1996.

**Patients are selected for number of involved nodes greater than or equal to 10 at the time of surgery for stage II or IIIA breast cancer, age under 56 years and completion of at least 4 months of study.

#Event-free and overall survival are reported from time of entry on study and are presented as 5 years data with 95% confidence intervals in parenthesis.

TABLE 13-2. Three-year Survival Data from Survey of American Transplant Center for Patients with Ten or More Axillary Lymph Nodes

	Number of Patients	Overall Survival	Event-free Survival
All patients	662	79%	66%
≥10 Lymph nodes	818	78%	70%
ER+, PR+ or both	389	82%	70%
ER–, PR–	273	70%	61%

DISCUSSION

The results of conventional-dose chemotherapy for high-risk primary breast cancer are unsatisfactory. When patients have multiple involved lymph nodes, the results of all trials indicate that the majority of patients will relapse within 5 years in randomized conventional-dose regimens in cooperative groups. Indeed, single-institutional data are similar for this treatment setting. The data summarized here for the use of high-dose intensification, particularly when applied to patients with high-risk primary breast cancer involving ten or more axillary lymph nodes, indicates an apparent value to the use of intensification.

Data from the single-institution trial presented above indicate that with extended follow-up, the results reported previously with a period of shorter follow-up have been maintained and the high-dose consolidation appears to be associated with an apparent improvement in both disease-free and overall survival in excess of 30% compared to 17 years of experience with conventional-dose therapy for similar patients. The results apparent from data obtained from a survey of the American transplant experience are consistent with the single-institution data. Overall, approximately 80% of patients are alive at a follow-up period of 5 years.

These data are subject to the limitation that they do not represent results of randomized trials. Such trials are underway in the United States and Europe. In the United States, two trials are being conducted through the intergroup mechanisms. CALGB 9082/SWOG 9114/NCIC MA-13 has now accrued in excess of 700 patients to the randomized portion of the trial and is expected to complete accrual within the next 18 months. However, because of the similar failure curves that are associated with both conventional and high-dose therapy during the first 2 years after treatment initiation, the proper analysis of the high-dose trials will not occur until 3 years after the entry of the last randomized patient. Thus, results will not be available until near the turn of the century. A second randomized trial is being conducted by the ECOG group and has accrued approximately one-half of its projected total number with completion expected during 1997. The completion of these prospective randomized trials represents one of the most important goals in contemporary oncology.

The potential utility of high-dose therapy is being enhanced by the concomitant reduction in toxicity resulting from improvements in supportive care. The combination use of peripheral blood progenitor cells, prophylactic antibiotics, improved antiemetic regimens, and increased experience has resulted in therapy-related mortality in the best centers in the range of 1–3%. Further, the reduction in toxicity has permitted the treatment to be undertaken largely as an outpatient in some centers. These changes have resulted in a substantial reduction in the cost of the therapy and this will ultimately be essential for the more widespread use of this therapeutic approach.

New data from randomized trials in metastatic disease raise questions about the timing of high-dose therapy, or about the necessity or value of induction chemotherapy. These questions will only be resolved through the conduct of prospective randomized trials. Further, the importance of tumor-associated antigens identified on cells present in bone marrow needs to be resolved. Whether the reduced disease-free survival that has been reported in patients with antigen-positive cells identified in the marrow is a direct result of the infusion of these cells, or alternatively, the reflection of a larger overall tumor burden also remains an important question. Both sets of observations have important implications for the development of the field.

ACKNOWLEDGMENT

The very important contributions of all of my colleagues at the Duke University Bone Marrow Transplant Program and from the many bone marrow transplant programs around the country who provided data for the survey are gratefully acknowledged.

REFERENCES

1. Hryniuk W, Busch H: The importance of dose intensity in chemotherapy of metastatic breast cancer. J.Clin Oncol 1984;2:1281–8.
2. DeVita VT: Dose-response is alive and well. J. Clin Oncol 1986;4:1157–9.
3. Hryniuk W, Levine MN: Analysis of dose intensity for adjuvant chemotherapy trials in stage II breast cancer. J. Clin Oncol 1986;4:1162.
4. Henderson IC, Hayes DF, Gelman R: Dose-response in the treatment of breast cancer. J.Clin Oncol 1988; 6:1501–15.
5. Bezwoda WR, Seymour L, Dansey RD: High-dose chemotherapy with hematopoietic rescue as primary treatment for metastatic breast cancer: a randomized trial. J.Clin Oncol 1995;13:2483–9.
6. Peters WP, Jones RB, Vredenburgh J, Shpall EJ, Hussein A, Elkordy M, Rubin P, Ross M, Affronti ML, Moore S, Berry D: A large, prospective, randomized trial of high-dose combination alkylating agents (CPB) with autologous cellular support (ABMS) as consolidation for patients with metastatic breast cancer achieving complete remission after intensive doxorubicin-based induction therapy (AFM). Proc 18th San Antonio Breast Cancer Symposium 1995, Abst. 192.
7. Peters WP, Rogers M: Variation in approval of private health insurance coverage for autologous bone marrow transplantation for breast cancer. N Eng J Med 1994;330(7):473–7.
8. Peters WP, Fay JN, Holland HK et al. Autologous bone marrow transplantation as adjuvant therapy in primary breast cancer: The American experience. Proc UCLA Keystone Conference on Bone Marrow Transplantation 1995, ed R. Champlin and R Gale.
9. Peters WP: High-dose chemotherapy with autologous bone marrow transplantation for the treatment of breast cancer, Important Advances in Oncology 1995, ed DeVita VT, Hellman S, Rosenberg S, pp 215–30.
10. Peters WP, Ross M, Vredenburgh JJ, Wu K, Rosner G, Winer E, Meisenberg B, Hussein AM: High-dose chemotherapy and autologous bone marrow support as consolidation after standard dose adjuvant therapy for high-risk primary breast cancer. Adjuvant Therapy of Cancer VII 1993, eds Salmon SE. Philadelphia: Lippincott Co. pp 207–13.
11. Peters WP, Ross M, Vredenburgh JJ, Nadel S, Marks L, Kurtzburg J, Jones R, Shpall E, Petros W, Reisner E, Berlangeri SU, Hurd D, Norton L, Gilbert C, Mathias B, Coniglio D, Rosner G: High-dose chemotherapy and autologous bone marrow support as consolidation after standard dose adjuvant therapy for high-risk primary breast cancer. J Clin Oncol 1993;11:1132-43.

Adjuvant Therapy of Cancer VIII, edited by Sydney E. Salmon. Lippincott–Raven Publishers, Philadelphia © 1997.

14

High–Dose-Intensity Doxorubicin–Cyclophosphamide with rh-GCSF and Peripheral Blood Stem Cells: Outpatient Adjuvant Treatment for Premenopausal Patients with Breast Carcinoma

P. Viens, D. Genre, G. Gravis, M. A. Cappiello, J. Camerlo, D. Cowen, F. Bertucci, G. Houvenaeghel, F. Penault-Llorca, C. Chabannon, and D. Maraninchi

Dose and dose intensity are considered to be major factors for response, and perhaps cure, of cancer (1). Retrospective and prospective studies have investigated this concept in various tumors such as breast or ovarian tumors (2–5). Recently, a prospective randomized study from CALGB (6) showed the impact of dose intensity in conventional regimens. The wide use of hematopoietic growth factors, and more recently peripheral blood progenitors (7), has permitted an increase in dose intensity of chemotherapy regimens.

The aim of this study is to establish an outpatient, high-dose intensity chemotherapy regimen using doxorubicin and cyclophosphamide in conjunction with rh-GCSF (filgrastim) and peripheral blood progenitors for adjuvant treatment of breast cancer.

PATIENTS AND METHODS

Eligibility Criteria—Patient Characteristics

Patient eligibility requirements included women at least 18 years old, premenopausal status, with histologically proven breast cancer which is nonmetastatic with 4–10 involved axillary homolateral lymph nodes. There could not be significant impairment of Karnofsky performance status or hematologic, hepatic, renal, or cardiac functions, or prior treatment for breast cancer. Excluded were patients with inflammatory breast cancer, metastatic breast cancer, or contralateral or subclavicular involved lymph nodes and patients whose breast cancer had relapsed.

Treatment Regimen and Schedule

After surgery, the patients were treated with four cycles of high-dose chemotherapy (Figure 14-1). All courses of chemotherapy were done on an inpatient basis. Each

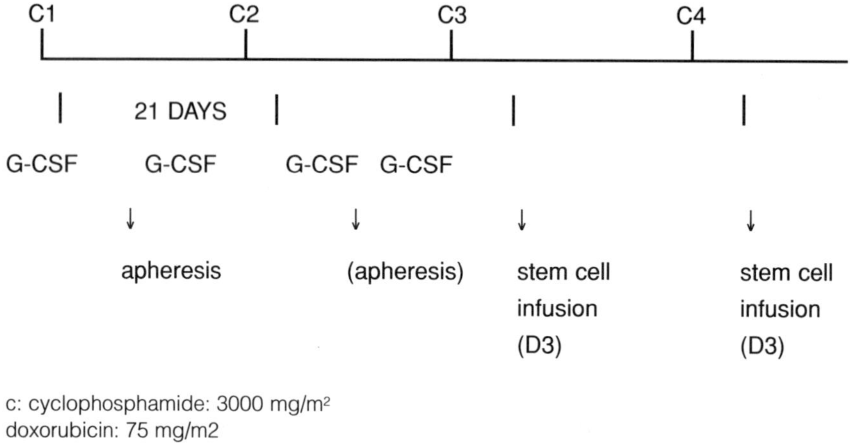

Figure 14-1. Chemotherapy schedule

cycle was repeated at interval of 21 days. If platelet count did not exceed 100 × 10^9/liter and neutrophil count 1.5 × 10^9/liter, a delay until hematologic recovery was possible. No chemotherapy reductions were allowed. One course consisted of cyclophosphamide = 3000 mg/m^2 and doxorubicin = 75 mg/m^2. These products were administered intravenously: cyclophosphamide during a 1-hr period and doxorubicin during a 25-min period with intravenous hydration (3 liters/m^2 of half-normal saline solution) during a 24-hr hospitalization.

For stem cell mobilization, each treatment was followed by a daily subcutaneous administration of 5 g/kg (maximum 300 g) hematopoietic growth factor G-CSF (filgrastim) initiated on day 3 after each cycle, continued for four cycles with apheresis until the day before the last leukapheresis and for the other cycles until the absolute neutrophil count exceeded 500/mm^3 on three consecutive days.

Peripheral blood progenitors were collected systematically after cycle 1 on day 13 and/or day 14 according to the number of CD 34+ cells × 10^6/kg harvested. The minimal number of CD 34+ cells × 10^6/kg required was 6 × 10^6/kg, which were divided into three bags. PBP also could be obtained after cycle 2 if it was necessary. A minimum of 2 × 10^6 CD 34+/kg were reinfused on day 3 of cycles 3 and 4.

After chemotherapy, surgery could be performed. Radiotherapy according to the protocol was begun as soon as possible after cycle 4.

Patient Evaluation

Baseline assessment prior to therapy included physical examination, Karnofsky performance status, vital signs, hemogram, coagulation profile, complete blood chemistries, tumor evaluation (chest x-ray, liver USS, bone nuclide scan, mammography and breast USS, ACE, CA 15-3), and cardiac evaluation (EKG, VEF). Once per course (day 1), physical examination, Karnofsky performance status, vital signs, and EKG were obtained, as were hemogram, liver function, creatinine determination, and coagulation profile. During the treatment, CBC and differential were obtained 3 times per week. All patients were assessed for toxicity, which was graded according to the World Health Organization (WHO) criteria, and assessed for cardiac toxicity according to the New York Heart Association (NYHA) classification.

Calculation of Dose Intensity

The calculation of dose intensity was done on the total population. The weekly dose intensity (DI) was calculated as the total dose received divided by body surface area, divided by the number of weeks that elapsed between the initial dose of treatment and 3 weeks after the last cycle of therapy. The relative dose intensity (RDI) was the result of delivered dose intensity divided by the theoretic dose intensity.

RESULTS

Treatment

From July 1993 to April 1995, 20 premenopausal women were enrolled in this trial and received four cycles of chemotherapy. A total of 80 cycles of chemotherapy were performed. Median age was 45 years (range, 27–52).

The majority of patients (95%) had undergone a tumorectomy with a homolateral axillary dissection; 5% underwent mastectomy. A median of five had axillary lymph node involvement (range, 4–8). Histologically, the majority had ductal carcinoma (90%) distributed in the SBR classification as 40% in Stages II and III versus 20% in stage I.

Hormonal receptors (ER and PR) were both positive in 50% of tumors, negative in 30%, and in 20% one was positive and one negative. The dose intensities for cyclophosphamide (CPM) and doxorubicin (DOX) were as follows: DI (mg/m^2/week): CPM = 1007 (range, 903.6–1065.4), DOX = 25.3 (range, 22.8–25.9); RDI: CPM = 1 (range, 0.9–1.0), DOX = 1 (range, 0.88–1.0).

Median number of apheresis after cycle 1 was two (range, 1–2) for the 20 patients. Median number of CD 34+ cells $\times 10^6$/kg harvested was 9.4 (range, 4.3–24.6). After cycle 2, leukapheresis was performed on only eight patients. Median number of apheresis after cycle 2 was one (range, 1–2) and median number of CD 34+ cells $\times 10^6$/kg harvested was 4.2 (range, 1.4–13.7). A sufficient number of CD 34+ cells $\times 10^6$/kg (6×10^6/kg) were collected after cycle 1 in 19 patients.

Hematologic Toxicity

Hematologic toxicity was frequent in terms of neutropenia grade IV (69%), and less important for thrombocytopenia grade III and/or IV (26%) and for thrombocytopenia grade IV (9%). No patient had a platelet count $<25 \times 10^9$/liter for the first cycle (Table 14-1). For patients with toxicity, the median duration of cytopenia is shown in Table 14-2. The median duration of neutropenia grade IV was 2 days

TABLE 14-1. Hematologic Toxicity

	Neutrophils <0.5 ×10⁹/l (%)	Platelets <25 ×10⁹/l (%)	Platelets <50 ×10⁹/l (%)
C 1	70	0	15
C 2	55	10	30
C 3	80	15	40
C 4	70	10	20
Total	69	9	26

C: Cycle

TABLE 14-2. Median Duration of Severe Cytopenia (days)

	NEUTROPHILS <0.5 × 0.5 0.5 × 10⁹/l Median [Range]	PLATELETS <25 × 10⁹/l Median [Range]
C 1	1 (1–4)	0
C 2	3 (1–5)	1.5 (1–2)
C 3	2.5 (1–5)	3 (1–3)
C 4	1.5 (1–5)	3
Total	2 (1–5)	2 (1–3)

C: Cycle

(range, 1–5). It seemed to be prolonged in cycle 2 (3 days; range, 1–5). The median duration of thrombocytopenia grade IV was 2 days (range, 1–3). The median duration of cytopenia per patient for the four cycles was as follows:

Neutropenia grade IV: 5 (range, 0–17)
Thrombocytopenia grade IV: 0 (range, 0–8)
Thrombocytopenia grade III and/or IV: 0 (range, 0–14)

One patient presented with delayed Grade II thrombocytopenia during radiotherapy and 43 days after the last course of chemotherapy. Effects of repeated cycles of high-dose chemotherapy on bone marrow recovery are summarized in the Table 14-3. The average initial level for the absolute neutrophil count was 5.4×10^9/liter and 3.7×10^9/liter 45 days after the last treatment, and for platelet count 312×10^9/liter and 221×10^9/liter. Of the 20 patients enrolled, 9 (45%) received packed red-cell transfusions and 1 (5%) received platelet transfusions. Platelet transfusions were only done after cycles 2 and 4. The majority of packed red-cell transfusions (45%) were performed after cycle 3 versus 10% for cycle 1, 15% for cycle 2, and 25% for cycle 4. The mean of packed red-cell transfusions per patient was two (2.6).

TABLE 14-3. Cumulative Bone Marrow Effect (mean ± 0)

	C 1 D 1	C 2 D 1	C 3 D 1	C 4 D 1	C 4 D 45
ANC	5.4	4.2	3.2	3.1	3.7
(× 10^9/l)	± 2.7	± 2.2	±1.6	± 1.2	± 1.9
PLATELETS	312	417	343	321	221
(× 10^9/l)	± 113	± 181	± 95	± 68	± 75

C: Cycle D: Day ANC: Absolute Neutrophil Count

Nonhematologic Toxicity

Table 14-4 shows proportion, reasons, and duration of rehospitalizations for toxicity. The median duration of stay for the patients who had been rehospitalized was 4 days (range, 1–5) after cycle 1, 4 days (range, 1–6) after cycle 2, 3 days (range, 1–6) after cycle 3, and 5 days (range, 3–7) after cycle 4. Mean days of hospitalization per patient for the 4 cycles was 3.3 (5.4, median 0, range 0–19). After cycles 3 and 4, all hospitalizations were for febrile aplasia. One septic fever (*Corynebacterium*) after cycle 4 was documented. Fever was always treated with intravenous antibiotics.

The most common and important toxicities (2) observed were vomiting (40%), asthenia (14%), and mucositis (9%). Vomiting was most frequent after the first administration of chemotherapy (65%), and it decreased during the treatment (45%, 30%, 20%). Asthenia increased after cycle 3 (25%) versus 5% (cycle 1), 10% (cycle 2), and 15% (cycle 4). Patients presented with other toxicities such as headaches, gastric discomfort, and bone pain.

TABLE 14-4 Nonhematological toxicity

	Hospitalization (% of patients)	Hospitalization with Febrile Aplasia (% of hospitalization)	Days of Hospitalization (Median)
C 1	25	80	4 (1–5)
C 2	20	75	4, 5 (1–6)
C 3	50	100	3 (1–6)
C 4	20	100*	5 (3–7)
Total	30	90	4 (1–7)

*One septicemia (Corynebacteria)

C: Cycle

Treatment after Protocol and Follow-Up

Off study, 30% of the 20 women enrolled in this trial had surgery, with a median delay of 48.5 days (range, 27–71) after the first day of cycle 4. All patients received radiotherapy, with a median delay of 38.5 days (range, 24–99). The median follow-up duration was 16 months (range, 9–33). One local relapse was noted. There were no deaths.

CONCLUSION

Twenty patients received 80 cycles of the high-dose cyclophosphamide–doxorubicin regimen. The dose intensities of cyclophosphamide and doxorubicin were 1007 $mg/m^2/week$ (range, 900–1065) and 25.3 $mg/m^2/week$ (range 22.8–25.9), respectively, with a median relative dose intensity of 1 for cyclophosphamide and doxorubicin. The main toxicity in our study was hematologic. However, neutropenia grade 4 was of short duration, and no cumulative thrombocytopenia was observed (8–10). The absence of cumulative thrombocytopenia in our study is probably related to reinfusion of peripheral blood progenitors and growth factors.

Increasing dose intensity or dose in chemotherapy for breast cancer, as in adjuvant programs or treatment for metastatic disease, is actually of major concern for the clinician. The following approaches are used: high-dose "single shot" treatment with hematopoietic stem cells (11) and sequential high-dose therapy (7,12). Most results are encouraging.

In our study, the goal was to establish an outpatient, high-dose intensity regimen associating doxorubicin and cyclophosphamide. The dose intensity achieved a low rate of hospitalization for toxicity, attesting to the feasibility of such an approach. However, this approach has to be compared in terms of efficacy, cost effectiveness, and quality of life to standard regimens without new drugs and to single-shot, high-dose treatments.

ACKNOWLEDGMENTS

This work was supported in part by Amgen France, Association pour la Recherche Contre le Cancer, and Fondation de France.

REFERENCES

1. Frei E, Canellos GP. Dose: A critical factor in cancer chemotherapy. Am J Med 1980;69:585.
2. Hryniuk W, Levine M. Analysis of dose intensity for adjuvant chemotherapy trials in stage II breast cancer. J Clin Oncol 1986;4:1162.
3. Bonadonna G, Valagussa P. Dose response effect of adjuvant chemotherapy in breast cancer. N Engl J Med 1981;304:10.
4. Hryniuk W, Bush H. The importance of dose intensity in chemotherapy of metastatic breast cancer. J Clin Oncol 1984;2:1281.
5. Kaye SB, Lewis CR, Paul J, et al. Randomized study of two doses of cisplatin and cyclophosphamide in epithelial ovarian cancer. Lancet 1992;340:329.
6. Wood WC, Budman DR, Korzun AH, et al. Dose and dose intensity of adjuvant chemotherapy for stage II, node-positive breast carcinoma. N Engl J Med 1994;330:1253.

7. Vahdat L, Raptis G, Fennelly D, et al. Rapidly cycled courses of high-dose alkylating agents supported by filgratim and peripheral blood progenitor cells in patients with metastatic breast cancer. Clin Cancer Res 1995;1:1267.
8. Trillet-Lenoir V, Green J, Manegold C, et al. Recombinant granulocyte colony stimulating factor reduces the infectious complications of cytotoxic chemotherapy. Eur J Cancer 1993;29A:319.
9. Honkoop AH, Hoekman K, Wagstaff J, et al. Dose-intensive chemotherapy with doxorubicin, cyclophosphamide and GM-CSF fails to improve survival of metastatic breast cancer patients. Ann Oncol 1996;7:35.
10. Shipp MA, Neuberg D, Janicek M, et al. High-dose CHOP as initial therapy for patients with poor-prognosis agressive non-Hodgkin's lymphoma: A dose-finding pilot study. J Clin Oncol 1995; 13:2916.
11. Peters W, Ross M, Vredenburgh J, et al. High dose chemotherapy and autologous bone marrow support as consolidation after standard dose adjuvant therapy for high risk primary breast cancer. J Clin Oncol 1993;11:1132.
12. Hudis C, Seidman A, Raptis G, et al. Sequential doxorubicin, paclitaxel and cyclophosphamide in women with resected breast cancer and >4 (+) lymph nodes: Preliminary results. Proc Am Soc Clin Oncol 1995;14:152.

III

Breast Cancer

Biologic Observations and Potential Clinical Relevance

Adjuvant Therapy of Cancer VIII, edited by Sydney E. Salmon. Lippincott–Raven Publishers, Philadelphia © 1997.

15

Breast Cancer, Surgery, and the Menstrual Cycle

William J. M. Hrushesky

The mammalian fertility cycle and cancer biology may be meaningfully linked. In 1836, A. P. Cooper observed that breast cancer growth waxes and wanes during the menstrual cycle (1). Six decades later, G. T. Beatson demonstrated that metastatic breast cancer may remit after resection of the premenopausal woman's ovaries (2). Ten years ago, we discovered that the timing of resection of a transplantable breast cancer within the mouse's estrous cycle affects whether or not the cancer metastasizes to the lungs and kills the animal or whether the operation cures the mouse (3). It was found that resection of the cancer during the vaginal cytology-defined proestrus phase cured two and a half times more frequently than when the same operation was performed during metestrus. Although the human and murine reproductive cycles differ substantially, this proestrus timing is associated with luteinizing hormone and follicle stimulating hormone and progesterone surges on the background of increasing estrogen concentrations corresponding roughly to the early luteal phase of the mammalian fertility cycle (4). Eight years ago, we discovered that this same relationship between surgical cure frequency and breast cancer resection timing holds true for young women with breast cancer (5). The 10-year disease-free survival of our patients was more than fourfold better when these young women were resected in the putative early luteal phase compared to the putative follicular phase of their menstrual cycles. To date, 10 retrospective studies of young women with breast cancer from one of three continents and six nations have confirmed our murine findings (5–16). About half as many retrospective studies have failed to detect a statistically significant relationship of surgery timing to outcome (17–19). A meta-analysis by Fentiman reveals an overall beneficial effect of early luteal resection, at least equal to the benefit conferred by adjuvant chemotherapy for premenopausal women (6). The case for prospective study has been made, with equal vigor, by those who have and those who have not found that the timing of surgery within the menstrual cycle affects breast cancer outcome (20,21).

CLINICAL OBSERVATIONS

Fifteen-year follow-up of our original breast cancer patients reveals no recurrence or death in any woman resected near to and up to seven days following putative ovulation. Nine subsequent studies, have confirmed our clinical observations (7–14,16). The three largest studies demonstrate, as would be expected, that the greatest benefit accrues to those young women at highest risk for recurrence (7,9,16). Several other series also demonstrate benefit of luteal resection timing for patients with stage I breast cancer. In five of these studies, multivariate analyses demonstrate that surgical timing is an independent predictor of both breast cancer recurrence and death, from breast cancer, second in prognostic power to primary tumor size and/or lymph node status.

Table 15-1 indicates the relative surgical curability of the breast cancer in each these clinical studies using a visual scale. The best possible clinical outcome is represented by ++++ and the worst possible is represented by +. The table arranges the likelihood of breast cancer control according to which quadrant of the menstrual cycle the operation was performed. Our murine study and the clinical study of Ville objectively document fertility cycle stage, while all other clinical studies rely entirely upon the menstrual history. The quarter cycle (7–10 days for humans and 1 day for mice) near and following putative ovulation, human early luteal phase, is consistently the most opportune time for resection. Although the least favorable time usually appears to be the quarter of the cycle following the first day of the menstrual flow, this does vary somewhat among these retrospective studies.

Non-confirmatory retrospective studies have recently been reviewed by both Davidson and Sharp (19,20). In the largest of these studies, treatment was not consistent within the study and many of the patients also underwent additional abdominal surgery for oophorectomy (17). Many irregularly cycling and/or perimenopausal patients were included. Few of these studies clearly excluded women consuming oral contraceptives. Subgroup comparability was rarely demonstrated nor were multivariate analyses usually performed. It is interesting that in the study of Powles, although statistical significance was not realized, women operated at the putative early luteal phase had a 10-year death rate of less than 20% while those resected at other times within the cycle had up to 45% death rates at 10 years (18). Other purportedly negative data are, unfortunately, not reported in a way that will permit evaluation of the behavior of breast cancer in women resected specifically in the early luteal phase of their cycles (17,19).

MECHANISMS RESPONSIBLE FOR THIS BIOLOGY

Menstrual Cycle Coordination of Cellular Immunity

To date, our laboratory has focused upon cyclic changes in the host's cellular immune capacity including splenocyte natural killer cell activity and interleukin-2 production. Cellular immune competence and, in particular, natural killer (NK) cell activity is potentially important in determining outcome in both murine and human cancer (22–24). These studies depicted in Figure 15-1 reveal that breast cancer surgical curability is optimal during the same estrous cycle stage, proestrus, when these measures of immunocompetence are most robust (25). More recently, we have observed that other aspects of the host-breast cancer balance change rhythmically and predictably during the mouse's estrous cycle. In our model system, this is reflected by a somewhat longer span to tumor palpability when high doses

TABLE 15-1. Summary of Positive Retrospective Results

	N of Patients	Optimal Span	End point	10 yr Comparative Advantage	Cycle Quarter: 1st	2nd	3rd	4th	Ref
Hrushesky	41	Mid-cycle/ Early Luteal	O.S.	95 % vs 78%	++++	+	+	+++	5
Senie	283	Luteal	D.F.S.	69 % vs 58%	++++	+++	++	+	7
Meyer	53	Mid-cycle/ Early Luteal	O.S.	78 % vs 52%	++++	+	+	++++	8
Badwe	249	Early Luteal	O.S.	84 % vs 54%	++++	+++	++	+	9
Powles	81	Early Luteal	D.F.S.	†80 % vs 55%	++++	++	++	+	14
*Ville	165	Early Luteal	D.F.S.	89 % vs 62%	++++	++	+	+	10
Saad	96	Early Luteal	O.S.	79 % vs 40%	++++	+++	++	+	12
Spratt	40	Mid-cycle/ Early Luteal	O.S.	71 % vs 20%	++++	+	+	++++	13
Marques	63	Luteal	O.S.	†72 % vs 49%	++++	++++	+	+	15
Veronesi	1279	Luteal	D.F.S.	§76 % vs 63%	++++	+++	++	+	16

△ Ovulation ▲ Mensus △ Ovulation

O.S. Overall Survival; D.F.S. Disease Free Survival

*Hormonal validation of menstrual cycle stage, 5 yr survival follow-up

†Did not reach statistical significance

§ Node positive patients

Reproduced with permission from Women's Health Issues (WHI) New York, NY: Elsevier Science Pub. Co. In press.

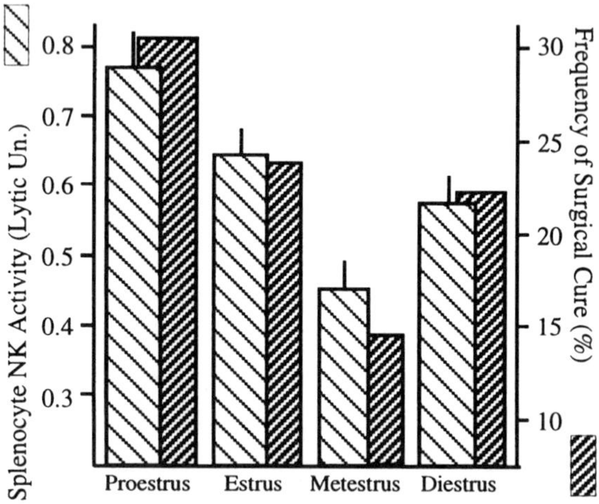

Figure 15-1. Covariation of breast cancer surgical curability and natural killer cell activity during the female reproductive cycle: Dark cross hatched bars represent the frequency of surgical cure. More than 80% of mice resected during proestrus (progesterone-rich "early luteal" phase of estrus cycle); fewer than 40% of mice resected during metestrus (follicular phase) were cured. Lighter cross hatched bars represent splenocyte natural killer cell activity, which is almost twice as robust in proestrus compared to metestrus.

of viable breast cancer cells are inoculated during the proestrus phase of the cycle (that associated with most frequent surgical cure of local disease). We also find rhythmic differences in actual tumor size during each estrous cycle. Very little tumor growth occurs during proestrus, and marked tumor growth occurs between metestrus and diestrus (26).

In women, lymphocyte helper/suppresser ratios vary predictably during the fertility cycle and are highest during the luteal phase (27). The negative impact of surgery upon the cellular immune function has been explored in both mice and cancer patients. Surgery adversely affects human NK activity for at least a month following operation (28,29). The menstrual cycle stage at the time of operation may modulate the subsequent depth and duration of cellular immune dysfunction in cycling women whose breast cancers are resected for cure.

Menstrual Cycle Coordination of DNA Synthesis, Cell Proliferation, Apoptosis, and Tissue Remodeling

During each fertility cycle, a complex dynamical network of hypothalamic, pituitary, and ovarian hormones coordinates profound and entirely predictable changes within the ovary. These changes include rhythmically enhanced DNA synthesis, cell division, blood vessel formation, and macroscopically obvious tissue remodeling.

The endometrium, even more obviously, undergoes profound rhythmic change in each of these processes during each fertility cycle. The ovarian cycle coordinates similar cell biology in the breast (30,31). The pathology literature documents that at least five stages of the ovarian cycle are clearly and reproducibly reflected in the histology of the breast (32,33). Breast epithelial DNA synthetic capacity, as measured by labeling index, changes rhythmically, several fold, during each menstrual cycle. Figure 15-2 displays the pattern of labeling index in the normal human endometrium and breast tissue throughout the menstrual cycle (30,31,33). The endometrium is rapidly built up following menses at about the same time the ovarian follicles are growing most rapidly. This follicular phase of the menstrual cycle is associated with most steeply rising and highest estrogen concentrations during the cycle. This first estrogen peak is unopposed by progesterone. Breast epithelial DNA synthesis gradually doubles during an entirely different phase of this cycle. Breast DNA synthesis is most prominent at the end of the luteal phase of the cycle, at a time associated with the highest but falling progesterone concentrations and the second estrogen peak. This rhythmic menstrual cycle phase-specific trebling of breast epithelial DNA content is associated with significant tissue and rhythmic new vessel formation. The premenopausal woman's breasts do not increase in size progressively throughout her reproductive life. Therefore, logic demands that this menstrual cycle-coordinated increase in cell proliferation is followed by a wave menstrual cycle-coordinated breast epithelial cell apoptosis during some other part(s) of this cycle. Since breast cancer cells are sensate of and potentially responsive to changes in circulating concentrations of estrogen and progesterone, these rhythmic hormone concentration changes potentially influence breast cancer cell growth, invasion, or spread.

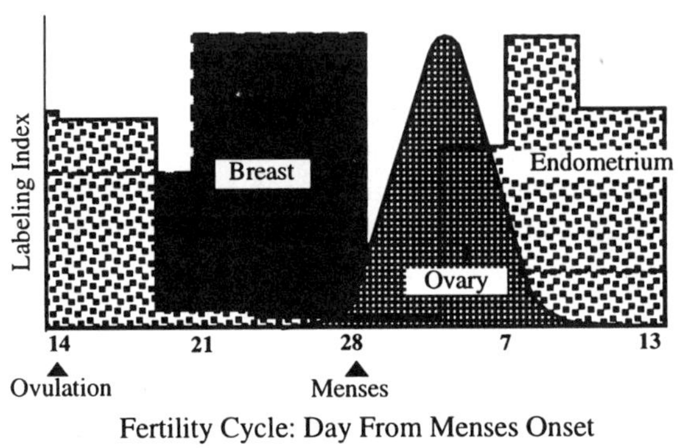

Figure 15-2. Labeling index of breast epithelium endometrial lining and ovary during the human menstrual cycle: Breast epithelium undergoes DNA synthesis rhythmically during the menstrual cycle. Greatest proportion of DNA synthesis occurring during the second half of the luteal phase. This same cycle coordinates DNA synthesis in other tissues disparately, e.g., endometrial cell DNA synthesis peaks in mid-follicular phase.

Menstrual Cycle Coordination of Cellular Sex Steroid Receptor Concentration in Breast Epithelium and Breast Cancer

Estrogen (ER) and progesterone (PR) receptors mediate the communication between the ovaries and other tissues including breast epithelium. Both breast and endometrial epithelial ER and PR concentrations change rhythmically during each ovarian cycle (34,35). Six separate studies have demonstrated that breast cancer ER positivity is more frequent and/or average ER concentrations are higher in breast cancer samples obtained during the follicular phase of the cycle (36–41). Three studies have shown that breast cancer PR positivity is more frequent, or that the average PR concentrations are higher in the early luteal phase of the menstrual cycle (38–40). One interesting study indicates that the likelihood of breast cancer tissues being both ER and PR positive is greater when that tissue is obtained in the early luteal phase and that both are most frequently negative when tissue has been obtained during the early follicular phase (42). Taken together, these data indicate that breast cancer cell ER and PR concentrations, like those of normal breast epithelial cells, are rhythmically affected by the menstrual cycle.

The Menstrual Cycle Coordinates Blood Vessel Formation, Arrest, and Destruction

Angiogenesis, new blood vessel formation, is essential for tumor growth beyond a few millimeters in diameter (43). The inhibition of vascular endothelial growth factor (VEGF)-induced angiogenesis suppresses tumor growth *in vivo* (44). The estrogen sensitive expression of VEGF and its receptor are each tightly hormonally regulated in various tissues by the ovarian cycle (45). VEGF causes increased vascular permeability at an early stage in the process of new vessel formation. VEGF is most prominently produced in and around the developing ovarian follicles and in the developing endometrium during the estrogen-rich and progesterone-poor early follicular phase of each cycle. Concurrent with the fall of unopposed estrogen toward the end of the follicular phase, the production of VEGF is abruptly switched off as vascularization in the ovarian follicle and the endometrium is completed. Following LH/FSH surges and ovulation, at mid-cycle, the corpus luteum secretes increasing amounts of progesterone. Progesterone enhances thrombospondin-1 transcription and translation by endometrial stromal cells both *in vivo* and *in vitro* (46). Benign and malignant breast tissues, like endometrium, are rich in thrombospondin-1 (47). This glycoprotein strongly inhibits further new vessel formation in the fully developed endometrium. The subsequent progesterone fall is tightly associated with endometrial breakdown and subsequent menses. Progesterone withdrawal induces transcription and translation of matrix metalloproteinase-2, which is, at least in part, responsible for the initiation of this cyclic endometrial breakdown (48).

Vascular permeability, as well as new vessel formation, is important for the successful growth and spread of cancer. Fascinating, companion literatures independently connect sex hormone mediated vascular permeability with the mammalian fertility cycle. Cerebral edema, brain herniation, and death are complications of postoperative hyponatremic encephalopathy. This syndrome is as likely to occur in men as well as in women. However, when it develops, menstruant (following physiologic progesterone withdrawal) women are 25 times more likely to either die or have permanent brain damage than either men or postmenopausal women. At autopsy, the brain is extremely edematous, indicating poorly restrained capillary permeability (49). A separate neurologic literature linking capillary permeability and hormones of the mammalian fertility cycle is even more provocative. Experimental head injury causes more capillary leak, brain edema, more severe behavioral depression, and more frequent death in female than male rats, but especially in female rats injured at times in the cycle when the circulating progesterone concentration is low (50). Progesterone pretreatment markedly attenuates head injury induced brain edema, behavioral dysfunction, and mortality (51).

Tumor cells must traverse capillary beds at least twice in order to successfully metastasize. Vascular permeability changes mediated by sex steroid regulated growth factors may be important both to whether cancer cells get into the blood from a primary cancer and whether they get from the blood into other tissues. The extensive literature documenting the reality of tumor cells in the blood of both mice or rats and human beings with cancer needs to be reconsidered in light of these connections between capillary integrity and the hormones of the fertility cycle, most prominently including progesterone. Proestrus in the mouse and rat is associated with a progesterone surge, and proestrus is the specific span in the estrous cycle when tumor growth is slowest and breast cancer metastatic potential lowest. The progesterone-rich early luteal phase is likewise the time within the menstrual cycle when human breast cancer resection results in the best long-term disease-free survival.

Menstrual Cycle and Circulating Tumor Cells

Circulating tumor cells have been found in the blood of patients with a wide variety of cancer types. Circulating tumor cell clumps are associated with higher metastatic efficiencies than single cells. Clotting factors promote the interactions required for tumor cell clumping (52). Cancer bearing is associated with abnormally high levels of most clotting factors. Treating patients with a variety of drugs that diminish the activated coagulatory state, associated with cancer bearing, enhances treatment efficacy, decreases the frequency of cancer spread, and improves survival duration (53). Sex steroids influence the interaction of platelets with one another and the endothelium and can activate platelets and mononuclear cells (54,55).

The aggregability of platelets changes rhythmically as a function of when in the menstrual cycle they have been obtained (56). The follicular phase of the menstrual cycle is associated with the highest concentrations of fibrinogen, higher blood viscosity, and less filterable, more stiff red blood cells. The progesterone-rich luteal phase of the cycle is associated with lower fibrinogen concentrations and lower blood viscosity, and more supple red blood cells (57). The possible interactions among platelets, fibrinogen, white blood cells, circulating cancer cells, and capillary endothelium, during the mammalian fertility cycle, may be relevant to our observations of better outcomes following operation in the progesterone-rich early luteal phase of the menstrual cycle.

Surgical Trauma, Cancer Spread, and Growth

"Athrepsia," as manifested by accelerated growth of metastatic cancer after excision of a primary tumor, suggested to Paul Ehrlich an intimate relationship of cancer at different sites in the same individual. He proposed that an actively growing tumor removed certain specific nutritive substances necessary for cancer growth. When a large primary tumor was removed, this provided more of these substances for the "daughter" tumors (58–60).

Early in this century, this observation of the timing and patterns of cancer spread in people was confirmed and experimentally expanded using mouse models (61,62). Later work demonstrated that a sham surgical procedure is also associated with the quickening of growth of metastases and can also result in increased growth of the primary cancer (63). Fisher and Fisher demonstrated elegantly and conclusively that resection of the primary tumor induces the formation and/or release of factors(s) responsible for ending apparent dormancy of tumor micro-metastases and increasing the growth of metastatic deposits (64). This work also demonstrated that the change in tumor dormancy, stimulated by resection of the primary tumor, is associated with a modulation of the capacity of the metastatic tumor cells to both bind estrogen and divide (65). Our data indicate that these effects of surgery differ depending upon when in the mammalian fertility cycle that operation is performed.

The Estrogen Hypothesis

Most scientists have focused upon "estrogen as an explanation" for the demographics, etiology, and outcome of breast cancer. A biodynamic point of view rejects single hormone perspectives such as the "estrogen hypothesis" as misleading oversimplifications. Cells, tissues, organisms, populations, and ecosystems do not sense, nor do they respond to, amounts of single stimuli. These hierarchical biological units sense and respond to rates of change among relationships (dynamic interactions). The favorable milieu for breast cancer resection is described by a network of rhythmically changing endocrine relationships. A quickening and sharpening of pulsatile FSH and LH surge patterns and rising progesterone concentration, on a background of rising estrogen characterize the early luteal phase of the menstrual cycle. Other hormone concentration trends also cued to these interactions (prolactin, TSH, ACTH, cortisone, and melatonin) may also be relevant to the creation of the most favorable milieu for breast cancer resection. Because of the rhythmic linkage of all of these endocrine networks, during each menstrual cycle, the possibility of pacing these changes endocrinologically with the carefully timed crescendo-decrescendo administration of a single hormone is real. Given the physiology and pathophysiology briefly outlined in this paper, I believe that appropriately modulating concentrations of progesterone provides the cleanest strategy for creating the most favorable endocrine milieu in which to resect cancer.

PROSPECTIVE STUDY IS ESSENTIAL

Provocative experimental and clinical data support the hypothesis that menstrual cycle resection timing affects outcome. Several retrospective series have, however, not confirmed the importance of surgery timing. In retrospective studies, it is difficult or impossible to accurately assess the extent of disease at diagnosis and whether or not irregularly cycling perimenopausal women or women using oral contraceptives have been rigorously excluded from study. The accuracy of retrospective menstrual cycle phase localization is always suspect. In fact, in several studies, women were asked to provide the date of the first day of their last menstrual period prior to that breast surgery, many weeks or even months following the operation. Because of necessary imprecision of these historical menstrual data, retrospective studies cannot tell us, with any degree of certainty, precisely the best time within the cycle for operation. Nor can they tell us accurately how long or widely this window of opportunity is open. The relative impact of the stage of disease at resection, and the relative impact of the extent of the operation performed, are likewise poorly assessable. These retrospective studies do not permit us to determine, when more than one surgical procedure is employed, the relative importance of the timing of an initial incisional or excisional biopsy or lumpectomy compared with follow-up "completion" surgical procedure and/or concurrent or later lymph node dissection. Each of these important questions can be adequately addressed only by a prospective clinical trial of breast cancer resection timing in regularly cycling premenopausal women. Regardless of the number of positive or negative retrospective results that might appear, oncologic practice will, apparently, not be altered without prospective studies confirming or refuting the impact of resection timing upon breast cancer outcome.

Surgical resection of primary breast cancer is the first step toward cure of this common disease in the majority of the 180,000 U.S., 20,000 Canadian, and 220,000 European women who develop breast cancer each year. Approximately one third of these women are premenopausal at the time of diagnosis and resection. If our discovery is confirmed by prospective study, the routine optimal timing of surgery, within the menstrual cycle, will save the lives of thousands young women around the world each year. This will be achieved without any added side effects or risks for these women and without any added costs. If carefully selected companion biologic studies of these women begin to elucidate mechanisms by which the luteal phase protects against metastases, this information will spur the development of pharmacoendocrinologic strategies to enhance the surgical curability of any potentially curative cancer resection.

REFERENCES

1. Cooper A. Practice and principles of surgery. London, 1836.
2. Beatson GT. On the treatment of inoperable cases of carcinoma of the mamma: Suggestions for a new method of treatment with illustrative cases. Lancet 1896;ii:104–107.
3. Ratajczak HV, Sothern RB, Hrushesky WJM. Estrous influence on surgical cure of a mouse breast cancer. J Exp Med 1988;168:88–96.
4. Butcher RL, Collins WE, Fugo NW. Plasma concentrations of LH, FSH, prolactin, progesterone and estradiol-17β throughout the 4-day estrous cycle of the rat. Endocrinology 1974;94:1704–1708.

5. Hrushesky WJM, Bluming AZ, Gruber SA, Sothern RA. Menstrual influence on surgical cure of breast cancer. Lancet 1989;ii:949–952.
6. Fentiman I, Gregory WM, Richards MA. Effects of menstrual phase on surgical treatment of breast cancer. Lancet 1994;344:402.
7. Senie R, Rosen P, Rhodes P, Lesser M. Timing of breast cancer excision during the menstrual cycle influences duration of disease-free survival. Ann Intern Med 1991;115:337–342.
8. Meyer K. Season and cycle: Variation in presentation and response to therapy in premenopausal breast cancer. 77th Ann Clin Congress, October 21–24, 1991, Chicago, IL.
9. Badwe RA, Gregory WM, Chaudary WM, et al. Timing of surgery during menstrual cycle and survival of premenopausal women with operable breast cancer. Lancet 1991;337:1261–1264.
10. Ville V, Lasry S, Spyratos F. Menstrual status and breast cancer surgery. Breast Cancer Res Treat 1990;16:119–121.
11. Ville V, Briere M, Lasry S, Spyratos F, Oglobine J, Brunet M. Timing of surgery in breast cancer. Lancet 1991;337:1604–1605.
12. Saad Z. Timing of surgery in relation to menstrual cycle in premenopausal woman and its effect on survival. Can J Surg 1992;35:438.
13. Spratt J, Zirnheld J, Yancey J. Breast cancer detection demonstration project data can determine whether the prognosis of breast cancer is affected by the time of surgery during the menstrual cycle. J Surg Oncol 1993;53:4–9.
14. Powles TJ, Jones AL, Ashley S, Tidy A. Menstrual effect on surgical cure of breast cancer. Lancet 1989;ii:1343–1344.
15. Marques L, Franco E, Torloni H, Bretani M, Silva-Neto J, Bretani R. Independent value of laminin receptor expression in breast cancer survival. Cancer Res 1990;50:1479–1483.
16. Veronesi U, Luini A, Mariani L, et al. Effect of menstrual phase of surgical treatment of breast cancer. Lancet 1994;343:1545–1547.
17. Gelber R, Goldhirsch A. Menstrual effect on surgical cure of breast cancer. Lancet 1989;2:1344.
18. Powles TJ, Ashley SE, Nash AG, Tidy A, Gazet J-C, Ford HT. Timing of surgery in breast cancer. Lancet 1991;337:164.
19. Davidson NE, Abeloff MD. Menstrual effects on surgical treatment for breast cancer. Cancer Treat Rev 1993;19:105–112.
20. Sharp D. Prospective look at breast surgery timing. Lancet 1994;344.
21. Hrushesky W. Menstrual cycle timing of breast cancer resection: Prospective study is overdue. J Natl Cancer Inst 1995;87(2).
22. Bariozzari T, Leonhardt J, Wiltrout RH, Heberman RB, Reynolds CW. Direct evidence for the role of LGL in the inhibition of experimental tumor metastasis. J Immunol 1985;134:2783–2789.
23. Wiltrout RH, Herberman RB, Zhang SR. Role of organ-associated NK cells in decreased formation of experimental metastases in lung and liver. J Immunol 1985;134:4267–4275.
24. Hanna N, Scheider M. Enhancement of tumor metastasis and suppression of natural killer cell activity by β-estradiol treatment. J Immunol 1982;130:974–980.
25. Hrushesky WJM, Gruber SA, Sothern RB, et al. Natural killer cell activity is age, estrous and circadian stage dependent and correlates inversely with metastatic potential. J Natl Cancer Inst 1988;80:1232–1237.
26. Torossov MT, Hrushesky WJM, Gupta H, Mann G, Vyzula R, Wood PA. Fertility cycle dependent tumor growth non-linearity unmasked. Proc Am Assoc Cancer Res 1995;36:38.
27. Krzanowski M. Low human T4:T8 lymphocyte ratios around ovulation time. Chronobiologia 1985;12:254.
28. Pollock RE, Babcock GF, Romsdahl M, Nishioka K. Surgical stress-mediated suppression of murine natural killer cell cytotoxicity. Cancer Res 1984;44:3888–3891.
29. Pollock RE, Lotzova E, Stanford SD. Effect of surgical stress on murine natural killer cell cytotoxicity. J Immunol 1987;138:171–178.
30. Potten C, Watson RJ, Williams GT, Tickle S, Roberts SA, Harris M, Howell A. The effect of age and menstrual cycle upon proliferative activity of the normal human breast. Br J Cancer 1988;58:163–170.
31. Anderson T, Battersky S, King RJB, Going JJ. Oral contraceptive use influences resting breast proliferation. Hum Pathol 1989;20:1139–1144.
32. Vogel P, Georgiade NG, Fetter BF, et al. The correlation of histologic changes in the human breast with the menstrual cycle. Am J Pathol 1981;104:23–24.
33. Longacre T, Bartow SA. A correlative morphologic study of human breast and endometrium in the menstrual cycle. Am J Pathol 1986;255:58–61.
34. Silva JS, Georgiade GS, Dilley WG, McCarty KS, Wells S, McCarty KJ. Menstrual cycle-dependent variations of breast cyst fluid proteins and sex steroid receptors in the normal human breast. Cancer 1983;51:1297–1302.

35. Pollow K, Schmidt-Goldwitzer M, Nevinny-Stickel J. Progesterone receptors in normal human endometrium and endometrial carcinoma. In: McGuire W, Paynaud JP, Baulieu EE, eds. Progesterone receptors in normal and neoplastic tissues. New York: Raven Press, 1977. pp 313–338.
36. Heise E, Gorlich M. Estradiol receptor in human breast cancers throughout the menstrual cycle. Oncology 1982;39:340–344.
37. Saez S, Martin PM, Chouvet CD. Estradiol and progesterone receptor levels in human breast adenocarcinoma in relation to plasma estrogen and progesterone levels. Cancer Res 1978;38:3468–3473.
38. Axelrod D, Menendez-Botet C, Kinne D, Osborne M. Levels of estrogen and progesterone receptor proteins in patients with breast cancer during various phases of the menses. Cancer Invest 1988;6(1):7–14.
39. Coradini D, Cappelletti V, Miodini P, Ronchi E, Scavone G, Di Fronzo G. Variations in estrogen and progesterone receptor content in premenopausal breast cancer patients throughout the menstrual cycle. Tumori 1984;70:339–344.
40. Smyth CM, Benn DE, Reeve TS. Influence of the menstrual cycle on the concentrations of estrogen and progesterone receptors in primary breast cancer biopsies. Breast Cancer Res Treat 1988;11:45–50.
41. Battersby S, Robertson B, King R, McPherson K. Influence of menstrual cycle, parity and oral contraceptive use on steroid hormone receptors in normal breast. Br J Cancer 1992;65:601–607.
42. Weimer DA, Donegan WL. Changes in estrogen and progesterone receptor content of primary breast carcinoma during the menstrual cycle. Breast Cancer Res Treat 1987;10:273–278.
43. Folkman JM, Long D, Becker FF. Growth and metastasis of tumor in organ culture. Cancer 1963;16:453–467.
44. Kim KJ, Bing L, Winer J, et al. Inhibition of vascular endothelial growth factor-induced angiogenesis suppresses tumor growth *in vivo*. Nature 1993;362:841–844.
45. Schweike D, Hin A, Neufeld G, Gitay-Goren H, Keshet E. Patterns of expression of vascular endothelial growth hormone (VEGF) and VEGF receptors in mice suggest a role in hormonally regulated angiogenisis. J Clin Invest 1991;91:2235–2243.
46. Iruela-Arispe M, Porter P, Bornstein P, Sage E. Thrombospondin-1, an inhibitor of angiogenesis, is regulated by progestereone in the human endometrium. J Clin Invest 1996;97:403–412.
47. Pratt D, Miller W, Dawes J. Thrombospondin in malignant and non-malignant breast tissue. Eur J Cancer Clin Oncol 1989;25:343–350.
48. Irwin J, Kirk D, Gwatkin BL, Navre M, Cannon P, Guidice LC. Human endometrial matrix metalloproteinase-2, a putative menstrual proteinase. J Clin Invest 1996;97:438–447.
49. Ayus J, Wheeler J, Arieff A. Postoperative hypoatremic encephalopathy in menstruant women. Ann Intern Med 1992;117:891–897.
50. Roof R, Duvdevani R, Stein DG. Gender influences outcome of brain injury: Progesterone plays a protective role. Brain Res 1993;607:333–335.
51. Roof R, Duvdevani R, Stein DG. Progesterone treatment attenuates brain edema following contusion injury in male and female rats. Restor Neurol Neurosci 1992;4:425–427.
52. Liotta L, Kleinerman J, Saidel GM. Quantitative relationships of intravascular tumor cells, tumor vessels, and pulmonary metastases following tumor implantation. Cancer Res 1974;34:997–1004.
53. Zacharski LR, Moritz TE, Baczek LA, et al. Effect of mopidamole on survival in carcinoma of the lung and colon: Final report of Veterans Administration Cooperative Study No.188. J Natl Cancer Inst 1988;80:90–97.
54. Orchard M, Botting JH. The influence of sex hormones on rat platelet sensitivity to adenosinediphosphate. Endocrinology 1981:106–109.
55. Rosen S, Berk M, Popp D, et al. B2- and A2-adrenergic receptors and receptor coupling to adenylate cyclase in human mononuclear leukocytes and platelets in relation to physiological variations of sex steroids. J Clin Endocrinol Metab 1984;58:1068–1076.
56. Yamazaki H, Motomiya T, Kikutani N, Saakaakibaara C, Watanabe S, Numata M, Noguchi K. Platelet aggregation during the menstrual cycle and pregnancy. Thromb Res 1979;14(2–3):333–340.
57. Solerte S, Fioravanti M, Spinillo A, Ferrari E, Guaschino S. Association between hormonal and haemorheological changes during the menstrual cycle in healthy women. Br J Obstet Gynecol 1988;95:1305–1308.
58. Ehrlich P. Referat uber die Genese des Carcinoms. Verh Dtsch Pathol Ges 1908;12:13–32.
59. Ehrlich P, Apolant H. Beobachtungen uber maligne Mausetumoren. J Med Res 1905;28:309–322.
60. Apolant H. The question of immunity. J Exp Med 1911;14:316.
61. Marie P, Clunet J. Frequence de metastases viscerales chez les souris cancereuses apres ablation chiruricale de leur tumeur. Bull Assoc Fr Etude Cancer 1910;3:19–23.
62. Tyzzer E. Factors in production and growth of tumor metastates. J Med Res 1913;28:309–322.
63. Simpson-Herron L, Sanford AH, Holmquist JP. Effects of surgery on the cell kinetics of residual tumor. Cancer Treat Rep 1976;60:1749–1760.

64. Fisher B, Fisher ER. Experimental evidence in support of the dormant tumor cell. Science 1959;130:918–919.
65. Fisher BG, Coyle J, Rudock C, Saffer E. Presence of a growth-stimulating factor in serum following primary tumor removal in mice. Cancer Res 1989;49:1996–2001.

Adjuvant Therapy of Cancer VIII, edited by Sydney E. Salmon. Lippincott–Raven Publishers, Philadelphia © 1997.

16

Rationale for Combined Antiestrogen–Somatostatin Analogue Therapy of Breast Cancer

M. Pollak, J. Ingle, V. Suman, and J. Kugler

The efficacy of antiestrogens in the adjuvant treatment of breast cancer is well documented for patients of many prognostic groups but is modest in magnitude, as shown both by individual trials and by meta-analysis of worldwide clinical experience (1). Although the benefits of adjuvant tamoxifen therapy are important enough to justify its widespread use, relapse of breast cancer despite such therapy is common. There is a clear clinical need to improve the efficacy of adjuvant antiestrogen therapy.

An initial approach to this challenge was to study the combination of tamoxifen and cytotoxic agents. Recent laboratory observations concerning the mechanisms of antineoplastic action of antiestrogens and of somatostatin analogues have provided clues that may lead to the development of novel strategies to enhance the antineoplastic action of antiestrogens.

BACKGROUND

Antiestrogens and Insulin-like Growth Factor I (IGF-I) Physiology

The precise mechanisms of action of tamoxifen remain incompletely understood (2). The classic view that the drug acts simply by antagonizing estrogen-stimulated growth is now known to be incomplete. Direct evidence for this comes from simple experiments that show that antiestrogens inhibit breast cancer proliferation even in the absence of estrogens (3–5). This suggests that so-called "antiestrogens" actually act at least in part as direct growth inhibitors, rather than as mere antagonists of estrogens.

IGF-I is a potent mitogen (6–9), inhibitor of apoptosis (10), and stimulator of cell motility (11). Human breast cancer xenografts grow less rapidly in hosts with a genetically determined IGF-I deficiency than in controls (12). It is known that antiestrogens interfere with IGF-I action at several levels, and this may contribute to their antineoplastic action. At the level of the malignant breast epithelial cell, it has been known for some time that antiestrogens upregulate autocrine growth inhibitory pathways involving production of TGF-β (13). More recent results show similar upregulation of autocrine growth inhibitory loops involving IGF binding protein 3 by antiestrogens (14). There is evidence that IGF binding protein 3 acts at least in part by interfering with the binding of IGFs to the IGF-I receptor.

It is further recognized that tamoxifen has important effects on IGF physiology of the host (as distinct from direct effects on tumor cells) that may contribute to its antineoplastic action. Examples are the suppressive effects of tamoxifen on growth hormone secretion (15,16), on serum IGF-I level (17,18), and on expression of the IGF-I gene in target organs for metastasis (19). These data raise the possibility that the IGF-I suppressive activity of tamoxifen may make target organs less fertile "soil" for the growth of metastases.

There is a positive correlation between the presence of estrogen receptors and IGF-I receptors on human breast cancer cells (20). Therefore, cancers predicted to be responsive to tamoxifen on the basis of high estrogen receptor level may also be those that would be growth-inhibited by reduction in local IGF bioactivity. Moreover, it is recognized that there are complex interactions between the growth stimulatory actions of IGFs and those of estrogens. For example, estrogens upregulate (21) and antiestrogens downregulate (22) IGF-I receptor levels on breast cancer cells, raising the possibility that estrogens act in part by enhancing responsivity to IGFs. The data in Figure 16-1 are consistent with this possibility, as they show that the proliferative response of MCF-7 human breast cancer cells (which are IGF-I receptor-positive and estrogen receptor-positive) to IGF-I is enhanced in the presence of estradiol. This implies that antiestrogens may act on estrogen-receptor positive cells in overlapping ways to reduce proliferation: not only do they

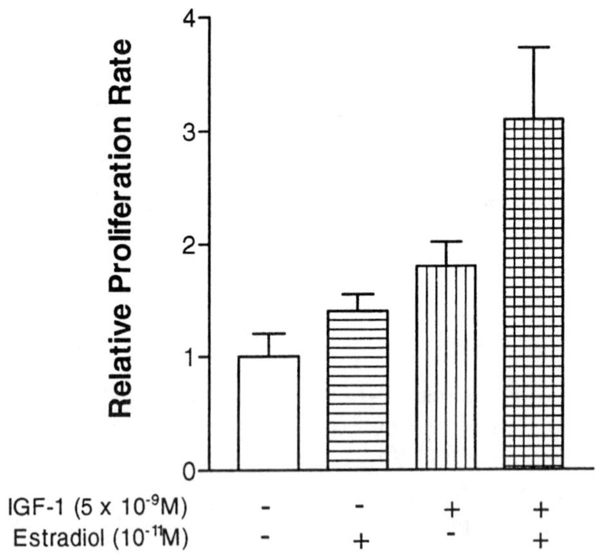

Figure 16-1. Mitogenic effect of estradiol and IGF-I singly and in combination on MCF-7 breast cancer cell proliferation. Assays were conducted using methods as described in reference (5). Combined treatment was associated with proliferation rate higher than estradiol or IGF-1 alone ($P \leq 0.05$, Mann-Whitney U test).

block estrogen-stimulated growth, but they also: (a) reduce circulating IGF-I levels, (b) reduce IGF-I expression in target organs for metastasis, and (c) reduce responsivity to IGFs by downregulating IGF-I receptors and upregulating IGFBP-3 expression.

Somatostatin Analogues and IGF-I Physiology

Expression of IGF-I is upregulated by growth hormone (23). Somatostatin analogues such as octreotide and RC-160 are known to suppress IGF-I levels (24). This involves both suppression of growth hormone secretion and direct suppression of IGF-I gene expression (25). In addition, there are data to support the view that somatostatin analogues also reduce IGF-I bioactivity by upregulating expression of IGF binding protein 1 (26,27).

Direct Effects of Somatostatin Analogues on Breast Cancer Cells

Apart from their action on IGF-I physiology of the host, somatostatin analogues have the potential to act directly on neoplasms that express somatostatin receptors (28–30). Recent studies have shown that most breast cancers have cell surface somatostatin receptors (31). Five distinct subtypes of somatostatin receptors have been described (32,33), and there is evidence that binding of somatostatin (or a somatostatin analogue) to receptor subtype 2 and/or subtype 5 is associated with direct growth inhibition (34–36).

COMBINING SOMATOSTATIN ANALOGUES AND ANTIESTROGENS

Preclinical Data

In standard *in vivo* and *in vitro* experimental systems, somatostatin analogues have been shown to have significant antineoplastic activity against breast cancer (37,38), although in general the single agent activity of somatostatin analogues is not greater than that seen with endocrine treatments already in clinical use. Of particular interest, however, is a report showing that in the DMBA mammary breast cancer model, combined antiestrogen-octreotide treatment has greater antineoplastic activity than either single agent tamoxifen or single agent octreotide (39) (Figure 16-2).

The basis for the favorable interaction in the DMBA model remains uncertain. It has been shown *in vitro* that the direct antiproliferative action of octreotide on breast cancer cells is maximized in the absence of estrogens (40), suggesting the possibility that *in vivo*, the direct antiproliferative effect of octreotide might be maximized in the presence of an antiestrogen. It has also been shown that the inhibitory effects of co-administered antiestrogens and octreotide on IGF-I expression are greater than the effects of either agent alone (41), suggesting the possibility that "indirect" mechanisms may be important. These two proposed mechanisms are not mutually exclusive. There is also a possibility of additive antiangiogenic effects (42,43) or other as yet uncharacterized additive actions.

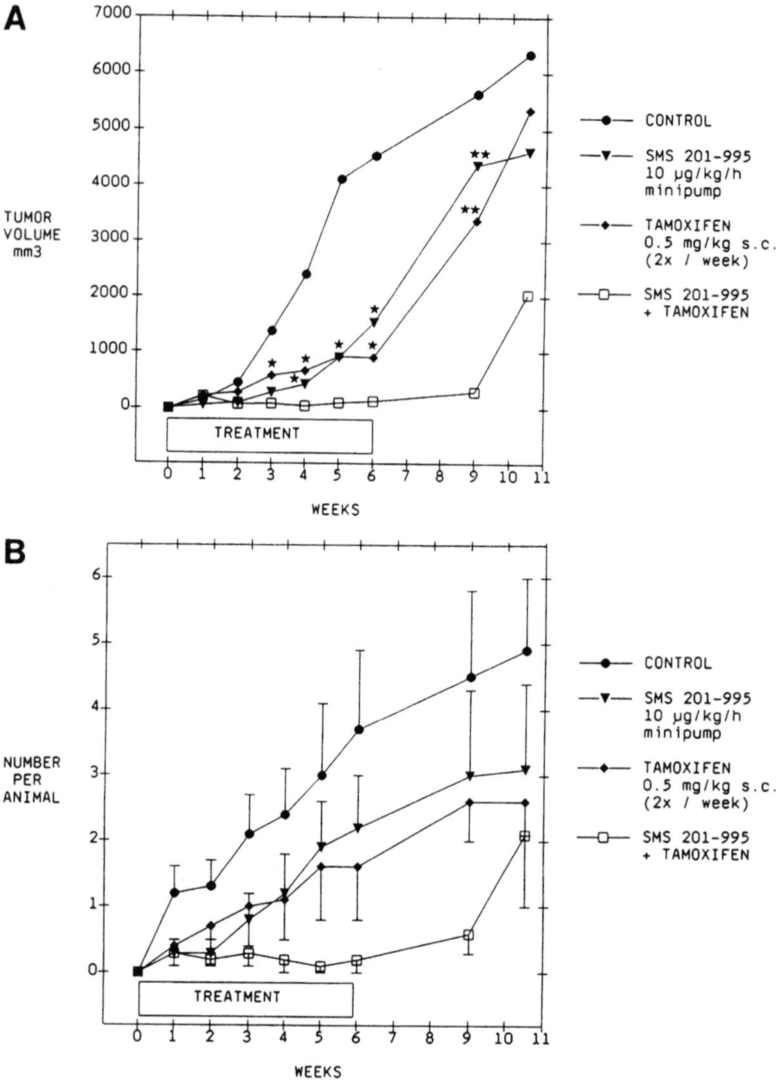

Figure 16-2. Effect of combination tamoxifen (0.5 mg/kg SC twice weekly) and octreotide (minipump infusion SC, 10 μg/kg/h) on tumor growth (A) and appearance (B) of tumors (tumor number) in rats bearing DMBA-induced mammary carcinomas. Note that treatment was stopped at 6 weeks. Points, mean tumor volume and number for 10 rats/group; bars, SE. For clarity SE omitted in A. The SE in A and B were similar. In A, comparison of the combination group with the single agent groups resulted in significant differences in tumor growth: $^{*}P \leq 0.05$; $^{**}P \leq 0.01$, t test. Pooled data for tumor number comparisons (B) gave a significant difference between the tamoxifen and combination group for weeks 4-6; $P \leq 0.02$. (From ref. 39)

Clinical Experience

There is extensive literature documenting the clinical use of tamoxifen in the adjuvant treatment of breast cancer (1), and considerable experience in long-term use of octreotide for conditions such as carcinoid syndrome and acromegaly (44). There are no reports of phase II trials of octreotide in breast cancer that demonstrate activity similar to or greater than that seen with currently available hormonal agents. The major controlled clinical trial of combined octreotide–tamoxifen therapy is the North Central Cancer Treatment Group 893253 study. This trial randomized women with metastatic estrogen receptor positive breast cancer to treatment with tamoxifen, 10 mg PO b.i.d., or to this dose of tamoxifen combined with octreotide, 150μg SC t.i.d. Analysis of clinical response endpoints is not expected prior to the fall of 1996. However, in a subset of 18 patients followed for treatment-related changes in serum IGF-I level, we observed (45) that: (a) there was no significant difference between arms with respect to baseline IGF-I level, (b) both treatments resulted in significant declines in serum IGF-I, and (c) the treatment-related percent decline of IGF-I between baseline and 3–6 weeks was significantly greater ($p = 0.004$, Wilcoxon rank sum test) in the combination arm than in the tamoxifen alone arm (medians −38.9%, −16.4%, respectively). These data demonstrate a difference between treatment arms with respect to a biological endpoint. However, the hypothesis that degree of decline of IGF-I can be used as a surrogate marker of treatment efficacy has not been proven, so further studies are clearly needed to follow-up this finding.

DISCUSSION

The worldwide experience with adjuvant tamoxifen therapy has shown that while this treatment improves prognosis for many women following a diagnosis of breast cancer, there is an obvious need to develop adjuvant therapies with improved efficacy. One response to this clinical need has been research in the direction of more aggressive cytotoxic treatments. A separate approach is to improve noncytotoxic treatments (46), and one example of research in this direction is the search for ways to enhance the activity of tamoxifen. The data reviewed here suggest that one possible way to achieve this may be to co-administer tamoxifen with somatostatin analogues such as octreotide.

In the development of novel adjuvant therapies for breast cancer, safety is an important consideration, even more so than in the case of novel treatments for patients with metastatic disease. This has made it difficult to bring novel agents to clinical trial for adjuvant treatment. However, available data concerning the toxicity profiles of tamoxifen and octreotide suggest that an adjuvant trial of this combination would be feasible, although careful follow-up (e.g., with respect to the risk of increased cholelithiasis) would be necessary.

In preclinical models, many noncytotoxic therapies, including octreotide, appear to be more active in preventing the growth of small tumors than in causing regression of existing large lesions. In the DMBA model, for example, octreotide appears more active when assayed in a way that involves measuring reduction of development of palpable lesions (39) than when it is assayed in a way that involves measurement of regression of large tumors (47). This implies that there may well exist novel approaches that could lead to improved adjuvant therapies, even if these do not demonstrate improved outcome in metastatic disease. Agents that act primarily by inhibiting angiogenesis are representative of compounds that might reasonably be expected to prevent growth of micrometastases to large lesions, while causing little or no regression of established metastases. (Both octreotide (42) and tamoxifen (43) have antiangiogenic properties, but it is not known to what extent these properties contribute to their antineoplastic actions.) Therefore, while it is obviously of importance to determine the activity in the adjuvant setting of all therapies that are useful in metastatic disease, it is possible that efficacious therapies for adjuvant treatment could be missed if adjuvant trials are conducted only on agents that cause regression of macrometastases.

Further clinical trials of the octreotide–tamoxifen combination are now being planned. These will be facilitated by the newly available monthly depot formulation of octreotide, which should enhance compliance and patient acceptability relative to the t.i.d. subcutaneous injections that have been needed until now. In addition to conventional clinical outcome endpoints, it will be important to use these trials to obtain serum and tumor samples for translational research that will generate new data relevant not only to the particular therapies under study, but also to broader goals of improving our understanding of breast cancer biology.

ACKNOWLEDGMENT

We thank Bonnie Deroo for assistance in preparing this manuscript.

REFERENCES

1. Early Breast Cancer Trialists' Collaborative Group. Systemic treatment of early breast cancer by hormonal, cytotoxic, or immune therapy. Lancet 1992;339:1–15, 71–85.
2. Jordan VC, Murphy CS. Endocrine pharmacology of antiestrogens as antitumor agents. Endocrinol Rev 1990;11:578–611.
3. Vignon F, Bouton MM, Rochefort H. Antiestrogens inhibit the mitogenic effect of growth factors on breast cancer cells in the total absence of estrogens. Biochem Biophys Res Commun 1987;146:1502–1508.
4. Wakeling AE, Bowler J. Novel antioestrogens without partial agonist activity. J Steroid Biochem Mol Biol 1988;31:645–653.
5. Pratt SE, Pollak M. Estrogen and antiestrogen modulation of MCF7 human breast cancer cell proliferation is associated with specific alterations in accumulation of IGF binding proteins in conditioned media. Cancer Res 1993;53:5193–5198.
6. Macaulay VM. Insulin-like growth factors and cancer. Br J Cancer 1992;65:311–320.
7. Pollak M, Polychronakos C, Yousefi S, Richard M. Characterization of insulin-like growth factor (IGF-I) receptors of human breast cancer cells. Biochem Biophys Res Commun 1988;154:326–331.
8. Arteaga CL, Osborne CK. Growth inhibition of human breast cancer cells *in vitro* with an antibody against the type l somatomedin receptor. Cancer Res 1989;49:6237–6241.
9. Furlanetto R, DeCarlo J. Somatomedin-C receptors and growth effect in human breast cells maintained in long term tissue culture. Cancer Res 1992;44:2122–2128.
10. Resnicoff M, Abraham D, Yutanawiboonchai W, Rotman HL, Kajstura J, Rubin R, Zoltick P, Baserga R. The insulin-like growth factor I receptor protects tumor cells from apoptosis *in vivo*. Cancer Res 1995;55:2463–2469.
11. Stracke ML, Engel JD, Wilson LW, Rechler MM, Liotta LA, Schiffmann E. The type I insulin-like growth factor receptor is a motility receptor in human melanoma cells. J Biol Chem 1989;264:21544–21549.
12. Yang XF, Beamer W, Huynh HT, Pollak M. Reduced growth of human breast cancer xenografts in hosts homozygous for the *lit* mutation. Cancer Res. 1996;56:1509–1511.

13. Butta A, MacLennan K, Flanders KC, Sacks NPM, Smith I, McKinna A, Dowsett M, Wakefield LM, Sporn MB, Baum M, Coletta AA. Induction of transforming growth factor β1 in human breast cancer *in vivo* following tamoxifen treatment. Cancer Res 1992;52:4261–4264.
14. Huynh HT, Yang X, Pollak M. Estradiol and antiestrogens regulate a growth inhibitory insulin-like growth factor binding protein 3 autocrine loop in human breast cancer cells. J Biol Chem 1996;271:1016–1021.
15. Tannenbaum GS, Gurd W, Lapointe M, Pollak M. Tamoxifen attenuates pulsatile growth hormone secretion: Mediation in part by somatostatin. Endocrinology 1992;130:3395–3401.
16. Malaab SA, Pollak M, Goodyer CG. Direct effects of tamoxifen on growth hormone secretion by pituitary cells *in vitro*. Eur J Cancer 1992;28A:788–793.
17. Pollak M, Costantino J, Polychronakos C, Blauer S, Guyda H, Redmond C, Fisher B, Margolese R. Effect of tamoxifen on serum insulin-like growth factor I levels in stage I breast cancer patients. J Natl Cancer Inst 1990;82:1693–1697.
18. Pollak M. Effects of adjuvant tamoxifen therapy on growth hormone and insulin-like growth factor I (IGF-I) physiology. In: Salmon SE, ed. Adjuvant therapy of cancer VII. Philadelphia: J. B. Lippincott Company, 1993.
19. Huynh HT, Tetenes E, Wallace L, Pollak, M. *In vivo* inhibition of insulin-like growth factor-I gene expression by tamoxifen. Cancer Res 1993;53:1727–1730.
20. Pekonen F, Partanen S, Makinen T, Rutanen EM. Receptors for epidermal growth factor and insulin-like growth factor I and their relation to steroid receptors in human breast cancer. Cancer Res 1988;48:1343–1347.
21. Stewart AJ, Johnson MD, May FEB, Westley BR. Role of insulin-like growth factors and the type I insulin-like growth factor receptor in the estrogen-stimulated proliferation of human breast cancer cells. J Biol Chem 1990;265:21172–21178. [Abstr. 1506.]
22. Nickerson T, Yang XF, Pollak M, Huynh HT. Post-transcriptional regulation of insulin-like growth factor I receptor by the pure antiestrogen ICI 182,780. Am Assoc Cancer Res Annual Mtg, Washington, DC, 1996. [Abstr. 1506.]
23. Roberts CT, Brown AL, Graham DE, Seelig S, Berry S, Gabbay KH, Rechler MM. Growth hormone regulates the abundance of insulin-like growth factor I RNA in adult rat liver. J Biol Chem 1986;261:10025–10028.
24. Pollak M, Polychronakos C, Guyda H. Somatostatin analogue SMS 201-995 reduces serum IGF-I levels in patients with neoplasms potentially dependent on IGF-I. Anticancer Res 1989;9:889–892.
25. Serri O, Brazeau P, Kachra Z, Posner B. Octreotide inhibits insulin-like growth factor-I hepatic gene expression in the hypophysectomized rat: Evidence for a direct and indirect mechanism of action. Endocrinology 1992;130:1816–1821.
26. Ezzat S, Ren SG, Braunstein GD, Melmed S. Octreotide stimulates insulin-like growth factor-binding protein-1: A potential pituitary-independent mechanism for drug action. J Clin Endocrinol Metab 1992;75:1459–1463.
27. Frystyk J, Skjaerbaek C, Alexander N, Foegh M, Orskov H. Tonic increase in serum IGFBP-1 and reduction in free and total IGF-1 during somatostatin analogue treatment in patients undergoing PTCA. Proc Third Int Symp IGF Binding Proteins, Tuebingen, Germany, 1995. [Abstr. 218.]
28. Schally AV. Oncological applications of somatostatin analogues. Cancer Res 1988;48:6977–6985.
29. Szepeshazi K, Milovanovic S, Lapis K, Groot K, Schally AV. Growth inhibition of estrogen independent MXT mouse mammary carcinomas in mice treated with an agonist or antagonist of LH-RH, an analog of somatostatin, or a combination. Breast Cancer Res Treat 1992;21:181–192.
30. Schally AV. Hypothalamic hormones: From neuroendocrinology to cancer therapy. Anti-Cancer Drugs 1994;5:115–130.
31. van Eijck CH, Krenning EP, Bootsma A, Lindemans J, Jeekel J, Reubi JC, Lamberts SW. Somatostatin-receptor scintigraphy in primary breast cancer. Lancet 1994;343:640–643.
32. Patel YC, Greenwood MT, Panetta R, Demchyshyn L, Niznik H, Srikant CB. The somatostatin receptor family. Life Sci 1995;57:1249–1265.
33. Hoyer D, Bell GI, Berelowitz M, Epelbaum J, Feniuk W, Humphrey PP, O'Carroll AM, Patel YC, Schonbrunn A, Taylor JE, et al. Classification and nomenclature of somatostatin receptors. Trends Pharmacol Sci 1995;16:86–88.
34. Patel YC, Srikant CB. Subtype selectivity of peptide analogs for all five cloned human somatostatin receptors (hSSTR 1–5). Endocrinology 1994;135:2814–2817.
35. Buscail L, Esteve JP, Saint-Laurent N, Bertrand V, Reisine T, O'Carroll AM, Bell GI, Schally AV, Vaysse N, Susini C. Inhibition of cell proliferation by the somatostatin analogue RC-160 is mediated by somatostatin receptor subtypes SSTR2 and SSTR5 through different mechanisms. Proc Natl Acad Sci USA 1995;92:1580–1584.

36. Buscail L, Delesque N, Esteve JP, Saint-Laurent N, Prats H, Clerc P, Robberecht P, Bell GI, Liebow C, Schally AV, et al. Stimulation of tyrosine phosphatase and inhibition of cell proliferation by somatostatin analogues: Mediation by human somatostatin receptor subtypes SSTR1 and SSTR2. Proc Natl Acad Sci USA 1994;91:2315–2319.
37. Weckbecker G, Raulf F, Stolz B, Bruns C. Somatostatin analogs for diagnosis and treatment of cancer. Pharmacol Ther 1993;60:245–264.
38. Weckbecker G, Liu R, Tolcsvai L, Bruns C. Antiproliferative effects of the somatostatin analogue octreotide (SMS 201-995) on ZR-75-1 human breast cancer cells *in vivo* and *in vitro*. Cancer Res 1992;52:4973–4978.
39. Weckbecker G, Tolcsvai L, Stolz B, Pollak M, Bruns C. Somatostatin analogue octreotide enhances the antineoplastic effects of tamoxifen and ovariectomy on 7,12-dimethylbenz(*a*)anthracene-induced rat mammary carcinomas. Cancer Res 1994;54:6334–6337.
40. Setyono-Han B, Henkelman MS, Foekens JA, Klijn GM. Direct inhibitory effects of somatostatin (analogues) on the growth of human breast cancer cells. Cancer Res 1987;47:1566–1570.
41. Huynh HT, Pollak M. Enhancement of tamoxifen-induced suppression of insulin-like growth factor I gene expression and serum level by a somatostatin analogue. Biochem Biophys Res Commun 1994;203:253–259.
42. Patel PC, Barrie R, Hill N, Landeck S, Kurozawa D, Woltering EA. Postreceptor signal transduction mechanisms involved in octreotide-induced inhibition of angiogenesis. Surgery 1994; 116:1148–1152.
43. Gagliardi A, Collins DC. Inhibition of angiogenesis by antiestrogens. Cancer Res 1993;53:533–535.
44. Lamberts SWJ, Vanderlely AJ, Deherder WW, Hofland LJ. Drug therapy—Octreotide. N Engl J Med 1996;334:246–254.
45. Pollak M, Ingle JN, Suman VJ, Kugler JW, Nickerson T, Deroo B. Enhancement of tamoxifen-induced suppression of serum IGF-1 levels in metastatic breast cancer patients by coadministration of the somatostatin analogue octreotide. Am Assoc Cancer Res Annual Mtg, Washington, DC, 1996. [Abstr. 1167.]
46. Schipper H, Goh CR, Wang TL. Shifting the cancer paradigm: Must we kill to cure? J Clin Oncol 1995;13:801–807.
47. Bakker GH, Setyono-Han B, Foekens JA, Portengen H, van Putten WL, de Jong FH, Lamberts SW, Reubi JC, Klijn JG. The somatostatin analog sandostatin (SMS 201-995) in treatment of DMBA-induced rat mammary tumors. Breast Cancer Res Treat 1990;17:23–32.

Adjuvant Therapy of Cancer VIII, edited by Sydney E. Salmon. Lippincott–Raven Publishers, Philadelphia © 1997.

17

Clodronate as an Adjuvant to Hormone and Chemotherapy in Patients with Breast Cancer

Alexander H. G. Paterson, John A. Kanis, Trevor Powles, Eugene V. McCloskey, and Susan Ashley

Despite recent advances in the hormone therapy and chemotherapy of breast cancer, bone pain, fractures, and hypercalcemia remain major causes of morbidity in patients. The problems of bone metastases may be compounded by the propensity in women to osteoporosis. Women have a lower total bone mass than men and the fracture threshold is reached at an earlier age. Additionally, the increased use of cytotoxic chemotherapy in premenopausal women with breast cancer leads to ovarian involution at an earlier age with consequent increased time for bone loss to occur.

The mechanisms underlying the appearance and growth of metastases in bone are poorly understood. It is presumed that tumor emboli from the primary tumor are arrested within the vascular network of the bone and secondary invasion through the sinusoids occurs.

Once a tumor embolus has its "foot in the door," subsequent growth results not only from its own genetic capacity for cell replication and invasion, but also depends on its ability to breakdown compartment-restricting materials such as bone trabeculae by the action of products secreted which have a direct effect on the osteoclast. In breast cancer, cytokines such as transforming growth factor (α) may be secreted, which stimulate host lymphoid cells, which themselves secrete osteoclast activating factors (1). It is also possible that breast cancer cells secrete pro-cathepsin D which has a direct stimulatory effect on osteoclast activity. Whatever the mechanism, the tumor cell embolus grows to a size capable of giving characteristic radiological appearances in bone—osteolytic or mixed osteolytic/osteoblastic lesions in the case of breast cancer or purely osteolytic lesions in the case of multiple myeloma.

Skeletal complications of bone metastases from breast cancer and other malignancies arise because of progressive focal or generalized osteolysis occurring as a result of osteoclast activation, either directly by tumor products or indirectly by products secreted by nearby host cells in response to tumor cell products (2). Since the osteoclast plays a central role in both focal and generalized osteolysis, we have postulated that inhibitors of osteoclast function may give useful palliation in patients with established bone metastases, and in some patients where clinically evident metastases are not present, they may inhibit their appearances (3).

A number of inhibitors of bone resorption have been assessed in patients with malignant disease. These agents include mithromycin, nonsteroidal anti-inflammatory drugs, gallium nitrate, and calcitonin. These have been found to have been either of limited efficacy or unacceptably toxic (4,5). Calcitonin appears to have a short to medium term effect only on malignant osteolytic bone disease. Mithramycin has additional affects on the bone marrow such as thrombocytopenia and is unacceptably toxic for routine use. Interest in the long-term therapy of bone metastases has therefore focused on the use of bisphosphonates.

Several bisphosphonates have been assessed in the management of hypercalcemia. These include etidronate, pamidronate, clodronate, residronate, mildronate, neridronate, alendronate, and more recently ibandronate. Etidronate, pamidronate, and clodronate have been the most extensively tested bisphosphonates and are widely available for the treatment of hypercalcemia and Paget's disease of bone. We have previously demonstrated the action of etidronate in the treatment of hypercalcemia (6). Pamidronate, clodronate, and etidronate lead to an effective lowering of serum calcium, which is attributable to decreased bone resorption, but etidronate appears to impair the mineralization of bone and must be given intermittently to allow normal bone formation to occur. Pamidronate may not be ideal for oral use because of dose-related gastrointestinal toxicity. There is some evidence that long-term pamidronate administered orally may also induce osteomalacia. Clodronate is effective when given intravenously for hypercalcemia and bone pain and can be used orally. Its long-term administration is not associated with a defect in bone mineralization (8).

In general, bisphosphonates are agents derived from a stable P-C-P bond. They bind with high affinity to hydroxyapatite crystals in bone and affect the activity of osteoclasts. Another action may be to reduce the numbers of osteoclasts by decreasing the recruitment of osteoclast precursors to the osteoclast cell pool.

In contrast to our negative results with etidronate, we have demonstrated in a double-blind, placebo-controlled trial of crossover design that intravenous clodronate can reduce bone pain and improve mobility in a proportion of patients with pain secondary to bone metastases (9).

We therefore performed two simultaneous studies of clodronate as an adjuvant. The first, a double-blind, placebo-controlled trial in patients with recurrent breast cancer involving bone, was designed to determine whether oral clodronate 1600 mg taken daily for 3 years could reduce the morbidity from skeletal metastases compared to a similarly treated placebo-control group of patients. Specifically, we looked at hypercalcemic episodes, fracture rate, and treatment courses of radiotherapy given for bone pain. In the second study, patients who had histologically proven recurrent breast cancer but no clinical, radiological, or bone scintigraphic evidence of bone metastases were similarly allocated to clodronate 1600 mg orally daily for 3 years or a placebo. In this study we not only assessed skeletal morbidity from subsequently developing bone metastases but also assessed the number and rate of development of newly appearing bone metastases in the two groups.

Finally, we have completed the accrual of 1000 patients to a trial of adjuvant oral clodronate 1600 mg daily for 2 years compared to placebo in patients presenting with operable breast cancer. This trial is currently under analysis.

METHODS

Trial 1: Patients with Bone Metastases

Patients with breast cancer and metastatic skeletal disease assessable according to UICC/NCI (US) (10,11) were eligible for trial entry. No specific chemotherapeutic or hormone regimen was stipulated, since the end points chosen did not include tumor response or remission length in bone. On progression of disease at any site, a change in chemotherapy or hormone therapy was allowed at the discretion of the treating physician, but patients were continued on the clodronate or placebo capsules. Treatment of intercurrent hypercalcemia excluded the use of bisphosphonates. A total of 173 patients were entered into the study at two cancer centres. All patients gave written, informed consent. The patients were randomly allocated to receive 18 months of oral clodronate 1600 mg/day or an identical capsule containing an inactive placebo (manufactured and supplied by Hutamaki Oy Leiras, Helsinki, Finland). The randomization process was controlled at an independent centre (Helsinki, Finland) using a prerandomized numbering system whereby patients, allocated a number of the order in which they presented, were prescribed the corresponding numbered medication package at each center at 3-month intervals. The clinicians, nursing staff, and pharmacy staff at each participating hospital were unaware of the treatment allocation of patients. A decision was made after 2 years to extend the treatment time to 3 years, and approval was obtained from the patients and from the ethics committees at each centre.

Patients were instructed to take the 4 × 400 mg capsules in the morning before eating or consuming milk-containing liquids. If gastrointestinal intolerance developed, patients took the capsules in two daily doses of 800 mg. The patients were assessed clinical at intervals of at least 3 months. A blood count, serum biochemistry, 10 mL of serum for storage, and a fasting urine specimen were taken every 3 months; every 6 months, bone scintigraphy, liver ultrasound, and x-rays of the hands, pelvis, skull, lumbar spine, and thoracic spine were taken. Clodronate concentrations were measured in serum and urine in patients at 3-month intervals.

The primary study end points for efficacy were hypercalcemia, the incidence of vertebral and nonvertebral fracture, and radiotherapy requirements for bone pain.

Serum Calcium, Hypercalcemia, and Hypercalciuria. Serum calcium levels were measured every 3 months. The serum value was adjusted for albumin by the addition or subtraction of 0.02 mmol/L for every 1 g/L that the albumin was less than or greater than 40 g/L, respectively. Hypercalcemia was defined as an adjusted calcium value of 2.6 mmol/L or greater. The number of hypercalcemic episodes was documented in each patient.

Fasting urinary calcium excretion (expressed as a ratio to urinary creatinine) was used as an index of net efflux of calcium from the skeleton. At study entry, hypercalciuria was defined as a fasting urinary calcium to creatinine ratio of greater than 0.4 mmol/mmol.

Fractures. Nonvertebral fractures were diagnosed and recorded by the trial radiologists at each center. A research assistant based at the University of Sheffield traveled to each center to perform vertebral and metacarpal morphometry.

Vertebral Morphometry Anteroposterior and lateral x-rays of the thoracic spine (taken during inspiration) and lumbar spine were obtained at a standard target to a film distance of 105 cm, with the thoracic and lumbar films centred on T-7 and L-3, respectively. The anterior, posterior, and central heights of each vertebra from T-4 to L-5 were recorded by a semi-automated technique using a rear-illuminated digitizing tablet and a fine cross-hair cursor. Vertebral deformities identified by an algorithm were characterized into four types, each of which was assigned a deformity score—central collapse (score 1), anterior wedge (score 2), posterior wedge (score 2), and total collapse (score 3). The total spine deformity score was then recorded for each patient. The technique has a high specificity for the detection of vertebral osteoporosis.

The incidence of new vertebral fractures during the study was determined by analyzing paired vertebrae in all subsequent radiographs as described above (point prevalence). A new fracture was counted if an abnormality was detected at one or more of the vertebral sites (anterior, central, or posterior) in a previously normal vertebra. The change in deformity score between paired radiographs was also recorded, i.e., the sum of deformity scores in the new vertebral fractures in each individual.

Radiotherapy Requirements No formal assessment of bone pain was made due to the inadequacy of pain assessment methodology for patients with bone metastases. An indirect assessment was made using radiotherapy requirements for bone pain in patients. Radiotherapy was undertaken as clinically required.

Statistics. Follow-up clinical data were entered onto computer files at both centers. Survival curves were constructed and the curves obtained were compared for significance using log-rank analysis. Episodes of hypercalcemia, radiotherapy, fractures, and all morbid events were compared in the two groups using the test of proportions. For each type of event, the event rate was calculated from the cumulative number of events occurring over the cumulative duration of follow-up and expressed as events per 100 patient-years.

Trial 2: Patients with Recurrent Breast Cancer But No Evidence of Bone Metastases

Patients with histologically proven breast cancer and recurrent disease diagnosed according to standard criteria were eligible for entry into the study. The absence of skeletal metastases was determined by skeletal x-rays and scintigraphy. No specific chemotherapeutic or hormone regimen was stipulated since the primary end points chosen did not include tumor response or remission. Where disease progressed at any site, a change in chemotherapy or hormone therapy was permitted at the discretion of the treating physician, but patients were continued on clodronate or placebo capsules. Radiotherapy and medication for bone pain were allowed. Treatment of intercurrent hypercalcemia excluded the use of bisphosphonates.

One hundred and thirty-three women were entered into the study. All patients gave written informed consent and the study had the prior approval of the local Ethics Committees. Patients were randomly allocated to receive clodronate by mouth 1600 mg daily as four capsules, or an identical placebo, for 3 years (supplied by Leiras Oy, Helsinki, Finland).

Patients were instructed to take four capsules daily in the morning, 1 hr before meals and away from calcium-containing liquids. If gastrointestinal intolerance was reported, the patient was asked to take the same daily dose divided on two occasions.

At each visit, blood was taken for a full blood count and serum and urinary biochemistry. Bone scintigraphy and skeletal x-rays (hands, pelvis, skull, and lateral lumbar and thoracic spine) were obtained at 6-monthly intervals.

Assessment of Patients The primary end point of the study was to assess the effects of clodronate on the incidence and number of skeletal metastases. Skeletal metastases were diagnosed by the presence of characteristic lesions evident on scintigraphy and skeletal x-rays. Secondary end points included an assessment of the complications arising from skeletal disease, comprising hypercalcemia, bone pain, and fractures.

The combined cortical width was computed from the radiographs of both hands as the sum of the radial ulnar cortical width of all six metacarpals at the midpoint of their length. The reproducibility error of the measurement is 1.5%. For each patient the combined cortical width measured at 6 months and at 1 year was compared to that at entry, and the rate of change calculated as a percentage change from values at entry.

Statistics were performed as in Trial 1.

RESULTS

Trial 1

The clinical and biochemical characteristics of patients at study entry showed a good distribution of patients in each arm of the study. There was no significant difference in side effects and toxicity in the two groups. A summary table showing the events related to bone metastases (fractures, episodes of hypercalcemia, and radiotherapy for bone pain) in both trials is shown in Table 17-1. Figure 17-1 shows the mean change in urinary calcium excretion assessed in mmol/mmol creatinine in clodronate and placebo patients at 6 months and 1 year. Figure 17-2 shows the cumulative skeletal events in patients receiving clodronate compared to placebo.

Trial 2

One hundred and thirty-three women were entered into the trial. Sixty-six were allocated to clodronate and 67 to placebo. There was no significant difference between the two treatment groups at the study entry with respect to age, previous or concurrent treatment for cancer, and sites of soft tissue metastases.

No significant differences in side effects were noted between the treatment groups. Hypocalcemia was not observed.

At the time of analysis, 98 women (74%) had died: 47 in the clodronate group and 51 on placebo. Of the remaining patients, five in each group were still taking

TABLE 17-1. The Incidence of Skeletal Complications in Patients According to Treatment and Stratum Expressed as Events/100 Patient Years[a]

	Trial 1			Trial 2		
	Clodronate	**Placebo**	**%[a]**	**Clodronate**	**Placebo**	**%[a]**
Number of patients	85	88		66	67	
Follow-up (months)	1158	1198		1695	1742	
Morbid events						
Radiotherapy	74.8	89.1	84	14.9	18.6	78
Nonvertebral fractures	31.9	39.8	80	1.4	5.5[g]	25
Vertebral fractures	84.0	124.1[c]	68	47.6	60.7	79
Hypercalcemia	27.9	51.8[d]	54	7.1	11.7[b]	61
Any of the above	218.6	304.8[f]	72	73.0	96.5[d]	72
Bone metastases				22.	43.4[e]	53

[a]The third column from each study shows the incidence of events in clodronate treated patients as a percentage of those in placebo-treated patients.

[b]$P < 0.05$
[c]$P < 0.025$
[d]$P < 0.01$
[e]$P < 0.005$
[f]$P < 0.001$
[g]borderline $P < 0.1$

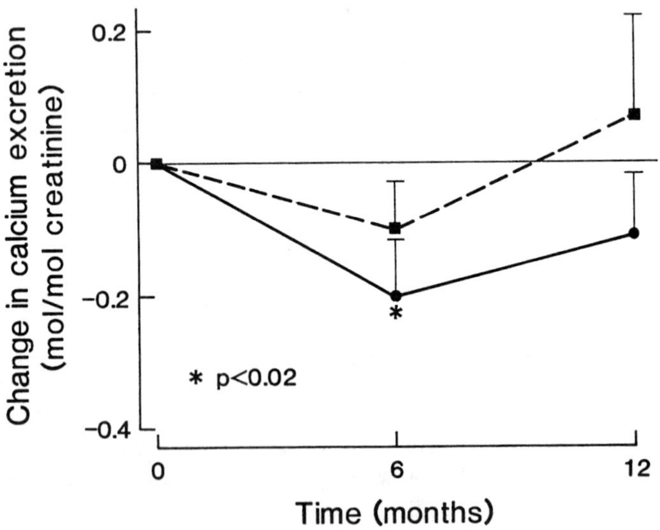

Figure 17-1. Mean change in urinary calcium excretion expressed in mmol/mmol creatinine in clodronate-treated patients (•——•) and placebo-treated patients (•- - -•). The reduction from baseline in clodronate-treated patients is statistically significant ($P < .02$).

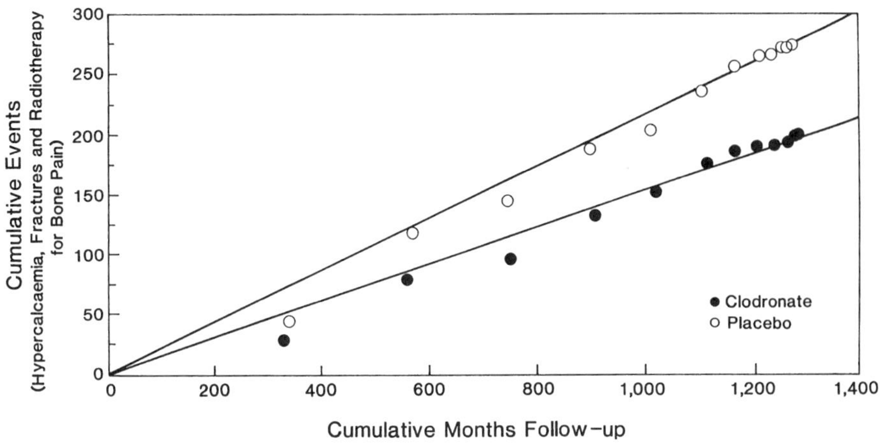

Figure 17-2. Skeletal events: clodronate vs placebo.

medication. In total, there were 282 patient-years of follow-up (138 for clodronate, 144 for placebo; NS).

The end points examined are summarized in Table 17-1. The use of clodronate was associated with a small and nonsignificant decrease in the number of patients who developed skeletal metastases compared with placebo treated patients. There was, however, a marked and significant decrease in the number of skeletal lesions observed (Figure 17-1). Clodronate treatment reduced the numbers of skeletal metastases by 48% when adjusted for duration of treatment.

Consistent trends were observed in favour of clodronate for the frequency of hypercalcemia, radiotherapy for bone pain, and vertebral and nonvertebral fractures. The cumulative incidence of skeletal morbid events was significantly reduced in the clodronate group (Figure 17-3). Combined cortical width of the metacarpals increased by 4.3% (SEM) ± 2.3% at 6 months and remained increased at 12 months in the clodronate group whereas in the placebo group combined cortical width decreased.

There were no significant differences seen in survival in either trial.

DISCUSSION

In the first study in patients with bone metastases secondary to breast cancer we demonstrated a significant reduction in overall skeletal morbidity, specifically in the rate of development of hypercalcemic episodes, fractures (particularly, serious vertebral deformities), and bone pain as measured by radiotherapy requirements (14). This effect has been also reported with pamidronate given orally (12). There was a significant reduction in urinary calcium excretion in the clodronate treated patients indicating a beneficial effect on bone loss.

In the second study in patients with recurrent breast cancer but no evidence of bone metastases at presentation of recurrence we have shown that fewer fractures occurred in patients receiving clodronate compared to patients in the placebo group.

There was a reduction in hypercalcemic events although the total number of events was lower than in patients with bone metastases. Of major interest is that there appears to be a reduction in the number of new bone metastases diagnosed in the clodronate patients compared to placebo patients.

This trial, therefore, showed a similar (though not as marked) reduction in skeletal events in patients who presented with recurrent breast cancer without bone metastases. There appeared to be an effect on the development of new bone metastases.

Currently, we have completed accrual of 1000 patients in a placebo-controlled adjuvant trial in patients with T1, T2, T3, N1, N2, or M0 breast cancer who are being treated with local and systemic therapy.

Bisphosphonates are useful in reducing skeletal complications in patients with bone metastases in breast cancer. They may also reduce the incidence of new bone metastases (either by delaying the appearance or preventing the development of bone metastases) and reduce the skeletal complications of the disease in patients presenting with recurrent breast cancer and no radiological evidence of skeletal disease.

Systemic adjuvant chemotherapy and hormone therapy, while producing significant advances in survival and disease-free recurrence rates, have a predominant effect by reducing recurrence rates of local and regional disease (13). The effect of these treatments on the reduction of bone metastases as a site of first recurrence has

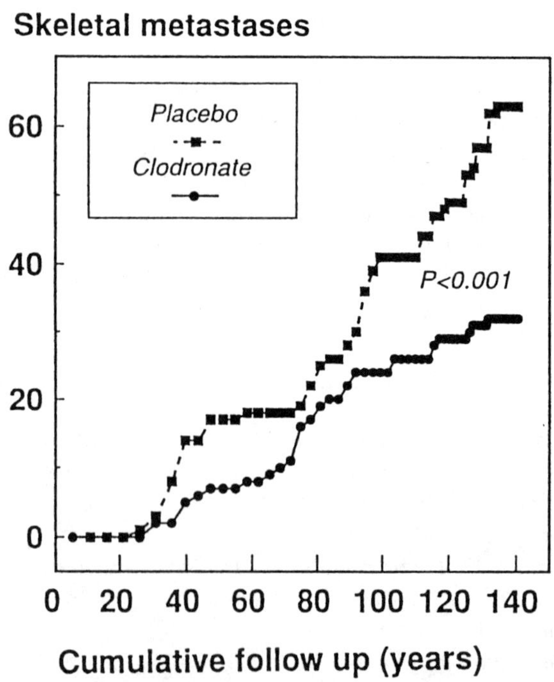

Figure 17-3. Skeletal metastases.

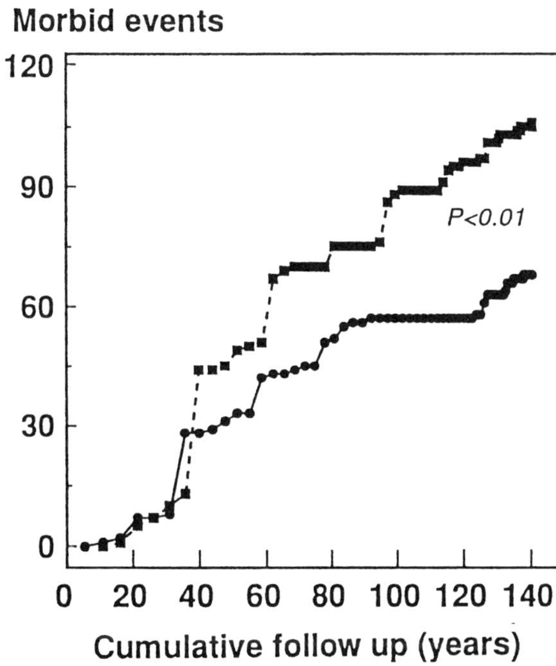

Figure 17-4. Morbid events.

been less impressive. This provides a rationale for exploring the use of bisphosphonates as an adjunct to systemic hormone therapy and chemotherapy in women with operable breast cancer who are at risk of developing metastases in the future.

ACKNOWLEDGMENTS

Capsules and placebo were supplied by Leiras Oy, and the study was supported by Leiras Oy and Boehringer Mannheim GmbH. We acknowledge the assistance of Mrs. Alwyn Tidy, Mrs. Linda Reaney, Ms. Seija Karinkanta, Mrs. Carla Danbrook, Dr. Kari Aranko, and others who collected data for this study.

REFERENCES

1. Mundy GR. Hypercalcemia of malignancy revisited. J Clin Invest 1988;82:1–6.
2. Mundy GR, Ibbotson KJ, DeSouza SM, Simpson EL, Jacobs JW, Martin TJ. The hypercalcemia of cancer. Clinical implication and pathogenic mechanisms. N Engl J Med 1984;310:1718.
3. Taube T, Elomaa I, Blomqvist C, Beneton MNC, Kanis JA. Histomorphometric evidence for osteoclast medicated bone resorption in metastatic breast cancer. Bone 1994;15(2):161–166.
4. Mundy GR. Calcium homeostasis: Hypercalcaemia and hypocalcaemia. London: Martin Dunitz, 1990.
5. Warrell RP, Israel R, Frisone M, Snyder T, Gaynor JJ, Beckman, RS. Gallium nitrate for acute treatment of cancer-related hypercalcemia. A randomized, double-blind comparison of calcitonin. Ann Intern Med 1988;108:669–674.

6. Ryzon B, Martodam RR, Troxell M, Benson A, Paterson A, Shepard K, Hicks R. Intravenous etidronate in the management of malignant hypercalcemia. Arch Intern Med 1985;145:449–452.
7. Taube T, Elomaa I, Blomqvist C, Beneton MNC, Kanis JA. Comparative effects of clodronate and calcitonin in metastatic breast cancer. Eur J Clin Oncol 1993;29:1677–1681.
8. Kanis JA. The pathophysiology and treatment of Paget's disease of bone. London: Martin Dunitz, 1991.
9. Ernst DS, MacDonald N, Paterson AHG, Jensen J, Brasher P, Bruera E. A double-blind, crossover trial of intravenous clodronate in metastatic bone pain. J Pain & Symptom Manage 1992;7:4–11.
10. Hayward JL, Meakin JW, Stewart HJ. Assessment of response and recurrence in breast cancer. Semin Oncol 1978;5:445–449.
11. Breast Cancer Task Force, Treatment Committee, National Cancer Institute. Breast cancer. Suggested protocol guidelines for combination chemotherapy trials and for combined modality trials. Washington, DC: US Department of Health, Education and Welfare, Publication No (NIH) 77-1192, 1977.
12. van Holten-Verzantvoort AT, Bijvoet OLM, Mermans J, et al. Reduced morbidity from skeletal metastases in breast cancer patients during long-term bisphosphonate (APD) treatment. Lancet 1987;2:983–985.
13. Pritchard KI. Adjuvant systemic therapy for breast cancer: A tale of relapse and survival [editorial]. Lancet 1994;343:370.
14. Paterson AHG, Powles TJ, Kanis JA, McCloskey EV, Hanson J, Ashley S. Double-blind controlled trial of oral clodronate in patients with bone metastases from breast cancer. J Clin Oncol 1993;11:59–65.

Adjuvant Therapy of Cancer VIII, edited by Sydney E. Salmon. Lippincott–Raven Publishers, Philadelphia © 1997.

18
Breast Cancer Roundtable*

Moderator: Emil Frei III
Panel members: Karen H. Antman, Bernard Fisher, William P. Peters, Sydney E. Salmon, and Pinuccia Valagussa, with audience participation

Dr. Frei: We've had a series of excellent presentations including mature data on adjuvant and neoadjuvant therapy for breast cancer as well as issues related to high-dose chemotherapy. We also heard about some new biological approaches and insights. At this point, I'd first like some comments from the panelists, and then we'll open up the discussion more broadly. I'd like to address the first question to Dr. Peters and to the others. Based on relapse-free survival curves we've seen at this conference, there is the issue of whether the risk of relapse after 3 years has diminished as much as we think as based on some of the reported studies. Bill, in your high-dose chemotherapy autotransplant study with a 9-year follow-up, if I read that correctly, there was only one relapse after 3 years. And that's been consistent with some other studies that do not have that kind of durability. In the NSABP studies presented by Dr. Fisher on patients with micrometastatic disease in the adjuvant situation, the hazard function appears to continue over a long period of time, but gradually diminishes. So there seems to be a difference. Is there really a difference, Bill? Do you think your data is predictive, and why is there a difference?

Dr. Peters: The majority, though not all of the relapses in the study I presented occurred during the first 3 years. There are few relapses that occur out later, and I think that if one looks at the data, the majority of the hazard occurs in the first 3 years and thereafter the curves begin to plateau or flatten out and achieve a similar pattern to others. I don't know why we don't see much later.

Dr. Frei: Does anything characterize the few late relapses such as CNS involvement?

Dr. Peters: I have to say that I haven't examined that question.

Dr. Salmon: I'd like to ask Dr. Peters about his strategy of using stem cells and bone marrow. It is impressive that, while you have a flat curve after 3 years, even in the patients in complete remission, there were nonetheless a number of relapses during the first 3 years. From what you said, very few deaths were due to toxicity and so most were due to recurrence. You've given both blood and bone marrow progenitors to patients who probably have micrometastatic disease in the bone marrow. And so, the real question is: we don't know whether

*Transcript edited by Sydney E. Salmon.

recurrence is due to residual disease in patients or in the returned hematopoietic progenitor cell population. There are several techniques available to deplete stem cell populations: on the one hand of tumor cells by using anti-keratin antibodies, or on the other hand by positive selection of hematopoietic progenitors using an anti-CD34 column. Do you have comments on efforts in that direction?

Dr. Peters: As you probably know, our group has done a large number of patients in the study exploring various collection techniques. To my knowledge, there is not a randomized comparative trial in breast cancer, which explores the question of whether taking these cells out is valuable or not. There are two ways of looking at it. Firstly, if you remove the tumor cells you have to be persuaded that, in fact, you can remove them sufficiently well enough that you're not still leaving some tumor cells in the autograft that could cause relapse. And secondly, that if you use the reverse strategy with a positive selection approach, that you're not removing something that might be a value to the patient. There has been some concern raised that as one selects only the hemopoietic stem cell, you're losing a lot of the lymphoid cells that may, in fact, contribute to a host response against the tumor. We must be very careful to evaluate the effect of what normal immune reconstitution represents. We need to learn how to use negative and positive selection strategies in an important way. And there may be other strategies that might be utilized in this fashion. Dr. Antman may want to comment on the use of gene therapy approaches that might enable some additional power to be gained by the manipulation of stem cells in this patient population.

Dr. Antman: At Columbia University, we have started a gene marking study wherein we transfect the autograft with a molecular marker after cell harvesting and prior to reinfusion. Currently we have about eight patients on the trial. We can get molecular marker bands in the marrow and peripheral blood of patients whose cells had been transduced and then autotransplanted. We won't know the clinical significance of this finding for several years, but it is an ongoing study that may help determine whether recurrence of breast cancer is from contaminating tumor cells present in the autograft (in which case they should be marked) or residual disease in the patient.

Dr. Salmon: I thought one of the most provocative observations that Dr. Frei made earlier today was based on Dr. Valagussa's presentation of the original CMF study from Milan. He pointed out that there was a clear flattening of the relapse curve for CMF treated patients that occurred late in the 20-year period of observation. And the question he raised was, "How can something that you did 20 years ago affect outcome that much later?" In thinking of various explanations, I would speculate that adjuvant chemotherapy might not only inactivate or kill malignant cells in breast cancer, but might also irreparably damage additional premalignant cells also present in the patient's breast that had not yet completed the stochastic process of multiple mutations required for full malignant transformation. Such mutated but still premalignant cells could be thought of as being at various steps along a transformation process such as that described by Vogelstein for colorectal cancer. In colon cancer, the complete process to malignant transformation can take decades. Premalignant cells are apparently less able to excise mutations (or else they wouldn't accumulate). DNA damage induced by CMF to premalignant cells might therefore have a greater chance of being lethal to such cells than it would in fully transformed breast cancer cells. My speculation is that late relapses in women with breast cancer might be due to eventual transformation of residual premalignant cells, and that such late recurrences might be eliminated with adjuvant chemotherapy. At least that's one possible answer to Dr. Frei's question.

Dr. Frei: Dr. Fisher, we haven't heard from you.

Dr. Fisher: I think this whole area is very speculative. I don't have a better explanation, I'll tell you that. The whole question of dormancy I think is one that still is a biological enigma. And yet, probably, there is an answer that's staring us in the face and we just don't know how to ... the penny hasn't dropped yet as to what's going on. There also may be host factors, the location of these cells vis-à-vis the milieu that they're located in, liver, for example, and suddenly there's damage to the liver with a cascade of growth factors which stimulates who knows what ... I don't.

Dr. Frei: Could we get some inference on this with failure analysis? For example, is there a difference between patients who relapse at 15 years after adjuvant therapy as compared to 5 years?

Dr. Fisher: I think that's something that we should be looking at. I think it would be a good idea to look at that. I don't know of any information.

Dr. Frei: Dr. Valagussa, do you want to comment on that or anything that's gone on so far or ask a question?

Dr. Valagussa: We failed to observe any difference in the nature of relapse over the years and some women receiving CMF developed skeletal metastasis within the first 3 years, within the first 5 years, from the 5th to the 10th year, and so on and so forth. So, I don't know exactly how one can go back and identify a difference that influences the shape of the relapse curves.

Dr. Antman: In sarcomas, we, and others, have published that when patients relapse after chemotherapy, the grade of the tumor is sometimes lower. And, therefore, if that's also happening in breast cancer, not only would you have some subset where patients didn't relapse at all (and obviously that's good) but in patients who were not cured by the adjuvant chemotherapy, the tumor that remains might be less aggressive and therefore you would have further separation curves if, in fact, this situation is the same as in sarcomas.

Dr. Frei: That's an appealing hypothesis because chemotherapy may, well, get rid of the more aggressive cells and leave you with a more indolent tumor cell population which would produce fewer late relapses.

Dr. Antman: It might account for the separation in the curves.

Dr. Fisher: I think one of the things that you've got to be aware of and very cautious about is that when you're showing these plateaus in survival curves, you don't show the number of patients which are out at these levels. I think that's something that needs to be taken into account.

Dr. Frei: We have someone in the audience who is a real pioneer in medical oncology, who's been around quite a bit of time, Dr. Ezra Greenspan. And he is going to say something.

Dr. Greenspan (audience): I think that the problem may be that we don't stage the patients ahead of time for their host immune factors. In a minority of cases, like 10 or 15%, patients might have better immune systems and live with larger tumors prior to treatment and nonetheless get rid of it, and then it doesn't come back after adjuvant treatment. It might be pure hocus-pocus postulation that they have macrophage factors and other factors that effect the morphology of the residual microscopic cells that must be in those patients. Now, Karen Antman says that when sarcomas recur, the recurrent cells are more well differentiated. Perhaps it's a macrophage differentiation factor these people have, and therefore, their tumors come out looking differently and a bit more slowly growing. When I look at ovarian cancer and find some psammoma bodies, I think I'm dealing with a much different type of a host. Not only a different tumor but a different type of host. There will be little subtle things we're not looking at in this group of long-time survivors. And I think we should.

Dr. Frei: Thank you, Ezra. Could we go to the audience, now, for questions?

Audience: I had a question for Dr. Peters concerning the metastatic disease study. How are the patients observed? Were they followed rigidly, with every 3-month CT scans or the like, or did they discover their own metastatic disease?

Dr. Peters: Patients were followed the same way on both randomized arms. They were followed with every 6 weeks physical examination, and CT scans every 12 weeks for the first 2 years. The CT scans were repeated at 6-month intervals between years 2 and 5 and then yearly thereafter, as long as they were alive.

Audience: Do you have any data as to whether which relapses were detected by the routine physical exams and scans or which ones were patient driven?

Dr. Peters: I don't have that off the top of my head in its precise form. I'll tell you that probably 60–70% were radiologically discovered first because of the intensity of the scanning. It was the minority, I'd say, that were discovered by the patients by themselves.

Audience: Results of Dr. Peters' metastatic disease study with high-dose chemotherapy are extremely fascinating. Are there any factors that could explain this unexpected outcome?

Dr. Peters: I don't think that the fact that we wait until relapse is the magic. I think it's the fact that we left some interval between induction therapy and the time when the transplant is done. The median time to failure in the study is 4 months on the observation arms, so it's relatively short. And as Tom Frei has suggested, resistance which develops after initial chemotherapy may in some cases be reversible over a period of time. Then, in fact, we might be observing transient resistance after initial remission induction chemotherapy for breast cancer. We've been trying to approach this problem for 4 years in the Cancer and Acute Leukemia Group B—and beating our head against a brick wall. I'd like to see us get a study under way where we randomly compare induction therapy plus transplant versus induction therapy alone versus transplant alone. And that, I think, would begin to give some final assessment of the quantitative importance of each of the components. I'm not sure, at this point, whether the induction therapy offers us any advantage. My gut says, "yes." My head says, "I'm not sure at all." And I think, in this day and age, with what we know and the ability to do simpler trials, we ought to be able to address such questions.

Dr. Antman: One caveat to this, however, is that when we look at the registry data on patients with metastatic disease, those who were transplanted in the first 6 months after their diagnosis of metastatic disease did significantly better than those where they were transplanted later in their course.

Dr. Peters: It doesn't address the same question and, really, those observations would be contaminated by the use of induction therapy.

Dr. Antman: That's exactly it. If you had four cycles of induction treatment in your transplant then you presumably would do better than someone who had a longer interval with more chemotherapy. But, in any case, it wasn't exactly the outcome I would expect based on the randomized trial.

Audience: How does bone involvement impact survival in the transplant patients?

Dr. Peters: Well, the registry data suggests that women with bone involvement actually do a little bit better and our data would argue the same. The trouble with the registry data is that it's not well controlled for other variables. Additionally there's a correlation between the development of the bone metastases and the presence of hormone-sensitive disease. And so, that may represent different biological subset and I think we have to be careful about drawing too many conclusions.

Dr. Antman: On the other hand, it's 4000 women. So you gain in numbers what you lose in randomization.

Dr. Peters: Well, it may be true. I mean, our data would point in the same direction that women with bone metastases do better but what does that mean in and of itself? It may just be a selection phenomenon of biologically different disease.

Audience: So that the patients that relapse have a higher percentage of bone involvement than patients that did not.

Dr. Peters: That's right. And, you know, the corollary of this is, does the contamination of the marrow or peripheral blood make a difference? If women with bone metastases do better in transplant settings (as they do with chemotherapy), what does it mean?

Dr. Antman: My impression is that such patients are the ones with the indolent disease and therefore they take longer to relapse.

Audience: In the relapse group, is anyone looking into repetitive transplants? Also, how are the taxanes being incorporated into the transplant setting with respect to dose intensity?

Dr. Antman: In our current studies, patients receive three transplants, including two as an outpatient. The first utilizes taxol, the second uses melphalan, and the third utilizes cyclophosphamide plus thiotepa and carboplatin. Thereafter, the patients are offered randomization between immunological treatments. This latter aspect compares IL-2 to interferon plus cyclosporine. These immunological treatments were piloted at the Dana-Farber Cancer Center and the Johns Hopkins Oncology Center, respectively.

Dr. Peters: There is a study that is ongoing in Colorado where taxol has been escalated down to a maximum tolerated dose of 725 mg/m^2. However, after such high doses of taxol, some patients can't walk. I have to say that I don't see much sense in it. That from a biochemical point of view it doesn't make a lot of sense to me to be utilizing taxol in that fashion. Dr. Frei may wish to comment on this. I mean, the reason the alkylating agents were chosen in this setting is because there is a linear dose response curve over an extended period of time. And from a mechanistic point of view, I don't understand why the taxane should be used in that fashion. And so, in our program, we're using taxol (though we planned to use taxatere) as part of the induction regimen because the dose-limiting toxicity really isn't myelosuppression in the range we think the taxanes will be effective.

Dr. Frei: I think that's correct, Bill. I'd like to ask about the Bezwoda study (1). That primarily involves mitoxantrone. The dose of cyclophosphamide is relatively low as compared to a usual transplant dose, and the third agent is etoposide. I'm not sure how important that is, but it does suggest that another agent like adriamycin may be very important if it's escalatable—which mitoxantrone is and adriamycin is not.

Dr. Peters: Well, there is no doubt that anthracyclines are somewhat escalatable, as they're not generally limited by myelosuppression. I mean, one can administer AFM or you can give doxorubicin at 90 mg/m^2 as was done by Dr. James Holland and his group. While there is some myelosuppression, that isn't what prevents further escalation. It's the mucositis and the other nonmyelosuppressive toxicities of the anthracyclines that limit its escalation.

Dr. Frei: But standard doses of mitoxantrone go from 10–12 mg/m^2 (which is standard dose) up to 100–120 mg/m^2, etc., which are alkylating agent-like proportional escalating doses.

Audience: I have a question for Dr. Peters. You show very outstanding data. My question is: For those patients with metastatic disease, what selection criteria were used to pick patients to be entered on the trial?

Dr. Peters: The only selection criteria that were used for the 423 patients were that they had to have metastatic disease, that they had to have biopsy-proven breast cancer, and they could not have received prior chemotherapy for metastatic disease. Moreover, they had to be hormone insensitive (that is to say biopsy-proven estrogen receptor and progesterone receptor negative or have failed prior hormonal therapy). They could not have received CMF for metastatic disease or have more than three metastatic sites on bone scan.

The primary reason that women were excluded was because they had received prior chemotherapy. The presence of metastatic disease in the CNS was probably less than 3%. Organ system dysfunction was not a significant problem for the patients who were in the study. The average age was in the mid-40s so that I took the total denominator. An important aspect of my presentation was that I only discussed the data on patients achieving complete remission. We have not finished the analysis of the patients who only achieved partial remission. What I was trying to communicate in this presentation was not how many patients had long-term survival but rather to point out that the strategy of using high-dose therapy tripled disease-free survival compared to that observed in patients not receiving high-dose chemotherapy.

Dr. Frei: If there are no further questions, I would like to thank the panel and the audience for your active participation in this roundtable.

REFERENCE

1. Bezwoda WR, Seymour L, Dansey RD. High-dose chemotherapy with hematopoietic rescue as primary treatment for metastatic breast cancer: A randomized trial. J Clin Oncol 1995;13:2483–2489.

IV

Gastrointestinal Cancer

Adjuvant Therapy of Cancer VIII, edited by Sydney E. Salmon. Lippincott–Raven Publishers, Philadelphia © 1997.

19
Adjuvant Therapy of Upper Gastrointestinal Tract Cancers

David Kelsen

ADJUVANT THERAPY OF ESOPHAGEAL CANCER

Cancer of the esophagus is a highly virulent malignancy with an exceedingly poor prognosis. Esophageal carcinoma has gradually become more common, with an estimated 12,000 new cases per year (an approximately 12% increase in the last 15 years) (1). Overall 5-year survival rates are poor (<10%).

For esophageal carcinoma, surgery alone remains one potentially curative option. Radiation therapy as a single modality has been supplanted (most clearly for patients with epidermoid carcinoma) by a combination of radiation and concurrent chemotherapy. Combined modality therapy including systemic chemotherapy in addition to a local modality (either surgery or radiation) is an attractive concept in this tumor, because it has both a high distant failure rate as well as a significant risk for local recurrence. Further, many patients present with such extensive local regional tumor that resection is impossible and outcome with radiation alone is unsatisfactory. This paper will review the rationale for the use of neoadjuvant and postoperative adjuvant therapy for esophageal carcinomas, summarizing the results of trials involving these approaches, with a focus on those performed during the last 5 years. Earlier studies have been reviewed in detail elsewhere (1).

Failure Pattern

Knowing the potential failure pattern of a solid tumor (localized or disseminated recurrence) is crucial to best plan adjuvant therapy. Tumors with a high local failure rate but a low risk of distant metastases (e.g., low grade sarcomas) may best be treated by extensive resection with or without postoperative radiation therapy (either external beam or brachytherapy). On the other hand, for tumors likely to metastasize to distant organs, systemic therapy early in the treatment plan is rational. Neoadjuvant chemotherapy (also known as preoperative or primary chemotherapy) is particularly attractive if complete resection of the primary tumor is difficult or impossible, or when radiation alone is frequently unable to sterilize the target volume. The recurrent patterns of esophageal cancer has been assessed by autopsies, and (less reliably) clinically. These data have been previously reported in detail (1). The results of several autopsy studies are summarized in Table 19-1. The median duration of survival in two of these trials was brief, and in a third trial approximately 25% of patients died in the immediate postoperative period. Thus, the finding of

TABLE 19-1 Esophageal Cancer Failure Pattern: Autopsy Data

	Anderson*	**Bosch(20)**	**Mandard****	**Sugimachi*****
Site				
Patient Number	79	82	111	303
Local Only %	9	27	—	—
Distal Only %	2	7	—	—
Local + Distant %	82	50	75	—
"Tumor Sites" (%)				
Local	91	77	61	13
Lung	52	20	31	33
Liver	47	28	23	27
Lymph Nodes	73	61	74	57
Adrenal	20	12	9	—
Trachea-Bronchus	17	33	16	—

*Autopsy performed a median of 4 months from diagnosis (21).

**Autopsy performed a median of 6.3 months from diagnosis (22).

***Includes seven patients with autopsy, 23 clinical first site of failure (23).

disseminated disease to lung, liver, and lymph nodes is even more impressive. In addition, a substantial number of patients had residual local regional disease despite attempted resection. In summary, esophageal cancer is a systemic disease even soon after diagnosis. Combined modality therapy may have an influence on the recurrence pattern. Gill et al. (2) described the failure pattern in patients having received cisplatin and fluorouracil plus radiation either alone or after prior operation. In a cohort of 49 patients, local regional failure was seen in only 20%. Thirty-nine patients had distant disease primarily in liver or lung. In another study, Kavanaugh et al. (3) reviewed sites of failure in a group of 103 patients receiving potentially curative chemotherapy plus radiation. Crude patterns of failure demonstrated lung metastasis in 28, liver metastasis in 21, bone in 13, lymph nodes in 19, and brain in 4. Local regional failure was seen in approximately one-third of these patients. While such widely metastatic disease has been seen in these Western studies, patients in high-risk areas who are found in an asymptomatic state after screening may have a lower risk for disseminated metastasis. These patients frequently have carcinoma *in situ* or T_1N_0 tumors.

The rationale for neoadjuvant therapy is thus suggested both by the fact that widespread metastasis are common soon after diagnosis as well as by the difficulty in achieving local control. This approach has been supported by a variety of animal models, data for which have been summarized in earlier reviews. The theoretical considerations for this approach have also been summarized by Muggia and McGill. The theoretical rationale for use of chemotherapy and concurrent radiation has been reviewed by Vokes (4) and by Steel and Peckham (5).

Chemotherapy might delay the regrowth of tumor cell subpopulations that are sensitive to radiation, and delay in regrowth may increase total cell kill when fractionated radiation treatment is given. Chemotherapy causes cell cycle synchronization, increasing the fraction of tumor cells in a radiation therapy-responsive phase of the cycle. By destroying cells in cycle, the recruitment of additional tumor populations from the G_0 phase (which is resistant to either radiation or chemotherapy) will occur. Chemotherapy-radiation interactions may improve as tumor masses decrease in size. Better oxygenation of the central portions of a smaller mass may improve radiation cell kill. Steel and Peckham proposed three additional mechanisms that resulted in enhanced activity of chemotherapy and radiation when delivered concomitantly (5). Spatial cooperation means that radiation can have a high degree of local regional tumor cell kill, while chemotherapy can be effective both locally and systemically. Spatial cooperation does not necessarily require that the two modalities be given simultaneously. Independence of toxicity profiles may allow full doses of each modality to be given concurrently. Finally, the goal of normal tissue protection is a theoretical one, which could be achieved either by technical improvements in radiation (3-D treatment planning) or by the development of pharmacologic agents that protect normal tissue while leaving the tumor vulnerable.

Choosing the Appropriate Patient for Adjuvant or Neoadjuvant Therapy

The staging system for esophageal tumors is based on the depth of penetration through the wall, the presence or absence of regional nodal metastasis, and the presence of distant metastasis. "High-risk" patients have tumors that are stage $T_{3\text{–}4}N_{any}M_0$. Definitive staging currently is obtained postoperatively, using pathological evaluation of the resected specimen, or intraoperative findings. Even patients with T_3N_0 have a 50% chance of dying within 5 years of resection. Nodal metastasis has an even more ominous implication. In China and Japan, where esophageal cancers are extremely common, large-scale screening programs have been employed in selected areas. Cure rates with surgery alone in early-stage patients are high (>80% 5-year survival). However, in the United States only a small proportion (5–10%) of patients will have early-stage disease. Still, until adjuvant programs of proven effectiveness for these diseases have been identified, sparing patients with a favorable outcome with surgery alone from the potential toxicities of such programs is appropriate. Thus, while 80–90% of American patients fall in the high-risk group, preoperative staging techniques available to identify patients at low risk are still in the developmental stage. CT or MRI scans of the abdomen and chest, do not have high accuracy in staging depth of tumor invasion (T stage) or in identifying regional nodal involvement (N stage). Thus, using standard staging techniques, the low-risk patient cannot be identified preoperatively. Two new techniques seem to be superior. Endoscopic ultrasonography is more accurate than conventional CT for T stage, and, less impressively, for nodal stage. In a comparison of the accuracy of dynamic CT scanning (using CT technology for the late 1980s) versus endoscopic ultrasonography (EUS), Lightdale et al. demonstrated in patients with gastric and esophageal cancer that EUS is significantly more accurate than CT in predicting T and N stage (6). Similar data in esophageal cancer have been reported by Tio (7). EUS thus is a promising tool in staging esophageal tumors. Recently there has been renewed interest in the use of laparoscopy as a staging technique for abdominal malignancies. Technical improvements in equipment and the introduction of laparoscopic ultrasonography probes have expanded the potential usefulness of this technique. A major potential advantage of laparoscopy with laparoscopic ultrasound over endoscopic ultrasonography is the ability to identify small volume peritoneal metastasis or small volume hepatic metastasis.

A recent study indicates, however, that location and cell type are important factors: laparoscopy had a low yield for upper and middle esophageal squamous cell cancers, but was much more useful for distal-third and GE junction adenocarcinoma (8). The more traditional approach to adjuvant therapy is the use of postoperative systemic treatment. There are a few esophageal cancer studies summarized below. In this case, chemotherapy has been given following surgery.

There are currently three major approaches using combined modality therapy for patients with localized esophageal cancers: preoperative chemotherapy (also called neoadjuvant therapy) followed by an operation, a combination of chemotherapy and concurrent radiation followed by surgery, or chemotherapy and radiation without an operative procedure. The results of trials using preoperative radiation (without chemotherapy) have been disappointing, and this topic will not be further discussed. A recent study has investigated postoperative chemotherapy without preoperative treatment.

Phase II nonrandomized trials using concurrent chemotherapy and radiation followed by resection have been disappointing; these data have been summarized elsewhere (1).

Very recently, two phase III trials comparing preoperative chemoradiation with surgery alone have been reported. In a preliminary communication submitted in abstract form by investigators from the University of Michigan (9), 50 patients were randomized to each arm of the study. The chemotherapy regimen was the same as that used in their phase II trial (cisplatin/fluorouracil/vinblastine): 4500 cGy were given using 150 cGy b.i.d. in 15 fractions. The two groups appeared to be well balanced for the usual prognostic factors. A strength of this study was that the same surgical (transhiatal esophagectomy) was used in all patients. No difference in operability, resectability, or survival was noted. This is the first large-scale trial using aggressive concurrent chemotherapy and radiation followed by operation versus operation alone. Pending the long-term results of this trial, the use of chemotherapy plus concurrent radiation prior to operation should be considered an experimental approach.

In a second random assignment trial, using sequential chemotherapy followed by radiation, Le Prise et al. compared surgery alone to preoperative chemotherapy plus radiation using cisplatin and fluorouracil (10). All patients had squamous cell cancers. The dose schedule used involved a single course of cisplatin and fluorouracil given during the first week of therapy. Radiation was given on days 8–19; a total of 20 Gy given in 10 treatment fractions over 12 elapsed days was used. A second course of cisplatin and fluorouracil was begun on days 21–25 with surgery planned for day 42. In this trial, 41 patients were randomized to receive chemoradiation prior to operation and 45 to surgery alone. There was no significant difference in median survival (1-year survival 46.6% chemo-RT, 46.7% surgery alone). Similarly, at 3 years, 19.2% of the chemo-RT and 13.8% of the surgery only patients were alive. Disease-free survival was a median of 7.6 months for chemo-RT and 5 months for surgery only. It should be noted that the doses of chemotherapy given were lower than in other series and the total dose of radiation was modest. Lastly, therapy was not concurrent.

Phase II studies involving the use of chemotherapy alone prior to surgery (neoadjuvant chemotherapy) have also been reviewed in detail (1). There are no data currently available to indicate that, for all patients, one cisplatin-containing combination is markedly superior to another.

Several small-scale phase III trials have been reported. Roth et al. treated 39 patients in a small phase III trial in which patients were randomly assigned to surgery only or to cisplatin/vindesine/bleomycin chemotherapy followed by exploration (11). There were no differences in resection rates, in operative morbidity (which was less for the chemotherapy arm), or in operative mortality. The response rate to cisplatin/vindesine/bleomycin was 47%. While there were no differences in overall survival between the two arms, a subgroup analysis indicated that patients responding to preoperative chemotherapy had a substantial improvement in median survival compared to those undergoing surgery only (>20 months versus 8.6 months, $p = 0.05$). As is the case for the other phase III studies reported so far, because of the small number of patients in the study, definitive conclusions could not be made.

Using a different approach, Kelsen et al. compared two preoperative techniques for patients with epidermoid carcinoma of the esophagus: preoperative radiation (RT) versus preoperative chemotherapy (CT) (12). A high dose of radiation (5500 cGy delivered in 5.5–6 weeks by multiple field techniques) was compared to a cisplatin/vindesine/bleomycin chemotherapy regimen. Ninety-six patients were included in this trial. Both modalities induced major objective responses prior to surgery (CT 55%, RT 64%), and both had equal operability and resectability rates. Treatment-related mortality was slightly less for the chemotherapy arm. Since the study allowed a postoperative crossover, and since most patients received both chemotherapy and radiation with only the sequence around surgery varying, it was not possible to determine long-term survival by arm of initial assignment. The overall long-term survival rate was approximately 20%. The authors concluded that since chemotherapy was equally efficacious at causing regression of local regional disease but also offered the opportunity to treat systemic metastasis, it was a logical path to pursue in combined modality regimens as opposed to preoperative radiation.

Nygaard et al. (13) performed a random assignment trial comparing surgery to preoperative chemotherapy using cisplatin/bleomycin, preoperative radiation, or the combination of radiation and chemotherapy prior to operation. The study had 40–50 patients per arm. There was no significant difference in outcome. Of note, the chemotherapy employed in this study, however, has among the lowest reported response rates for advanced esophageal cancer. There was no significant difference in survival for patients receiving preoperative cisplatin/bleomycin compared to those receiving surgery alone.

Schlag et al. (14) randomly assigned patients to undergo operation immediately or to undergo surgery after receiving three cycles of preoperative chemotherapy with fluorouracil and cisplatin. In this study, which involved a group of 40 patients receiving surgery and 29 receiving preoperative chemotherapy, there was no significant difference in operability or resectability rates. There was an increased operative mortality (21% for chemotherapy followed by surgery versus 12% for those undergoing surgery alone). No difference in median survival was seen. Long-term survival outcome was not stated.

All of these studies have involved relatively small groups of patients severely limiting the power of their observations. In order to more definitively address this issue, a large-scale national intergroup trial has been recently completed in the United States. The design of this trial and its current status are described below. In addition, a similar trial is currently under way in Great Britain under the auspices of the Medical Research Council.

Postoperative Systemic Adjuvant Therapy

Until recently, there have been few data addressing the issue of postoperative systemic chemotherapy in the resected patient. Pouliquen et al. (15) recently reported the results of a phase III random assignment trial in patients undergoing palliative surgical resection of squamous cell carcinomas of the esophagus. Two groups were stratified. The first were those who underwent resection of all gross disease but were found to have positive margins, and the second had either positive margins or distant metastasis. Both groups were randomized to receive or not receive cisplatin and fluorouracil chemotherapy for a maximum of eight cycles. Thirty-eight patients who had metastatic lymph nodes only (no distant metastases, negative margins) were observed and 24 received chemotherapy. In a second group of patients who had incomplete resection, 30 were observed and 28 treated. There were no significant differences in median or long-term survival, whether patients received or did not receive additional chemotherapy. Although not discussed in detail, some patients also received radiation. Four chemotherapy patients (8%) had treatment-related deaths. Thus, this small study does not support the routine use of postoperative adjuvant cisplatin/fluorouracil in lymph node positive patients.

Chemotherapy Plus Radiation Therapy without Surgery

Chemotherapy and radiotherapy have been combined in two ways. The first involves giving chemotherapy (usually for one or two cycles) prior to definitive radiotherapy (usually 50–60 Gy). The second gives concurrent chemotherapy and radiation therapy. While most trials reported to date are single-arm, phase II pilot studies, involving less than 50 patients, there are several recent prospective randomized studies, which are summarized below.

Chemotherapy Plus Concurrent Radiation

Phase II pilot studies have been previously reviewed.

More recently, several prospective random assignment controlled trials have been completed. These have tested the hypothesis that systemic chemotherapy plus concurrent radiation is superior to radiation therapy alone. The ECOG completed a trial of systemic therapy using mitomycin and 5-fluorouracil plus concurrent radiation versus radiation alone (16). In this study, patients could undergo surgery following completion of chemotherapy and 40 Gy of radiation or after 40 Gy of radiation alone at the discretion of the attending physician. The introduction of surgery in a nonrandomized fashion makes interpretation of the data more difficult. In a preliminary report, a survival advantage has been noted for the chemotherapy-RT arm.

In 1992, Herskovic et al. reported the results of an important study comparing chemotherapy plus concurrent radiation with radiation alone; surgery was not part of the treatment plan (17). The design of the trial involved giving radiation alone to one group of patients; the treatment plan was 5000 cGy with a boost of 1400 cGy to a total dose of 6400 cGy delivered over 6.4 weeks. Patients randomized to receive chemotherapy plus radiation were given a lower total dose of 5000 cGy over 5 weeks. The chemotherapy regimen was fluorouracil by continuous infusion at 1 g/m^2 per day for 4 consequent days plus cisplatin 75 mg/m^2 on day 1 of each 5-FU course. At the initial report with the median follow-up of 18 months, a highly significant survival advantage for chemo-radiation versus radiation alone was demonstrated. A recent update of this study published in abstract form showed that 31% of patients receiving chemo-radiation were alive at 3 years compared to no patients randomized to receive radiation alone (18). Toxicity of chemo-radiotherapy was, however, substantial, with 64% of patients experiencing grade 3 or 4 toxicity.

Two recent phase II studies involving the use of induction chemotherapy followed by chemo-radiation (using the same dose and schedule of chemo-radiation as that employed in the initial RTOG study) have recently been reported. An unexpected increase in toxicity including a treatment-related mortality of approximately 10% has been seen in these trials. In the second study, reported only in abstract form, chemo-radiation plus brachytherapy also had an unacceptable risk of toxicity (19).

Chemotherapy Followed by Radiation Therapy

In general, cisplatin-based multi-drug chemotherapy has been employed in treatment regimens involving sequential chemotherapy and radiation. Response to chemotherapy using this approach ranges from 20 to 60% with no evidence of additive toxicity. However, most studies have not involved postradiation chemotherapy; many have not analyzed failure patterns, so the percentage of patients relapsing first in the local field is difficult to interpret. An attempt to use induction chemotherapy followed by chemo-radiation encountered unacceptable toxicity as described above.

Intergroup Trials

The large number of phase II trials performed to date have demonstrated that preoperative chemotherapy for esophageal carcinoma can be performed safely. Tumor regression is seen in 50–60% of patients, with no increase in operative morbidity or mortality. Most regimens are based on cisplatin, with no compelling evidence that one cisplatin-containing regimen is markedly superior to another. Only one Japanese study has addressed the issue of purely postoperative adjuvant chemotherapy; no change in outcome was seen. A large-scale intergroup trial, 113, has closed recently to accrual. It addresses the issue of whether or not preoperative and postoperative adjuvant chemotherapy improves outcome for patients with operable esophageal cancers. The study design involved three cycles of cisplatin and fluorouracil given at 1-month intervals. Following surgery, resected patients received two additional cycles of chemotherapy. Patients randomly assigned to standard therapy undergo surgery alone. The study is now being analyzed. A similar study is under way in England.

As noted above, there is strong evidence that concurrent chemotherapy plus radiation is superior to radiation alone. A second intergroup trial will soon start comparing the superior arm of RTOG 85-01 (in which a total of 5040 cGy was given with four cycles of cisplatin and fluorouracil) to the same chemotherapy plus a higher dose of radiation (6400 cGy). The aim of the study is to determine if the higher dose of radiation will translate into an improvement in local control.

CONCLUSIONS

Important progress has been made in the treatment of esophageal cancer, with recent data indicating that combined modality therapy involving chemotherapy and concurrent radiation is superior to radiation alone. The intergroup trials of chemotherapy plus surgery versus surgery alone will address the population of patients who have potentially resectable disease. Should this study also demonstrate that combined modality treatment is superior to surgery only, a future intergroup trial should address the question of best local treatment allowing for the first time a major comparison of surgery versus radiation as local therapy. In addition to the demonstration that concurrent chemotherapy plus radiation is superior to radiation alone, at least for patients with squamous cell cancers of the esophagus, the identification of paclitaxel as an active drug in the treatment of this disease has increased the therapeutic armamentarium of medical oncologists. Paclitaxel as a single agent has been demonstrated to cause objective regressions in approximately one-third of patients both with adenocarcinoma and epidermoid cancer in a joint study performed by Memorial Sloan-Kettering Cancer Center and the M. D. Anderson Cancer Center. In follow-up trials, paclitaxel has been added to cisplatin and fluorouracil, a combination that appears to have a higher response rate than paclitaxel alone but with substantial toxicity. Newer studies involving paclitaxel and cisplatin without fluorouracil and paclitaxel plus radiation therapy (with or without the use of cisplatin) are now under way at several institutions. The aim of these trials is to assess whether the addition of this new agent will improve both local control and decrease distant failure rates. A number of other agents which have substantial activity in GI malignancies will shortly begin their trials in esophageal cancer, including irinotecan. Thus, a fairly large number of avenues of clinical research have opened using new agents plus radiation therapy or given in the preoperative setting.

In addition, there is intense interest in the development of genetic data which will predict outcome. These studies, involving cytogenetic abnormalities, oncogene amplification, or expression, are all a high priority. Preliminary data regarding cytogenetic abnormalities in gastric cancer and gene amplification are being amassed. Comparison of biological data between Japanese and American patients will be of great interest in addressing the issue of better outcome in Japanese patients being related to a different biology of the disease.

ACKNOWLEDGMENT

The authors gratefully acknowledge the expert assistance of Ann Martin in the preparation of the manuscript.

REFERENCES

1. Kelsen DP. Adjuvant therapy of upper gastrointestinal tract cancers. Semin Oncol 1995;22:582–599.
2. Gill PG, Denham JW, Jamieson GG, Devitt PG, Yeoh E, Olweny C. Patterns of treament failure and prognostic factors associated with the treatment of esophageal carcinoma with chemotherapy and radiotherapy either as sole treatment or followed by surgery [corrected; erratum to be published; see comments]. J Clin Oncol 1992;10:1037–1043.
3. Kavanagh B, Anscher M, Leopold K, et al. Patterns of failure following combined modality therapy for esophageal cancer, 1984–1990. Int J Radiat Oncol Biol Phys 1992;24:633–642.
4. Vokes EE. Interactions of chemotherapy and radiation. Semin Oncol 1993;20:70–79.
5. Steel GG, Peckham MJ. Exploitable mechanisms in combined radiotherapy-chemotherapy: The concept of additivity. Int J Radiat Oncol Biol Phys 1979;5:85–91.
6. Lightdale C, Botet J, Brennan M, et al. Endoscopic ultrasonography compared to computerized tomography for preoperative staging of gastric cancer. Gastrointest Endosc 1989;35:154.
7. Tio TL, Coene PP, Luiken GJ, Tytgat GN. Endosonography in the clinical staging of esophagogastric carcinoma. Gastrointest Endosc 1990;36:s2–s10.
8. Bemelman WA, vanLanschot JJB, VanDelden OM, deWit LTH, Smits NJ, Fockens P, et al. Guidelines for laparoscopy and laparoscopic sonography in preoperative staging of esophageal cancer. Presented at the Sixth World Congress of the International Society for Diseases of the Esophagus, Milan, Italy, ISDE, August 23–26, 1995.
9. Urba S, Orringer M, Turrisi A, Whyte R, Natale R, Iannettoni M, et al. A randomized trial comparing transhiatal esophagectomy (THE) to preoperative concurrent chemoradiation followed by esophagectomy in locoregional esophageal carcinoma. Proc Am Soc Clin Oncol 1995;14:199. [Abstr.]
10. Leprise E, Etienne PL, Meunier B, et al. A randomized study of chemotherapy, radiation therapy, and surgery versus surgery for localized squamous cell carcinoma of the esophagus. Cancer 1994;73:1779–1784.
11. Roth JA, Pass HI, Flanagan MM, Graeber GM, Rosenberg JC, Steinberg S. Randomized clinical trial of preoperative and postoperative adjuvant chemotherapy with cisplatin, vindesine, and bleomycin for carcinoma of the esophagus. J Thorac Cardiovasc Surg 1988;96:242–248.
12. Kelsen DP, Minsky B, Smith M, et al. Preoperative therapy for esophageal cancer: A randomized comparison of chemotherapy versus radiation therapy. J Clin Oncol 1990;8:1352–1361.
13. Nygaard K, Hagen S, Hansen HS, et al. Pre-operative radiotherapy prolongs survival in operable esophageal carcinoma: A randomized, multicenter study of pre-operative radiotherapy and chemotherapy. The second Scandinavian trial in esophageal cancer. World J Surg 1992;16:1104–1110.
14. Schlag P. Preoperative chemotherapy in localized squamous cell carcinoma of the esophagus: Results of a prospective randomized trial. Eur J Cancer 1991;27:426. [Abstr.]
15. Pouliquen X, Levard H, Hay JM, McGee K, Fingerhut A, Langlois-Zantin O, et al. 5-Fluorouracil and cisplatin therapy after palliative surgical resection of squamous cell carcinoma of the esophagus. A multicenter randomized trial. Ann Surg 1996;223:127–133.

16. Sischy B, Ryan L, Haller D, Smith T, Dayal Y, Schutt A, et al. Interim report of EST 1282 phase III protocol for the evaluation of combined modalities in the treatment of patients with carcinoma of the esophagus, stage I and II. Proc Am Soc Clin Oncol 1990;9:105. [Abstr.]
17. Herskovic A, Martz K, Al-Sarraf M, et al. Combined chemotherapy and radiotherapy compared with radiotherapy alone in patients with cancer of the esophagus [see comments]. N Engl J Med 1992;326:1593–1598.
18. Al-Sarraf M, Pajak T, Herskovic A, et al. Progress report of combined chemo-radiotherapy (CT-RT) vs. radiotherapy (RT) alone in patients with esophageal cancer. An intergroup study. Proc Am Soc Clin Oncol 1993;12:197. [Abstr.]
19. Minsky BD, Neuberg D, Kelsen DP, Pisansky TM, Ginsberg R, Benson A. Neoadjuvant chemotherapy plus concurrent chemotherapy and high-dose radiation for squamous cell carcinoma of the esophagus: A preliminary analysis of the phase II intergroup trial 0122. J Clin Oncol 1996;14:149–155.
20. Bosch A, Frias Z, Caldwell WL, Jaeschke WH. Autopsy findings in carcinoma of the esophagus. Acta Radiol Oncol 1979;18:103–335.
21. Anderson LL, Lad TE. Autopsy findings in squamous-cell carcinoma of the esophagus. Cancer 1982;50:1587–1590.
22. Mandard AM, Chasle J, Marnay J, et al. Autopsy findings in 111 cases of esophageal cancer. Cancer 1981;48:329–335.
23. Sugimachi K, Inokuchi K, Kuwano H, Kai H, Okamura T, Okudaira Y. Patterns of recurrence after curative resection for carcinoma of the thoracic part of the esophagus. Surg Gynecol Obstet 1983;157:537–540.

Adjuvant Therapy of Cancer VIII, edited by Sydney E. Salmon. Lippincott–Raven Publishers, Philadelphia © 1997.

20

Adjuvant Therapy for Carcinoma of the Colon and Rectum: Review of the NSABP Clinical Trials

Norman Wolmark, and Bernard Fisher

At the time of the 7th International Conference on the Adjuvant Therapy of Cancer held in March of 1993, it was noted that the standard of care for adjuvant therapy of colorectal cancer had been strongly influenced by the recommendations of a consensus panel sponsored by the National Cancer Institute and convened in April of 1990 (1,2). Unfortunately, in the last 3 years there has been little inclination to significantly modify this influence despite an accumulating library of data from well-conducted randomized prospective clinical trials that are in conflict with the recommendations of this consensus statement. While the aim of the consensus development mechanism was to provide an overview of the standard of care at a particular point in time, there are major negative ramifications if the resulting authoritative document remains unmodified for an interval of time that is now approaching 7 years. In the current atmosphere of managed health care, any authoritative (or authoritarian) promulgation that purports to define "acceptable" therapy will have far-reaching consequences; the exploration of other therapeutic interventions will invariably be discouraged creating a situation favoring the entrenchment of lowest common denominator therapy. Accordingly, it is essential to review the conclusions of the 1990 consensus panel in light of the subsequently reported data from randomized prospective clinical trials. Some of the principal conclusions of the 1990 consensus panel on colorectal cancer may be summarized as follows

1. Adjuvant therapy for stage II (Dukes' B) patients cannot be recommended outside of clinical trials.
2. Patients with carcinoma of the colon and histologically positive nodes (stage III, Dukes' C) should be offered adjuvant 5-FU and levamisole.
3. Combined chemotherapy and radiation improves local control and survival in rectal cancer; this treatment is recommended.

It is evident that the results from the NSABP clinical trial experience have made some aspects of these statements anachronistic.

NSABP CLINICAL TRIALS ASSESSING ADJUVANT THERAPY FOR CARCINOMA OF THE COLON

NSABP Protocol C-02

The first NSABP protocols assessing adjuvant therapy in colorectal cancer were initiated in 1977, well after the NSABP had become an established group investigating the operative and adjuvant treatment of stage I and II breast cancer. Although the common theme that was explored by the series of studies in colorectal cancer involved the assessment of postoperative interventions, one trial, protocol C-02, is unique in that it evaluated regional continuous 5-FU infused into the portal vein immediately following the curative operation for patients with Dukes' A, B, and C lesions of the colon. The basis for studying chemotherapy delivered via the portal vein was grounded in the belief that the intraoperative manipulation of a colonic tumor by the surgeon would result in showers of emboli into the portal vein circulation that subsequently would lead to the development of clinically detectable metastases. This notion was particularly popular in the mid-1950s when a number of animal experiments were performed providing a rationale for subsequent studies carried out in humans with carcinoma of the colon. Since Taylor's initial study using portal vein 5-FU and heparin (3), numerous efforts to confirm the positive findings from this study have produced equivocal conclusions. Consequently, in March of 1984, protocol C-02 was initiated in which 896 eligible patients were available for analysis by the time of protocol conclusion in July of 1988. Patients with Dukes' A, B, and C carcinoma of the colon were randomized to receive either (a) no further treatment following curative resection or (b) 5-FU and heparin administered via the portal vein; therapy was started on the day of operation and consisted of a constant infusion for 7 successive days and the daily dose of 5-FU was 600 mg/m^2 together with 5000 units of sodium heparin. The results of this study were initially reported in 1990 after an average time on study of approximately 40 months (4) and subsequently updated at 65 months (2). At that time, there was a significant disease-free survival and survival advantage in favor of the group receiving portal vein 5-FU. The analysis presented herein utilizes data as of June 30, 1995, with a mean time on study of 9 years. Disease-free survival and survival curves are presented in Figure 20-1 and there continues to be a statistically significant prolongation in both disease-free survival and survival in favor of the group receiving portal vein 5-FU hepatic perfusion. At 5 years, for example, the proportion of patients who are disease free is 60% for the control arm and 69% for the cohort receiving portal vein 5-FU ($p = 0.005$, cumulative odds 1.34). There is a concomitant prolongation in overall survival favoring the portal vein 5-FU group: 78% versus 71% ($p = 0.02$, cumulative odds 1.33). The global *P* values presented in the figure relate to the entire period of observation and are one-sided; the data are adjusted for the number of positive nodes.

The benefit achieved in both disease-free survival and survival when a rather small dose of 5-FU is continuously infused into the portal vein cannot be lightly dismissed. Despite the fact that the mechanism of action remains unclear, the findings raise an obvious challenge to the conclusion that 5-FU and levamisole should

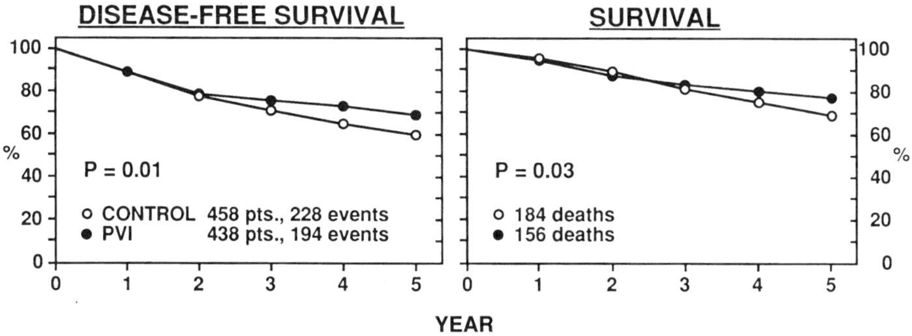

Figure 20-1. Disease free survival and survival in NSABP protocol C-02.

constitute the standard of care for patients with colon cancer and histologically positive nodes. The clinical trials commonly accepted as indicating a benefit for 5-FU and levamisole did not contain a control arm utilizing 5-FU alone and hence the conclusions are predicated on the assumption that 5-FU when administered as a single agent is without efficacy (5–7). Clearly, the results of NSABP protocol C-02 refute this assumption. Whether the benefit attributable to portal vein 5-FU hepatic perfusion is a result of the continuous administration, the result of giving the 5-FU in the perioperative setting or is a consequence of giving 5-FU via the portal vein remains enigmatic. Fortunately, there is an inter-group study in which the same doses of 5-FU and heparin that are used in protocol C-02 are given systemically via a peripheral vein in one of two treatment arms employing "conventional" postoperative 5-FU and levamisole (Int 0136).

NSABP Protocol C-03

NSABP protocol C-03 was initiated in August of 1987 and represents the first reported study to demonstrate a benefit for leucovorin-modulated 5-FU in Dukes' B and C (stage II and III) carcinoma of the colon. In this study, leucovorin-modulated 5-FU was compared to a combination of MeCCNU, vincristine and 5-FU. The reason for having chosen this latter regimen as a control arm was based on the results from a previous NSABP trial initiated in 1977. In that study, protocol C-01, the combination of MeCCNU, vincristine and 5-FU (MOF) was compared to an untreated control. Although at 10 years of follow-up, there is no statistically significant advantage for the MOF arm, at 5 and 6 years, just prior to the initiation of protocol C-03, there was a statistically significant advantage in disease-free survival and survival favoring chemotherapy, thus explaining why MOF was selected as the control arm for leucovorin-modulated 5-FU. NSABP protocol C-03 was of a two-arm study in which the MOF regimen from protocol C-01 was compared with a leucovorin-modulated 5-FU regimen consisting of the weekly administration of 500 mg/m^2 of 5-FU and 500 mg/m^2 of leucovorin for 6 consecutive weeks followed by a 2 week rest; this regimen was repeated for a total of six cycles. Between August of 1987 and April of 1989, 1081 patients with Dukes' B and C carcinoma of the colon were randomized. The results from this study were first published in 1993 and at that time, with a mean time on study of 47.6 months, there was a significant prolongation in disease-free survival and survival in favor of leucovorin-modulated 5-FU (8). The updated analysis presented in this report is with a mean time approaching 7 years. There continues to be a highly significant prolongation in disease-free survival and survival in favor of leucovorin-modulated 5-FU with a two-tailed global *P* value of <0.001 (Figure 20-2). At 5 years, for example, disease-free survival is 66% for leucovorin-modulated 5-FU compared with 54% for the MOF chemotherapy regimen ($P < 0.001$, cumulative odds 1.50); for survival there is a 75% versus 65% benefit in favor of leucovorin-modulated 5-FU ($P < 0.001$, cumulative odds 1.50). There have been 146 deaths for the leucovorin-modulated 5-FU treated patients compared to 202 deaths in the group treated with MOF. Further analyses indicated that there was no interaction between the benefit of treatment and whether the patients had Dukes' B or C tumors; both subsets responded in the same direction. It may be conjectured that the benefit attributable to leucovorin-modulated 5-FU in protocol C-03 is an underestimate of what may have been achieved had leucovorin-modulated 5-FU been compared to an untreated control since, as has already been noted, the combination of MeCCNU, 5-FU and vincristine did have some activity in the adjuvant setting at 5 years of follow-up.

The findings from this study could not be used to establish a new standard of therapy since the 5-FU and leucovorin regimen was not directly compared to the 5-FU and levamisole established as the preferred treatment by the Consensus Development Panel. Protocol C-03 did, however, demonstrate an unequivocal benefit for 5-FU and leucovorin and provided support for a pharmacologic interaction between 5-FU and leucovorin. The stage was therefore set for the initiation of protocol C-04 in which 5-FU and leucovorin was compared to 5-FU and levamisole as used in the North Central Intergroup Studies (6,7).

NSABP Protocol C-04

This protocol represented a continuation of the concepts evolved in protocols C-01 and C-03. This protocol was initiated with the intent to directly compare 5-FU and leucovorin as used in protocol C-03 to 5-FU and levamisole. Accrual was commenced in July of 1989 and completed in December 1990 after 2151 patients had been randomized to one of three treatment arms (Table 20-1): (a) 5-FU and leucovorin (LV) as used in protocol C-03, (b) 5-FU and leucovorin plus the addition of levamisole (LEV), or (c) 5-FU and levamisole as used in the North Central Study. The average time on study for this preliminary report of the results is 63.4 months with 49% of the patients having contributed survival information through 5 years. Grade III or higher toxicity was reported in 36% of FU-LV patients, in 38% of FU-LV-LEV patients and in 28% of patients receiving 5-FU with levamisole. The global *P* value for disease-free survival and survival among the three

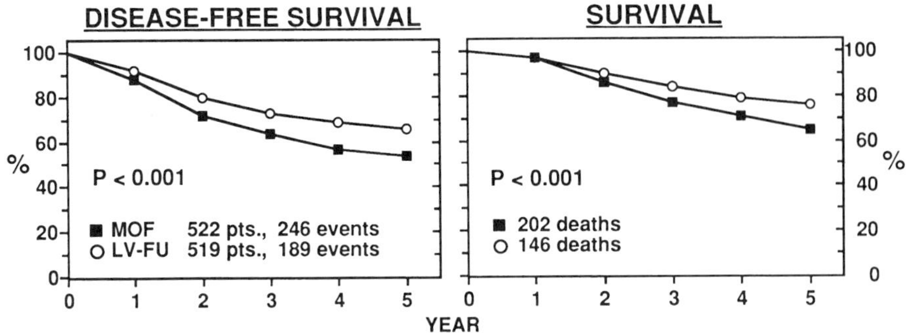

Figure 20-2. Disease free survival and survival in NSABP protocol C-03.

arms was 0.12 and 0.14, respectively. The pairwise comparison between the leucovorin-modulated 5-FU to the identical regimen to which levamisole had been added indicated that there is absolutely no advantage to adding levamisole to leucovorin-modulated 5-FU. When, however, leucovorin-modulated 5-FU was directly compared to 5-FU and levamisole, there was a small but significant advantage in disease-free survival in favor of leucovorin-modulated 5-FU. At 5 years, the percent disease free was 64% for leucovorin-modulated 5-FU compared to 60% for 5-FU and levamisole ($p = 0.05$). There was a concomitant prolongation in overall survival in favor of the leucovorin-modulated 5-FU treated group with an overall p value of 0.04. At 5 years, 74% of the leucovorin-modulated 5-FU treated group was alive compared to 69% for the 5-FU and levamisole treated cohort. There were 170 deaths in the leucovorin-modulated 5-FU group compared with 199 deaths in patients treated with 5-FU and levamisole. The results from this study indicate that leucovorin-modulated 5-FU as used in NSABP protocols C-03 and C-04 is at least as good as 5-FU and levamisole.

The next in the series of studies addressing the pharmacologic modulation of 5-FU was NSABP protocol C-05 which assessed the addition of α-interferon α-2a to 5-FU and leucovorin. This study was activated in October of 1991 and closed in February of 1994 after 2176 patients had been randomized. The average time on

TABLE 20-1 NSABP Protocol C-04

Arm	Treatment
FU-LV	FU: 500 mg/m² + LV: 500 mg/M² weekly × 6 for 6 cycles
FU-LV-LEV	FU: 500 mg/m² + LV: 500 mg/M² weekly × 6 for 6 cycles LEV:50 mg PO TID × 3 days, repeat every 14 days for 1 year
FU-LEV	FU: 450 mg/m² daily × 5 and weekly after 29 for 1 year LEV:50 mg PO TID × 3 days, repeat every 14 days for 1 year

study is 24 months, and no end results are as yet available. The currently proposed NSABP colon study, protocol C-06, continues to evolve the theme of pharmacologic modulation with a comparison between leucovorin-modulated 5-FU (using a regimen similar to that employed in protocol C-04) and UFT and leucovorin administered orally.

NSABP CLINICAL TRIALS ASSESSING ADJUVANT THERAPY FOR CARCINOMA OF THE RECTUM

The NSABP effort in rectal cancer has also generated studies that address and challenge the basic standard of care. Clearly, rectal cancer does not readily lend itself to testing the Halstedian or the "alternate" hypothesis as the NSABP has done for carcinoma of the breast. Accordingly, the Halstedian versus "alternate" hypothesis had to be addressed in a less dramatic manner, such as determining the effect of regional radiotherapy in rectal cancer, where regional radiotherapy may be regarded as the surrogate of an extended node dissection.

NSABP Protocols R-01 and R-02

NSABP protocol R-01 was initiated as a companion to the colon study, protocol C-01. Between 1977 and 1986, 574 patients with Dukes' B and C carcinoma of the rectum were randomized to one of three treatment arms: (a) no further therapy following curative operation, either abdomino-perineal resection or anterior resection, (b) MOF chemotherapy, or (c) postoperative radiotherapy. An opportunity thus became available to determine the effect of radiotherapy alone without chemotherapy. A pairwise comparison between the group treated with MOF and the control group receiving no further therapy after the operation, indicates that at 10 years there is a 31% versus 27% disease-free survival advantage in favor of MOF ($P = 0.01$), as well as a concomitant 39% versus 31% survival advantage ($P = 0.05$). The pairwise comparison between the group receiving postoperative radiation and the control group (receiving no adjuvant therapy) discloses that at 10 years, there is no significant difference between the two groups either for disease-free survival or survival ($P = 0.5$ and 0.9, respectively). There are 133 deaths for the operation alone arm compared with 138 deaths for the group receiving postoperative radiotherapy. Thus, the results from this study indicate that chemotherapy given alone without radiotherapy can prolong disease-free survival and survival, whereas radiotherapy given alone without chemotherapy has no effect on disease-free survival and survival. The studies that are commonly cited to support the use of the combination of radiotherapy and chemotherapy as a standard adjunct following resection of carcinoma of the rectum invariably compare the combination of chemoradiotherapy to radiotherapy alone without using the critical additional comparison arm of chemotherapy alone.

The next study undertaken for carcinoma of the rectum by the NSABP was designed to determine whether adding radiotherapy to a chemotherapy baseline provided an additional salutary effect. NSABP protocol R-02 was started in 1987 and completed in 1992 after 741 patients were randomized. All patients received chemotherapy; male patients were randomized to either MOF or leucovorin-modulated 5-FU and female patients received leucovorin-modulated 5-FU only. All patients were randomized to receive, in addition to the chemotherapy, either radiotherapy or no radiotherapy. The results of this study have only been reported in abstract form in 1994 with a mean time on study of 43 months (9). A pairwise comparison between the group receiving chemotherapy and radiation to the group receiving chemotherapy alone indicated no significant difference in disease-free survival. At 5 years the cumulative odds are 1.12 ($P = 0.2$). Similarly, there is no difference in overall survival with the cumulative odds being 1.07 ($P = 0.3$) at 5 years. There was a significant diminution in the cumulative incidence of loco-regional pelvic recurrent disease from 14.4% in the chemotherapy group to 8.9% in patients receiving the combination of chemotherapy and radiotherapy ($P = 0.03$). Despite this reduction in loco-regional recurrence, there was no influence on disease-free survival and survival.

Cumulatively, the data from protocols R-01 and R-02 demonstrate that although radiotherapy can decrease the incidence of loco-regional recurrence, it has no demonstrable effect on overall survival whether used by itself or when added to chemotherapy. In this regard there seem to be striking parallels between the behavior of carcinoma of the breast and rectal cancer. The findings have far-reaching biological implications and challenge the popular belief that nuances in the extent of operative resection for carcinoma of the rectum result in improved survival. In light of these results it would be difficult to substantiate a rationale for operations such as meso-rectal resection (10,11).

NSABP Protocol R-03

NSABP protocol R-03 represents one of the most challenging and provocative studies that this group has carried out. It is a companion trial to NSABP protocol B-18 that was designed to ascertain the role of preoperative chemotherapy in carcinoma of the breast. In carcinoma of the rectum, with the demonstration that adjuvant postoperative chemotherapy prolongs disease-free survival and survival and that radiotherapy decreases loco-regional recurrences without providing an additional salutary effect in overall survival, it became appropriate to address the concept as to whether the use of chemotherapy and radiotherapy in the preoperative setting could significantly reduce the size of the primary lesion and result in a less mutilating operative procedure (such as sphincter-sparing procedures or local excision). Also, this protocol was designed to determine whether preoperative chemo-radiotherapy has any overall disease-free survival and survival advantage compared to the same modalities given in the traditional postoperative setting. Accordingly, NSABP protocol R-03 was initiated in June of 1993 and to date 113 patients have been randomized to one of two treatment options: (a) three cycles of preoperative 5-FU and leucovorin together with radiotherapy followed by the operation and four cycles of additional postoperative chemotherapy and (b) seven cycles of 5-FU, leucovorin, and radiotherapy given in the traditional postoperative setting. Cycles 2 and 3 of chemotherapy are administered during the course of radiotherapy. Preliminary analysis indicates that there is a significant reduction in tumor size with preoperative chemoradiotherapy from 16.0 ± 14.2 cm^2 to 5.0 ± 7.0 cm^2. Surgical complication rates were no greater in the preoperative therapy group.

CONCLUSIONS

The NSABP effort in colorectal cancer has given rise to conclusions that are incongruent with those promulgated by the April 1990 consensus development panel. In the NSABP colorectal experience with adjuvant therapy, both classic Dukes' B (full thickness tumor penetration) and Dukes' C patients have benefitted from chemotherapy in that the differences have all been in the same direction and of similar magnitude (12). Consequently, the NSABP has not performed separate studies for the B and C subsets and has maintained that Dukes' B patients are candidates for adjuvant chemotherapy. Moreover, from the results of these studies, the survival of patients with lesions with full thickness penetration is not of the magnitude that would exclude this group from protocol randomization. The results from NSABP Protocol C-03 challenge the dictum that 5-FU and levamisole should represent the standard of therapy for Dukes' C colon patients. Preliminary results indicate that leucovorin-modulated 5-FU is at least equal to the 5-FU levamisole regimen and justify the NSABP effort to address 5-FU modulation in subsequent studies using 5-FU and leucovorin as the control group. We have come to regard 5-FU and levamisole as a regimen that will not lend itself to further optimization and, therefore, is not amenable to be exploited for additional gain. The NSABP rectal trials have also challenged the conclusion of the consensus panel in that the combination of chemotherapy and radiation, when compared to the same chemotherapy given without radiation, does not result in a survival benefit. There is no salutary interaction between chemotherapy and radiotherapy as inherently implied by the consensus recommendations. The current findings from the NSABP trials as well as studies from other cooperative groups provide compelling justification for the formulation of a new consensus; the major disadvantages inherent in allowing a document formulated in 1990 to remain unmodified are self-evident.

The NSABP is committed to evolve a program of translational research that is stimulated by clinically relevant hypotheses derived from the protocol process. A preliminary example of this effort is the demonstration that thymidilate synthase levels served as a prognostic discriminant independent of Dukes' class and that patients with higher levels of thymidilate synthase were those that showed the greatest benefit from chemotherapy in NSABP protocol R-0113. A number of other recently described genetic and biochemical markers may have implications for the determination of prognosis and the development of therapy for colorectal tumors. The assessment of various markers in the primary tumor may play an important role in identifying patients who will benefit from adjuvant chemotherapy and in determining which regimen is optimal. The NSABP has embarked on a collaborative research effort in which a panel of markers will be assessed in ongoing and future studies; these markers include mismatch repair phenotype, P53, 18q deletion, tumor cell proliferation, and thymidylate synthase.

The prospect for future gains in the adjuvant therapy of colorectal cancer is excellent. There has been significant progress in the development of new pharmacologic regimens which will be evaluated in the adjuvant setting. Some examples of these reagents include the class of pure thymidylate synthase inhibitors (Tomudex), inhibitors of topoisomerase 1, the class of 5-FU prodrugs, dihydropyrimidine dehydrogenase inhibitors such as 5-ethynyluracil and combinations such as FU-LV and oxaloplatin. There is clearly no shortage of compelling concepts to be assessed and progress will be forthcoming provided that the mechanism of carrying out randomized prospective trials remains unencumbered.

REFERENCES

1. National Institutes of Health Consensus Development Conference Statement. Adjuvant therapy for patients with colon and rectum cancer. Office of Medical Applications of Research, April 16–18, 1990.
2. Wolmark N, Rockette H, Fisher B. Adjuvant therapy for carcinoma of the colon: Review of NSABP clinical trials. In: Salmon S, ed. Adjuvant therapy of cancer VII. Philadelphia: J. B. Lippincott Company, 1993. pp 300–306.
3. Taylor I, Machin D, Mullee M, et al. A randomized controlled trial of adjuvant portal vein cytotoxic perfusion in colorectal cancer. Br J Surg 1985;72:359–363.
4. Wolmark N, Rockette H, Wickerham DL, Fisher B, Redmond C, Fisher ER, Potvin M, Davies RJ, Jones J, Robidoux A, Wexler M, Gordon P, Cruz AB, Horsley S, Nims TA, Thirlwell M, Phillips WA, Prager D, Stern HS, Lerner HJ, Frazier TG. Adjuvant therapy of Dukes' A, B, and C adenocarcinoma of the colon with portal-vein fluourouracil hepatic infusion: Preliminary results of National Surgical Adjuvant Breast and Bowel Project Protocol C-02. J Clin Oncol 1990;8:1466–1475.
5. Laurie JA, Moertel CG, Fleming TR, Wieand HS, Leigh JE, Malliard J, Twito DI, Morton RF, Tschetter LK, Barlow JF. Surgical adjuvant therapy of large-bowel carcinoma: An evaluation of levamisole and combination of levamisole and fluorouracil. J Clin Oncol 1989;7:1447–1456.
6. Moertel CG, Fleming TR, MacDonald JS, Haller DG, Laurie JA, Goodman PJ, Ungerleider JS, Emerson WA, Tormey DC, Click JH, Veedder MH, Maillard JA. Levamisole and fluorouracil for adjuvant therapy of resected colon cancer. N Engl J Med 1990;322:352–358.
7. Moertel CG, Fleming TR, MacDonald JS, et al. Fluorouracil plus levamisole after resection of stage III colon carcinoma: A final report. Ann Intern Med 1995;122:321–326.
8. Wolmark N, Rockette H, Fisher B, Wickerham DL, Redmond C, Fisher ER, Jones J, Mamounas EP, Ore L, Petrelli NJ, Spurr CL, Dimitrov N, Romond EH, Sutherland CM, Kardinal CG, DeFusco PA, Jochimsen P, other NSABP Investigators. The benefit of leucovorin-modulated 5-FU as postoperative adjuvant therapy for primary colon cancer. Results from NSABP protocol C-03. J Clin Oncol 1993;11:1879–1887.
9. Rockette H, Deutsch M, Petrelli N, Wolmark N, Mamounas E, Fisher B, Jones J, Hyams D, Romond E, Wexler M, Cruz A, Gordon P, Jochimsen P. Effect of postoperative radiation therapy when used with adjuvant chemotherapy in Dukes' B and C rectal cancer: Results from NSABP C-02. Proc Am Soc Clin Oncol 1994;13:193.
10. Heald RJ. The "Holy Plane" of rectal surgery. J R Soc Med 1988;81(9)503–509.
11. Heald RJ. Total mesorectal excision is optimal surgery for rectal cancer: A Scandinavian consensus. Br J Surg 1995;82:1297–1299.
12. Mamounas E, Rockette H, Jones J, Wieand S, Wickerham DL, Fisher B, Wolmark N. Comparative efficacy of adjuvant chemotherapy in patients with Dukes' B vs Dukes' C colon cancer: Results from four NSABP adjuvant studies (C-01, C-02, C-03, C-04). Proc Am Soc Clin Oncol 1996;15:205.
13. Johnston PG, Fisher ER, Rockette HE, Fisher B, Wolmark N, Drake JC, Chabner BA, Allegra CJ. The role of thymidylate synthase expression in prognosis and outcome of adjuvant chemotherapy in patients with rectal cancer. J Clin Oncol 1994;12:2640–2647.

Adjuvant Therapy of Cancer VIII, edited by Sydney E. Salmon. Lippincott–Raven Publishers, Philadelphia © 1997.

21

5-Fluorouracil Plus Levamisole with or without 6-S-Leucovorin as Adjuvant Treatment of Resected Colon Cancer

INTACC (Intergruppo Nazionale Terapia Adiuvante Carcinoma Colon)

Colon cancer is one of the most important causes of cancer death in Western countries; about half of the patients with colorectal cancer will die of disseminated disease. Surgical resection remains the main therapeutic approach for the cases in which cancer is limited to the colon and the regional lymph nodes. Nevertheless, more than 30% of patients show recurrent disease after radical surgical resection; the likelihood of recurrence is different according to pathological stage and other biological parameters (histological grading, venous or perineural invasion, preoperative level of CEA, ploidy, S-phase-cell fraction, p53 gene).

RATIONALE OF ADJUVANT THERAPY

Unlike rectal cancer, colon cancer is intraperitoneal and has less propensity to local recurrence, occurring only in 3–12% of cases, whereas distant recurrences—mainly in the liver—occur more frequently. The rationale for applying adjuvant therapy in colon cancer derives both from this observation of the frequent recurrences, which are probably the expression of cancer growth in micrometastases present *ab initio*, and from the concept that commonly available therapeutic modalities are more effective on minimal residual disease. In fact, in experimental models the likelihood of killing cancer cells by chemotherapeutic agents is inversely proportional to the tumor volume, as consequences of the reduced number of chemoresistent clones and of the altered cell kinetics. Also, for immunotherapy, some evidence exists that a small tumor mass is more susceptible to the available agents. Therefore, in the period following the radical removal of the primary tumor and in absence of clinically evident metastases, the number of residual cells is likely to be the smallest and the therapy is likely to be more effective (with respect to the same therapy applied on evident macrometastases).

The potential benefits of adjuvant therapy (prologation of overall or progression-free survival, improvement of quality of life) have to be balanced against the

The INTACC (Intergruppo Nazionale Terapia Adiuvante Carcinoma Colon, National Intergroup of Adjuvant Therapy for Colon Cancer) is made up of the following groups: IST, Genova; GOIRC; GONO; GOPTAD; and IOR.

potential risks both in terms of acute toxicity, worsening the quality of life during the treatment, and in terms of delayed toxicity, with negative consequences on survival. It should also be taken into consideration that in the adjuvant setting all the patients have to be treated, although most of them do not actually need the therapy, since some are already cured by surgery and others recur in spite of the treatment.

In the last two decades many randomized trials have been performed on the adjuvant treatment of resected colon cancer, and fluorouracil plus levamisole is now commonly considered the standard adjuvant treatment for patients with stage III (Dukes' C) resected colon cancer. In spite of the positive results obtained by this combination, many patients recur and die by metastases from colon cancer, so further studies are warranted to improve results of adjuvant treatments.

TRIALS OF ADJUVANT THERAPY

The earliest trials of adjuvant therapy of colon cancer were carried out employing single-agent chemotherapy. Nitrogen mustard, thiothepa, and fluorouracil proved ineffective in prolonging survival of patients with resected colon cancer.

A second generation of adjuvant trials regarded combinations including methyl-CCNU on the basis of superior results of the methyl-CCNU and fluorouracil combination with respect to fluorouracil alone in metastatic colon cancer. No survival advantage was seen in a series of large trials performed by the NSABP and other groups (1). Notably, the Gastrointestinal Tumor Study Group randomized patients to observation versus methanol extraction residue of BCG (MER) versus fluorouracil and methyl-CCNU versus fluorouracil, methyl-CCNU, and MER, finding no difference in survival but a significantly higher incidence of leukemias and myelodysplasia among the patients treated with methyl-CCNU (2).

In a series of trials, levamisole, an antihelmintic agent with immunostimulatory properties, has been evaluated. In the important trial of the North Central Cancer Treatment Group the value of addition of fluorouracil to levamisole was studied. In the whole group a statistically significant advantage in the progression-free survival, but not in the overall survival, was noted; furthermore, the subset analysis showed a survival advantage among Dukes' C patients (3). A confirmatory study performed by a North American intergroup considered a randomized comparison between observation and fluorouracil-levamisole combination in Dukes' B2 patients and a comparison among observation, levamisole, and fluorouracil-levamisole in Dukes' C patients. Again, a survival advantage was observed for Dukes' C patients treated with the combination (4).

Until now, three large studies have examined the role of addition of leucovorin to fluorouracil. The NSABP compared weekly fluorouracil and leucovorin with the combination MOF (5); the intergroup compared fluorouracil and leucovorin with a loading schedule versus no postoperative therapy (6); an international group compared the Machover schedule versus no postoperative therapy (7). Overall, these trials demonstrated the superiority of the biochemical modulation.

Other studies have examined the role of portal vein infusion of fluorouracil. The largest one was carried out by the NSABP and compared fluorouracil and heparin infusion versus no therapy. A significant improvement in survival in the treatment arm was not associated with a reduction in incidence of liver metastases, so the authors concluded that the advantage was due to a systemic effect of the perioperative administration of fluorouracil (8).

As far as the impact of adjuvant chemotherapy on different prognostic subgroups is concerned, a recent intergroup study showed no difference in recurrence and death rate in Dukes' B2 patients with or without an adjuvant treatment (fluorouracil and levamisole) (9).

THE INTACC STUDY

The main aim of the present study was to assess whether the addition of a high dose of 6-S-leucovorin to 5-fluorouracil and levamisole is able to prolong the survival of patients with colon adenocarcinoma (Dukes' stages B2-B3-C) after radical resection of the primary tumor. Disease-free survival and toxicity have been regarded as secondary end points.

The rationale of the study is based on the following considerations: (a) although more toxic, the combination of 5-fluorouracil and leucovorin has been shown to be more active than 5-fluorouracil alone in patients with advanced or metastatic disease; (b) the combination of 5-fluorouracil and leucovorin is at least as active as 5-fluorouracil and levamisole in the adjuvant setting; and (c) 6-S-leucovorin is at least as active as the racemic mixture in potentiating the clinical activity of 5-fluorouracil.

Based on these premises, we have designed a prospective randomized trial comparing the following two treatment arms: *arm A:* 5-fluorouracil 450 mg/m^2 IV bolus on days 1 through 5 every 28 days for six times, plus levamisole 50 mg orally three times daily on days 1 through 3 every 2 weeks for 24 weeks; *arm B:* 5-fluorouracil 370 mg/m^2 IV bolus on days 1 through 5 every 28 days for six times, plus 6-S-leucovorin 100 mg/m^2 IV bolus before each administration of 5-fluorouracil, plus levamisole 50 mg orally three times daily on days 1 through 3 every 2 weeks for 24 weeks.

For entering the trial, patients should have met the following eligibility criteria: histologically proven colon carcinoma; site of disease intraperitoneal; radical resection of the primary tumor; Dukes' stage B2, B3, or C; absence of metastases; start of therapy within 60 days from surgery; ECOG performance status ≤ 1; good clinical and hematological profile; no previous cancer at any site; no other antineoplastic treatments; and informed consent. When we started this trial we projected a study population of 1450 patients to be accrued over a period of 3 years. With an α error = 0.05 and a β error = 0.20, this was the sample size foreseen to detect a 20% reduction of mortality. The study accrual has been closed after entry of 1703 patients from March 1992 to February 1995.

Patient characteristics are the following: in arm A (5-fluorouracil and levamisole), median age 63 years; 53.6% males; stage B2/B3 in 45.8% and stage C in 53% of the patients; number of involved nodes 1–4 in 69.7% of stage C patients and >4 in 19.9% of stage C patients; ECOG performance status 0 in 88.4% and 1 in 11.6% of the patients; and in arm B (5-fluorouracil plus levamisole and 6-S-leucovorin), median age 63 years; 53.1% males; stage B2/B3 in 49.6% and stage C in 48.4% of the patients; number of involved nodes 1–4 in 67.8% of stage C patients and >4 in 22.2%

of stage C patients; ECOG performance status 0 in 88.5% and 1 in 11.3% of the patients.

At the time the present evaluation was performed, data on the compliance to treatment were available for 1468 patients. The median number of days between surgery and the start of chemotherapy was 31 days in both arms. Ten patients in arm A and 10 patients in arm B never started therapy; 389 (54.4%) patients in arm A and 362 (48.1%) patients in arm B had the full planned dose of drugs, while (30.4%) patients in arm A and 249 (33.1%) patients in arm B had some dose modification because of toxicity. Ninety-seven patients (13.5%) in arm A and 128 (17.1%) in arm B discontinued treatment.

A total of 1468 patients are evaluable for toxicity, with results as follows: in arm A (5-fluorouracil and levamisole), stomatitis grade 3–4 in 27/716 (3.8%) patients; leukopenia grade 3–4 in 19/716 (2.7%) patients; alopecia grade 3–4 in 6/716 (0.8%) patients; diarrhea grade 3–4 in 33/716 (4.7%) patients; nausea and vomiting grade 3–4 in 13/716 (1.8%) patients; and in arm B (5-fluorouracil plus levamisole and 6-S-leucovorin), stomatitis grade 3–4 in 70/752 (9.4%) patients; leukopenia grade 3–4 in 4/752 (0.5%) patients; alopecia grade 3–4 in 6/752 (0.8%) patients; diarrhea grade 3–4 in 74/752 (10.0%) patients; nausea and vomiting grade 3–4 in 25/752 (3.4%) patients. We observed four cases of treatment-related death: three in arm A and one in arm B.

Preliminary data on events (death or relapse) are also available. We have observed until now 66 deaths and 126 relapses in arm A (5-fluorouracil and levamisole); deaths were considered related to tumor progression in 54 cases. In arm B (5-fluorouracil plus levamisole and 6-S-leucovorin), 51 deaths and 116 deaths have been observed until now; in 42 cases, death was related to tumor progression.

Tumor progression occurred with a similar pattern in both arms. In arm A (5-fluorouracil and levamisole), we observed 43/127 (33.8%) relapses in the liver only; a local failure alone in 30/127 (23.6%) patients; a distant failure in 9/127 (7.1%) patients; and multiple sites of relapse in 38/127 (30.0%) patients. In arm B (5-fluorouracil plus levamisole and 6-S-leucovorin), we observed 36/116 (31.1%) relapses in the liver only; a local failure alone in 28/116 (24.1%) patients; a distant failure in 13/116 (11.2%) patients; and multiple sites of relapse in 28/116 (24.1%) patients.

In conclusion, chemotherapy including 5-fluorouracil plus levamisole and 6-S-leucovorin is feasible as adjuvant treatment of extraperitoneal colon carcinoma. The toxicity of the experimental arm was acceptable even though slightly higher than that of 5-fluorouracil plus levamisole. So far, the number of relapses and deaths in the two treatment arms is too limited for any reliable conclusion.

REFERENCES

1. Fuchs CS, Mayer RJ. Adjuvant chemotherapy for colon and rectal cancer. Semin Oncol 1995;22:472.
2. Gastrointestinal Study Group. Adjuvant therapy of colon cancer—Results of a prospective randomized trial. N Engl J Med 1984;312:737.
3. Laurie JA, Moertel CG, Fleming R, et al. Surgical adjuvant therapy of large bowel carcinoma: An evaluation of levamisole and the combination of levamisole and fluorouracil. J Clin Oncol 1989;7:1447.

4. Moertel CG, Fleming TR, McDonald JS, et al. Levamisole and fluorouracil for adjuvant therapy of resected colon carcinoma. N Engl J Med 1990;322:352.
5. Wolmark N, Rockette H, Fisher B, et al. The benefit of leucovorin modulated fluorouracil as post-operative adjuvant therapy for primary colon cancer: Results from National Surgical Adjuvant Breast and Bowel Project protocol C-03. J Clin Oncol 1993;11:1879.
6. O'Connell M, Maillard J, MacDonald J, et al. An intergroup trial of intensive course 5-FU and low dose leucovorin as surgical adjuvant therapy for high risk colon cancer. Proc Am Soc Clin Oncol 1993;12:552. [Abstr.]
7. Elrichman C, Marsoni S, Seitz J, et al. Event free and overall survival is increased by FUFA in resected B and C colon cancer: A prospective pooled analysis of 3 randomized trials. Proc Am Soc Clin Oncol 1994;13:562. [Abstr.]
8. Wolmark N, Rockette H, Wickerham DL, et al. Adjuvant therapy for Dukes' A, B and C adenocarcinoma of the colon with portal vein fluorouracil hepatic infusion: Preliminary results of National Surgical Adjuvant Breast and Bowel Project protocol C-02. J Clin Oncol 1990;8:1466.
9. Moertel CG, Fleming TR, MacDonald JS, et al. Intergroup study of fluorouracil plus levamisole as adjuvant therapy for stage II/Dukes' B2 colon cancer. J Clin Oncol 1995;13:2936.

Adjuvant Therapy of Cancer VIII, edited by Sydney E. Salmon. Lippincott–Raven Publishers, Philadelphia © 1997.

22

A Prospective Comparison of Fluorouracil/Folinic Acid Versus Levamisole/Fluorouracil as Adjuvant Therapy after Resection of Stage III Colon Carcinoma

Alfred Wong and Alexander Chan

Randomized clinical trials, started in the mid-1980s, have clearly established the survival benefit of postoperative adjuvant chemotherapy with fluorouracil plus levamisole in patients after resection of stage III colon carcinoma (1,2). This treatment regimen has also been endorsed by the NIH Consensus Development Conference (3). In addition, poorly differentiated tumor histology and tumor perforation of the visceral peritoneum or invasion of contiguous structure (T_4 lesion) were identified as features at increased risk of recurrence. However, fluorouracil plus levamisole had not demonstrated any superiority in terms of response rate in treatment of metastatic colorectal cancer as compared to fluorouracil-treated controls (4). Fluorouracil plus folinic acid has shown an increased response rate and may have survival benefit in patients with advanced colorectal cancer (5). In view of this apparent advantage of fluorouracil plus folinic acid, a prospective, nonrandomized cohort study was started in 1990 in which patients with resected stage III colon carcinoma exhibiting T_4 lesion or poorly differentiated tumor histology were treated with fluorouracil plus folinic acid as adjuvant therapy. Patients without these two adverse risk factors were treated with levamisole plus fluorouracil. The end point of the study is survival time of patients. This paper reports on the outcome of 103 patients accrued into these two treatment groups.

PATIENTS AND METHODS

All eligible patients underwent potentially curative resection of adenocarcinoma of the colon with metastases to regional lymph nodes (TNM stage III). They were also required to have normal postoperative studies including carcinoembryonic antigen, chest x-ray, and computed tomographic scan or ultrasound of the liver.

Patients whose resected tumor specimen showed one of two adverse risk factors (poorly differentiated tumor histology and tumor perforation of visceral peritoneum or direct invasion of contiguous structure [T_4 lesion]) were assigned to treatment with fluorouracil plus folinic acid. These patients received folinic acid 200 mg/m^2 and 5-fluorouracil 370 mg/m^2 bolus intravenous injections every 28 days for six cycles.

Patients with a resected tumor specimen showing moderately to well differentiated tumor histology and tumor invasion through the muscularis propria into subserosa or non-peritonealized pericolic tissue (T_3 lesion) were treated with levamisole plus fluorouracil. Treatment consisted of levamisole 50 mg orally three times per day for 3 days, repeated every 2 weeks for 1 year. 5-Fluorouracil 450 mg/m^2 bolus intravenous injection daily was given for 5 days. Twenty-eight days after starting the course, weekly treatment with 5-fluorouracil was begun at 450 mg/m^2 intravenously and continued for 48 weeks.

All patients were started on adjuvant chemotherapy between 35 and 70 days after surgery. The same calculated dose of 5-fluorouracil was administered without dose escalation during the entire treatment course. While on chemotherapy, carcinoembryonic antigen and liver function tests were monitored monthly. Chest x-ray and radiologic imaging of the liver were carried out at 6 and 12 months after initiation of chemotherapy. Subsequent follow-ups were continued at 6-month intervals with physical examination and carcinoembryonic antigen and liver function tests until at least 5 years after surgery. Survival was calculated from the date of registration with the Kaplan-Meier method (6). The log rank test was used to test the difference between survival curves.

RESULTS

Between 1990 and 1994, a total of 103 patients were entered into this study. Forty-six were treated with fluorouracil plus folinic acid and another 57 patients received levamisole plus fluorouracil. The clinical characteristics of patients according to treatment groups are shown in Table 22-1. Ninety-six patients completed their assigned chemotherapy treatment. Seven patients on the levamisole/fluorouracil arm did not complete chemotherapy. Five patients relapsed while receiving levamisole/fluorouracil, at 4, 5, 6, 9, and 11 months, respectively. Another two patients developed ataxia, and treatment was stopped after 5 and 8 months due to neurotoxicity. There were no treatment-related deaths, and all 103 patients were on follow-up.

As of February 1996, the median follow-up time for this study is 46 months (range 23–72 months). Table 22-2 summarizes the outcome of the two treatment groups. Kaplan-Meier relapse-free survival and survival curves are shown in Figures 22-1 and 22-2, respectively. Treatment with fluorouracil/folinic acid showed a prolongation of relapse-free interval over levamisole/fluorouracil ($P = 0.103$). At 3.5 years, 86% of patients treated with fluorouracil/folinic acid and 71% of patients receiving levamisole/fluorouracil were free of recurrence. Fluorouracil/folinic acid resulted in a significant survival benefit as compared to levamisole/fluorouracil ($P = 0.035$). The 3.5-year actuarial survival estimates were 91% for the fluorouracil/folinic acid group versus 79% for the levamisole/fluorouracil group.

Treatment-related toxicity was measured by WHO Toxicity Criteria and is shown in Table 22-3. Side-effects were clinically tolerable. The most common side-effect of the fluorouracil/folinic acid regimen was diarrhea. For patients receiving levamisole/fluorouracil, nausea and changes in taste perception were common. However, for both regimens, gastrointestinal toxicity was mild, with only 2–4% of

TABLE 22-1. Patient Characteristics According to Treatment Regimen

	5FU/Folinic Acid (n = 46)	**5FU/Levamisole (n = 57)**
Sex		
Male	24	38
Female	22	19
Age		
Median	60	62
Range	27–76	18–77
Location of primary tumour		
Cecum and right colon	22	17
Flexure and transverse colon	6	7
Left colon and sigmoid	18	33
$T_3N_1M_0$		
Well/moderately differentiated	—	57
Poorly differentiated	15	—
$T_4N_1M_0$		
Gross perforation	6	—
Perforated visceral peritoneum	19	—
Invaded contiguous structure	6	—
No of nodes involved		
1–4	41	53
>4	5	4

TABLE 22-2. Results according to treatment regimen

	5FU/Folinic Acid	**5FU/Levamisole**
Relapse of Cancer	8	17
Site of Relapse		
liver	4	10
lymph nodes	3	2
peritoneum	1	5
Cancer Death	3	12
3½ year actuarial relapse free rate	86%	71%
95% CI	76–96	59–83
3½ year actuarial survival	91%	79%
95% CI	81–100	67–91

patients experiencing grade 3 toxicity. Hematologic toxicity was minimal. Only one patient developed grade 3 neutropenia. Two patients on levamisole/fluorouracil experienced ataxia as a side-effect. Both patients recovered fully within 2 months after cessation of chemotherapy and remained free of relapse.

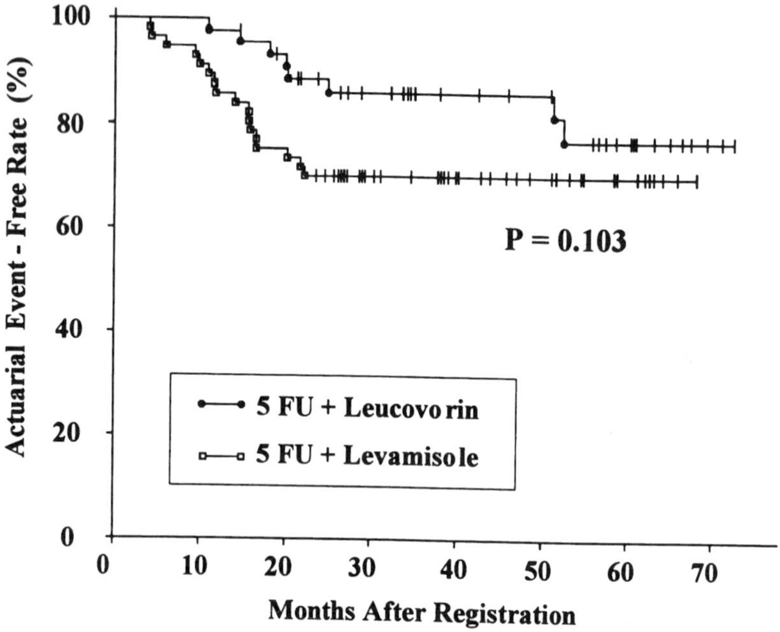

Figure 22-1. Kaplan-Meier relapse-free survival.

DISCUSSION

Since the NIH Consensus Development Conference in 1990, levamisole plus fluorouracil has been widely used as adjuvant treatment in North America for patients after resection of stage III colon cancer. Recent update of the intergroup study with 7 years follow-up reaffirmed the long-term survival benefit of this regimen. Mortality was reduced by 33% as compared to untreated surgical control (7). Results from the International Multicentre Pooled Analysis of Colon Cancer Trials (IMPACT) investigators also demonstrated a significant 22% reduction in mortality for patients receiving fluorouracil plus folinic acid (8). Results of our current study are in agreement with these reports. Both levamisole/fluorouracil and fluorouracil/folinic acid were effective adjuvant regimens for stage III colon cancer.

Our study attempted to compare the efficacy of fluorouracil/folinic acid versus levamisole/fluorouracil as adjuvant therapy for stage III colon cancer. It utilized a nonrandomized design with patients exhibiting one of two adverse prognostic features (poorly differiated tumor histology or T_4 lesion) who were assigned to fluorouracil/folinic acid regimen. Patients without these adverse prognostic features were treated with levamisole/fluorouracil. Otherwise, the clinical characteristics of patients were similar in both treatment groups. Our results suggested that 6-month fluorouracil/folinic acid postoperative chemotherapy significantly ($P = 0.035$) reduced the mortality of patients after resection of stage III colon adenocarcinoma

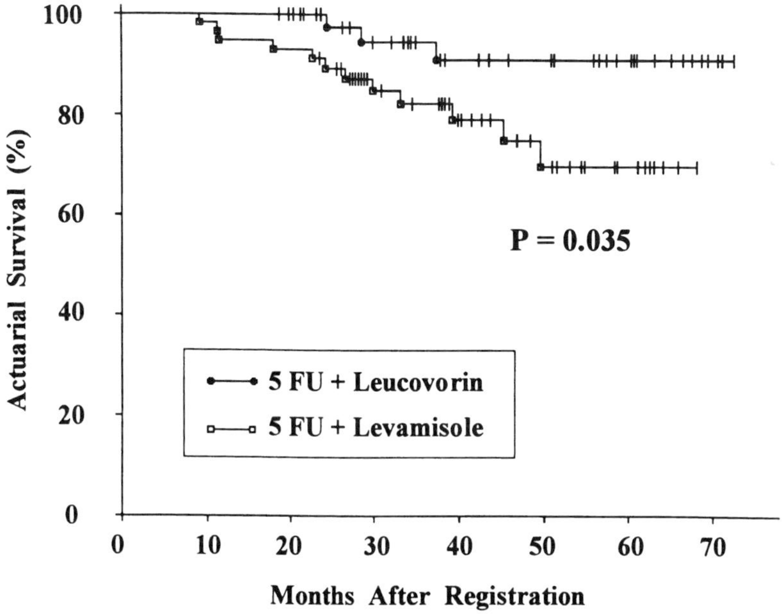

Figure 22-2. Kaplan-Meier actuarial survival.

TABLE 22–3. Treatment Related Toxicity

	5FU/Folinic Acid (n = 46)	**5FU/Levamisole (n = 57)**
Diarrhea		
All grades	16 (35%)	12 (21%)
≥ grade 3	1 (2%)	—
Mucositis		
All grades	6 (13%)	3 (5%)
≥ grade 3	—	—
Nausea		
All Grades	8 (17%)	22 (38%)
≥ grade 3	—	2 (4%)
Neutropenia		
All grades	4 (9%)	9 (16%)
≥ grade 3	—	1(2%)
Others		
Conjunctivitis	2 (5%)	—
Ataxia	—	3 (5%)
Skin Rash	—	5 (9%)
Arthralgia	—	4 (7%)
Taste Change	—	15 (26%)

as compared to 12-month levamisole/fluorouracil. At 3.5 years, the actuarial survival was 91% versus 79%. The fluorouracil/folinic acid regimen showed a trend favoring longer relapse-free interval over levamisole/fluorouracil ($P = 0.103$). This prolongation of the relapse-free interval may contribute to the survival benefit of patients receiving adjuvant fluorouracil and folinic acid.

REFERENCES

1. Laurie JA, Moertel CG, Fleming TR, et al. Surgical adjuvant therapy of large bowel carcinoma: An evaluation of levamisole and combination of levamisole and fluorouracil. J Clin Oncol 1989;7:1447.
2. Moertel CG, Fleming TR, MacDonald JS, et al. Levamisole and fluorouracil for adjuvant therapy of resected colon carcinoma. N Engl J Med 1990;322:352.
3. NIH Consensus Conference. Adjuvant therapy for patients with colon and rectal cancer. JAMA 1990;264:1444.
4. Buroker TR, Moertel CG, Fleming TR, et al. A controlled evaluation of recent approaches to biochemical modulation or enhancement of 5-fluorouracil therapy in colorectal carcinoma. J Clin Oncol 1985;3:1624.
5. Erlichman C, Fine S, Wong A, Elhakim T. A randomized trial of fluorouracil and folinic acid in patients with metastatic colorectal carcinoma. J Clin Oncol 1988;6:469.
6. Kaplan EL, Meier P. Nonparametric estimation from incomplete observation. J Am Stat Assoc 1958;53:457.
7. Moertel CG, Fleming TR, MacDonald JS, et al. Fluorouracil plus levamisole as effective adjuvant therapy after resection of stage III colon carcinoma: A final report. Ann Intern Med 1995;122:321.
8. International Multicentre Pooled Analysis of Colon Cancer Trials (IMPACT) Investigators. Efficacy of adjuvant fluorouracil and folinic acid in colon cancer. Lancet 1995;345:939.

V

GYNECOLOGIC AND GENITOURINARY CANCER

Adjuvant Therapy of Cancer VIII, edited by Sydney E. Salmon. Lippincott–Raven Publishers, Philadelphia © 1997.

23
Adjuvant Therapy of Ovarian Cancer—Is There Reason for Optimism?

David S. Alberts and Dava J. Garcia

EPIDEMIOLOGY AND STAGING

Ovarian cancer continues to be the leading cause of death from gynecologic cancers in the United States. There will be an estimated 26,700 new cases of ovarian cancer in 1996 and approximately 14,800 deaths (1). During an adult lifetime, 1 in 70 women will develop ovarian cancer.

Approximately 10% of patients will be diagnosed with stage I ovarian cancer and approximately 70% will have stage III disease at diagnosis. The 5-year survival rate for patients with stage I/II disease is approximately 80% and for those with stage III optimally debulked disease (i.e., less than 1 cm residual tumor mass) is approximately 40%.

The most important prognostic factors for survival in patients with stage I disease are the completeness of the exploratory laparotomy, the presence or absence of cytologically positive ascites, and tumor grade. For patients with stage III optimally debulked disease, important prognostic factors include the volume of residual disease (i.e., microscopic versus <0.5 cm versus <1 cm), performance status (i.e., SWOG 0–1 versus SWOG 2 or greater), patient age (i.e., less than 50 years versus 50 or more years), tumor grade (i.e., grade 1 versus grade 2/3), and histology (i.e., serous versus clear cell/mucinous).

ADJUVANT THERAPY OF EARLY-STAGE OVARIAN CANCER

Early-stage ovarian cancer can be stratified into two groups with markedly different long-term prognoses. Young et al. (2) reported that patients with a "favorable" prognosis were those with stage IA or IB disease and well or moderately well-differentiated tumors. In contrast, patients with an "unfavorable" prognosis were those with stage IA or IB disease with poorly differentiated cytologies, stage IC (tumor on the external surface of the ovary, a ruptured ovarian capsule, ascites, or positive peritoneal washings), or stage II disease. It is essential that clinical studies stratify patients according to these types of prognostic factors prior to randomization.

Because early-stage ovarian cancer represents a relatively small percentage of all ovarian cancer cases, it has been extremely difficult to accrue adequate numbers of patients to phase III clinical studies. Listed in Table 23-1 are the results of four of the most widely quoted phase III trials in patients with surgically documented

TABLE 23 1. Randomized Studies of Adjuvant Therapy in Stage I-II Ovarian Cancer

Investigator Group & Year	Stage	Histological Grade	Treatment Groups	Number of Evaluable Subjects	Number of Relapses (%)	5-Year Survival (%)
Young et al (2) OCSG/GOG 1990	Ia, Ib	1–2	Observation versus	38	4 (11)	94
			melphalan	43	1 (2)	98
Young et al (2) OCSG/GOG	I or II	3 or any Grade	Intraperitoneal ^{32}P versus	73	14 (19)	78
			melphalan	68	13 (19)	81
Walton et al (3)* OCSG/GOG	II	any	Intraperitoneal ^{32}P versus	48	10 (20)	~76
			melphalan	45	11 (24)	~80
Chiara et al. (4) NICR/Genova	I/II	2/3	Cisplatin/ cyclophosphamide versus	35	(74)	71
			whole abdominal radiation	35	(50)	53

*The report by Walton et al, is a subgroup analysis of the study by Young et al.

stage I and II epithelial type cancers. Young et al. (2) reported a study from the Ovarian Cancer Study Group (OCSG)–Gynecologic Oncology Group (GOG) which randomized patients with stage IA or IB, grade 1 or 2 ovarian cancer to observation versus intermittent oral melphalan (0.2 mg/kg/day for 5 days with repeat courses administered every 4–6 weeks for a total of 12 courses or 18 months of therapy, whichever came first). With a median follow-up of more than 5 years, there were four relapses in the observation group and only one in the melphalan-treated patients; however, there was no significant difference in survival with 5-year survival rates of 94% in the observation and 98% in the melphalan-treated patients. Based on these study results, the authors concluded that patients with stages IA and IB disease with well to moderately differentiated tumors do not require further treatment, if they have undergone thorough exploratory laparotomy.

A second study conducted simultaneously by Young et al. (2) evaluated patients with stage I, poorly differentiated tumors and patients with stage II disease. These patients with "unfavorable" prognostic factors were randomized to receive either a single intraperitoneal dose of ^{32}P (15 mCi of chromic phosphate) administered at the time of surgery or melphalan (0.2 mg/kg/day for 5 days every 4–6 weeks for a total of 12 courses or 18 months of therapy). After 5 years of follow-up, there was no significant difference in survival, with 78% of the ^{32}P-treated patients and 81% of the melphalan-treated patients still alive. Young et al. concluded that it was possible that neither treatment significantly affected survival and that the approximately 80% 5-year survival rate represents the natural history of the disease in thoroughly staged patients with "unfavorable" prognostic features. In 1992, Walton et al. (3) reanalyzed the study results of Young et al. (2) to determine the 5-year survival rates of patients with stage II disease who underwent comprehensive surgical staging and subsequent treatment with intraperitoneal ^{32}P or oral melphalan. Five-year survival rates were 76% for the ^{32}P-treated patients and 80% for the melphalan-treated patients, a nonsignificant difference.

Chiara et al. (4) have performed a small randomized trial of cisplatin (50 mg/m^2) plus cyclophosphamide (600 mg/m^2) administered every 28 days for six courses to 70 patients with high-risk stage I and II cancers. As shown in Table 23-1, 5-year survivals were 71% and 53% ($P = 0.16$) and relapse-free survivals were 74% and 50% ($P = 0.07$) for chemotherapy and whole abdominal radiation, respectively. Although this study obviously was underpowered to detect survival differences between the two treatments, the cisplatin-based therapy proved much safer than whole abdominal radiation (e.g., grade 3–4 diarrhea was experienced by 28% of the patients treated with radiation) and was, therefore, considered the better treatment.

More recently, three randomized European trials have tested cisplatin as an adjuvant treatment of early stage disease (5). In a study performed in Italy, patients with stage 1A and 1B, grade 2 and 3 cancers were randomized to cisplatin or observation. A second Italian study compared cisplatin to intraperitoneal ^{32}P in stage IC patients. Additionally, a Norwegian study randomized patients with stages I–III disease to cisplatin or intraperitoneal ^{32}P. In both Italian studies, disease-free survival was 30–40% longer in cisplatin-treated patients, but there was no evidence of overall survival prolongation in any of the three studies (6). These study results led to the design of the ongoing European-wide ACTION-ICON I trial in patients with stage I disease wherein patients are randomized to observation (with treatment at relapse) or at least four courses of either cisplatin (at least 75 mg/m^2) or carboplatin (at least 350 mg/m^2). If the observation group experiences equivalent survival duration, then a watch-and-treat approach to early stage disease may be adopted until the results of paclitaxel-platinum based studies are available.

STAGE III, OPTIMAL DISEASE ADJUVANT THERAPY STUDIES

There have been a limited number of randomized phase III trials of adjuvant chemotherapy in patients with optimally debulked stage III disease. Often, patients with stage III optimal disease were combined with patients with suboptimal stage III and stage IV disease in randomized treatment studies. As a result, it is difficult to separate the data for these two extremely different groups of patients. Listed in Table 23-2 are four studies wherein it was possible to separate out those patients with optimal disease for the purpose of analysis. Unfortunately, the majority of these studies had far too few patients to allow firm conclusions to be drawn.

In 1989, a Southwest Oncology Group (SWOG) study conducted by Alberts et al. (7) compared a combination of doxorubicin (40 mg/m^2) plus cyclophosphamide (600 mg/m^2) plus BCG to cisplatin (50 mg/m^2) plus doxorubicin (40 mg/m^2) plus cyclophosphamide (600 mg/m^2) with or without BCG in patients with stage III optimal disease ovarian cancer. Courses were repeated every 3–4 weeks for a total of 12 cycles. As shown in Table 23-2, there was a nonsignificant trend toward longer survival in patients receiving cisplatin. The results of this study and other larger trials in patients with suboptimal disease suggest that cisplatin is an important drug in the adjuvant treatment of patients with stage III optimal disease.

Omura et al. (8) reported the results of a GOG study in 1989 which compared cisplatin (50 mg/m^2) plus cyclophosphamide (1000 mg/m^2) to a regimen of cisplatin (50 mg/m^2) plus doxorubicin (50 mg/m^2) plus cyclophosphamide (500 mg/m^2) in patients with stage III optimal disease. Courses were repeated at 3-week intervals for a total of eight cycles. Pathologically proven complete response rates, median progression-free intervals and median survivals were not significantly different for the two treatment programs. Further follow-up of this study suggests that there was a trend toward improved survival in patients treated with the doxorubicin containing regimen; however, this was at the cost of significantly greater toxicity.

Recently, Kaye et al. (9,10) updated a phase III study which compared cisplatin (100 mg/m^2) plus cyclosphosphamide (750 mg/m^2) to cisplatin (50 mg/m^2) plus cyclophosphamide (750 mg/m^2) with courses repeated every 3 weeks for a total of six courses in patients with stage IC–IV ovarian cancer. The initial database was reanalyzed in 1995, after 115 of the original 159 patients had died. Overall, there was a significant survival advantage for those patients treated on the high-dose cisplatin regimen. In optimal disease patients (stages IC–III) the 4-year survival rate was 44% in the high-dose group and 41% in the low-dose group. Thus, the follow-up data from this study suggest that a 100% increase in cisplatin dose intensity does not lead to improved survival in patients with <2 cm residual tumor masses after primary surgery.

TABLE 23-2. Randomized Studies of Adjuvant Therapy in Optimally Debulked Ovarian Cancer

Investigator Group & Year	Stages	Treatment Groups*	Number of Evaluable Subjects	Pathological Complete Response (%)	Median Survival (Months)
Alberts et al (7)	III	DC + BCG VS	30	20	37
SWOG, 1989		CDP VS	22	23	48
		CDP + BCG	29	41	57
Omura et al (8)	III	CP VS	176	30	31
GOG, 1989		CDP	173	33	39
Kaye et al>+ (9,10)	IC-IV	P (low-dose)	37	—	41% at 4 yrs.
SOTG. 1992		P (high-dose)	35	—	44% at 4 yrs.
Alberts et al (11)	III	IP P/IV C	279	36	49[a]
		IV P/IV C	267	47	41

* Abbreviations: D-doxorubicin, C-cyclophosphamide, BCG-bacillus Calmette-Guerin, P-cisplatin.

[a] + $p = .02$

Results of a pivotal trial to evaluate the importance of the intraperitoneal route for cisplatin therapy in stage III optimal disease (i.e., <2 cm residual tumor masses) ovarian cancer have recently become available (11). This intergroup study (INT 0051) which was conducted by the SWOG, GOG, and Eastern Cooperative Oncology Group (ECOG) randomized 546 eligible patients to intraperitoneal cisplatin (100 mg/m^2) plus intravenous cyclophosphamide (600 mg/m^2) versus intravenous cisplatin (100 mg/m^2) plus cyclophosphamide (600 mg/m^2). Courses were repeated at 3-week intervals for six cycles. Second-look surgical procedures were mandatory in patients who had no clinical evidence of disease at the end of chemotherapy. Patients were stratified before randomization on the basis of size of residual tumor (i.e., 0 to <0.5 cm disease versus 0.5 to <2.0 cm disease). Eligible patients with no clinical evidence of disease at the completion of chemotherapy, who underwent an adequate second-look surgical procedure, had a pathological complete response rate of 36% on the intravenous arm and 47% on the intraperitoneal arm ($P = 0.06$). Survival of eligible patients on the intraperitoneal arm (estimated median = 49 months, 95% CI 42–56 months) was significantly longer ($P = 0.02$) than on the intravenous arm (estimated median = 41 months, 95% CI 34–47 months). The estimated intraperitoneal versus intravenous death hazard ratio is 0.76 (95% CI 0.61–0.96). Of considerable interest, moderate to severe oto-, neuro-, and myelotoxicities were significantly more frequent on the intravenous cisplatin arm. Thus, simply changing the administration route of cisplatin from intravenous to intraperitoneal resulted in superior patient survival and significantly less toxicity in patients with optimal stage III ovarian cancer.

ONGOING OVARIAN CANCER ADJUVANT THERAPY TRIALS

Listed in Table 23-3 are the ongoing or recently completed/unreported studies of adjuvant chemotherapy in patients with stage I–III ovarian cancer. An extremely important intergroup study in the GOG (GOG-95) with SWOG and North Central Cancer Treatment Group (NCCTG) participation randomly assigns patients with stage I (unfavorable prognostic factors) and II disease to a single dose of intraperitoneal ^{32}P versus intravenous cisplatin (100 mg/m^2) plus cyclophosphamide (1000 mg/m^2) every 3 weeks for three courses. This study was closed as of March 1994 with 251 patients entered. It will require an additional 3–5 years before the completed analysis will be available for discussion.

A replacement protocol for GOG-95 has been activated by the GOG with participation by the SWOG. This study, GOG-157, randomizes patients with stage IA/IB, high-grade tumors and stage IC/II, any tumor grade, to treatment with either three or six courses of carboplatin, dose based on a target AUC of 7.5 using the Calvert equation (12), plus paclitaxel 175 mg/m^2 by 3-hr infusion.

As stated above, the European community is conducting a study in patients with stage I ovarian cancer which should resolve whether adjuvant platinum-based therapy improves survival in this patient population. The ACTION-ICON study randomizes patients to observation (with treatment at relapse) versus at least four courses of cisplatin or carboplatin.

TABLE 23-3. Ongoing Ovarian Cancer Adjuvant Therapy Trials

Cooperative Group	Stage/Residual IP Tumor	Prior Therapy	Trial Design
ACTION-ICON	I/ None	None	Observation vs cisplatin × ≥4 or carboplatin × ≥4
GOG	I–II/ None	None	Paclitaxel/carboplatin x 3 vs × 6
GOG/SWOG	III/ <1 cm	None	High-dose carboplatin/IP cisplatin/ IV paclitaxel vs IV paclitaxel/IV cisplatin
GOG	III /<1 cm	None	IV paclitaxel (3 hr) /IV carboplatin vs IV paclitaxel (24 Hr) /IV cisplatin
SWOG	III/ none*	Platinum	IP α-interferon vs observation
GOG	III/ none*	Platinum	IP ^{32}P vs observation
EORTC	III/ none*	Platinum	IP ^{32}P vs observation

*No pathological evidence of disease at second-look surgery following platinum-based chemotherapy.

Current phase III studies in optimal disease, stage III ovarian cancer are evaluating the efficacy of paclitaxel, high-dose platinum, and intraperitoneal chemotherapy in this patient group. The GOG and SWOG have recently completed accrual to a study which evaluates high-dose carboplatin (AUC = 9 mg • min/ml or approximately 550 mg/m^2) for two courses prior to intraperitoneal cisplatin (100 mg/m^2) plus IV paclitaxel (135 mg/m^2 over 24 hr) plus intravenous cisplatin (75 mg/m^2) for six cycles. The major objective of the study is to evaluate the relative efficacy of dose-intensive carboplatin administered prior to intravenous paclitaxel plus intraperitoneal cisplatin compared to standard doses of paclitaxel/cisplatin. Final results of this study will not be available until 1998–1999.

The GOG is currently conducting a phase III study (GOG-158) which principally studies the relative efficacy of a 3-hr versus 24-hr infusion of paclitaxel. Patients with stage III optimal disease ovarian cancer are randomized to either cisplatin, 75 mg/m^2, plus paclitaxel, 135 mg/m^2 by 24-hr infusion versus carboplatin, AUC = 7.5 mg/ml • min, plus paclitaxel, 175 mg/m^2 by 3-hr infusion for six cycles.

In preparation for a possible phase III study, the SWOG is conducting a pilot phase II trial (SWOG-9619). Approximately 100 patients with stage III optimal disease ovarian cancer will receive combination chemotherapy with intravenous paclitaxel on day 1, intraperitoneal cisplatin on day 2, and intraperitoneal paclitaxel on days 8 and 15. The rationale for this study is based upon the SWOG's previous phase III study (INT-0051) which determined that the intraperitoneal route of cisplatin administration compared to intravenous delivery is associated with increased survival and decreased toxicity. Additionally, intriguing data suggest that the therapeutic index of paclitaxel might also be enhanced by intraperitoneal administration.

Three important phase III trials are being conducted in patients who have no pathologically proven evidence of disease in the intraperitoneal space at the time of second-look surgery following primary platinum-based chemotherapy. These are critical studies since more than 50% of patients with advanced ovarian cancer will relapse within 5 years following a pathologically negative second-look procedure. The study conducted by the SWOG randomly assigns patients to either intraperitoneal α-interferon (50 million units/m^2 weekly for 6 consecutive weeks) versus observation only. Approximately 50% of the number of patients necessary to complete this study have been accrued and the GOG is expected to join the study in the fall of 1996. A second study being performed by the GOG in this same patient population randomly assigns patients to receive intraperitoneal ^{32}P versus observation only. It is anticipated that this study will achieve its full accrual goals by the summer of 1996. Finally, the EORTC has an ongoing study to compare intraperitoneal cisplatin versus observation only in patients who have no pathological evidence of disease at the time of second-look surgery. All three of the trials are designed to evaluate whether the study treatment can prevent the long-term recurrence of the disease.

An increasing number of patients with advanced ovarian cancer who achieve a complete clinical response to primary chemotherapy do not undergo a second-look surgical restaging procedure. In that 70% of patients in this category will eventually recur, there is a somewhat controversial rationale for administering "adjuvant" therapy to this group. The SWOG is conducting a phase II trial of oral altretamine, 260 mg/m^2/day × 14 days every 28 days for 6 months. The primary study end point will be the 2-year overall survival rate.

CONCLUSIONS

Stage I Disease

On the basis of the report by Young et al. (2) survival of patients with "favorable" prognosis stage I disease (i.e., stages IA and IB with well to moderately well differentiated tumors) who have undergone comprehensive surgical staging probably is not improved by current adjuvant therapy programs. In contrast, patients with stage I disease with "unfavorable" prognostic factors are definite candidates for adjuvant therapy programs. Postsurgical treatment is recommended even though the results of a randomized study by the Gynecologic Oncology Group did not establish a definite benefit from either intraperitoneal ^{32}P or oral melphalan therapy. It is unclear whether the 80% 5-year survival rates for patients in both arms of the GOG study resulted from study treatment or the comprehensive surgical staging that was required prior to enrollment. Clearly, the results of the ongoing GOG-SWOG-NCCTG trial of intraperitoneal ^{32}P versus cisplatin-cyclophosphamide study will help to clarify the role of adjuvant therapy for this relatively high-risk group of stage I–II patients. Since patients with clear cell histology and those with stage II disease appear to have significantly poorer prognoses than those with stage I disease, if they are not entered into randomized clinical studies, they should be considered for more intensive platinum-based chemotherapy programs. The role of paclitaxel in the adjuvant therapy of early stage disease presently is being examined in the GOG through a comparison of three versus six courses of paclitaxel plus carboplatin.

Stage III Optimal Disease

The results of two recently completed trials in the SWOG and GOG will impact greatly on the future design of adjuvant therapy studies in stage III ovarian cancer. For example, since intraperitoneal cisplatin-cyclophosphamide is associated with a survival advantage over intravenous cisplatin-cyclophosphamide in the SWOG-GOG-ECOG Intergroup 0051 trial in patients with stage III optimal disease, future trials should consider the incorporation of intraperitoneal chemotherapy with either cisplatin or other promising agents, like paclitaxel. Furthermore, the positive results of GOG-111 require that paclitaxel be incorporated into the adjuvant treatment of patients with stage III optimal disease.

Disposition of the Patient with No Clinical or Pathological Evidence of Disease after Primary Chemotherapy

Advanced ovarian cancer patients who have no pathological evidence of disease at second-look surgery may have as high as a 50% recurrence rate over a period of 5 years. At this point, no therapy is indicated for this patient population outside of a clinical research trial. As mentioned previously, the GOG, SWOG, and EORTC all have ongoing phase III studies to evaluate either intraperitoneal ^{32}P, high-dose intraperitoneal α-interferon, or intraperitoneal cisplatin, respectively. The results of these studies will not be available for many years, because of the relatively prolonged survival of the study population.

Patients with stage III optimal or suboptimal disease have an approximately 70% risk of disease relapse if they have no clinical evidence of disease and do not undergo second-look surgery following primary platinum-based chemotherapy. An increasingly larger proportion of such patients do not undergo second-look surgery, because of either patient refusal or a lack of adequate insurance coverage for the surgical procedure. Thus, it is necessary to begin planning clinical studies to identify useful therapeutic strategies for this increasingly large patient population. The SWOG has initiated protocol SWOG-9326 to evaluate the activity of six courses of altretamine (260 mg/m^2/day × 14 every 28 days). A SWOG follow-up phase III study of 3 versus 12 consolidation courses of paclitaxel (3-hr infusion) has been reviewed recently by NCI-CTEP.

REFERENCES

1. Parker SL, Tong T, Bolden S, Wingo PA. Cancer statistics 1996. CA 1996;41:5–27.
2. Young RC, Walton LA, Ellenberg SS, et al. Adjuvant therapy in stage I and stage II epithelial ovarian cancer. Results of two prospective randomized trials. N Engl J Med 1990;322:1021–1027.
3. Walton LA, Yadusky A, Rubenstein L, et al. Stage II carcinoma of the ovary: An analysis of survival after comprehensive surgical staging and adjuvant therapy. Gynecol Oncol 1992;44:55–60.
4. Chiara S, Conte P, Franzone P, et al. High-risk early stage ovarian cancer. Randomized clinical trial comparing cisplatin plus cyclophosphamide versus whole abdominal radiotherapy. Am J Clin Oncol 1994;17:72–76.
5. Colombo N. Multimodality therapy of early-stage (FIGO I/II) ovarian cancer: Review of surgical management and postoperative adjuvant treatment. Proceedings of Current Concepts in the Management of Gynecologic Tumors Conference, International Gynecologic Cancer Society Congress, Philadelphia, 1995.
6. Percorelli S. Adjuvant therapy is effective in early-stage ovarian cancer—Yes/no. Proc Soc Gynecol Oncol 1995;5:13. [Abstr. 42.]
7. Alberts DS, Mason-Liddil N, O'Toole RV, et al. Randomized phase III trial of chemoimmunotherapy in patients with previously untreated stage III, optimal ovarian cancer: A Southwest Oncology Group Study. Gynecol Oncol 1989;32:16–21.
8. Omura GA, Bundy BN, Berek JS, et al. Randomized trial of cyclophosphamide plus cisplatin with or without doxorubicin in ovarian carcinoma: A Gynecologic Oncology Group study. J Clin Oncol 1989;7:457–465.
9. Kaye SB, Lewis CR, Paul J, et al. Randomized study of two doses of cisplatin with cyclophosphamide in epithelial ovarian cancer. Lancet 1992;340:329–333.
10. Kaye S. Long-term follow-up of a randomized trial of cisplatin dose in advanced ovarian cancer. Intl J Gynecol Cancer 1995;5(Suppl 1):11. [Abstr. 38.]
11. Alberts DS, Liu PY, Hannigan EV, et al. Phase III study of intraperitoneal cisplatin/intravenous cyclophosphamide versus intravenous cisplatin/intravenous cyclophosphamide in patients with optimal disease stage III ovarian cancer: A SWOG-GOG-ECOG Intergroup study (INT 0051). Proc Am Soc Clin Oncol 1995;14:273. [Abstr. 760.]
12. Calvert AH, Jones TR, Jackman AL, et al. Carboplatin dosage: Prospective evaluation of a simple formula based on renal function. J Clin Oncol 1989;7:1748–1756.

Adjuvant Therapy of Cancer VIII, edited by Sydney E. Salmon. Lippincott–Raven Publishers, Philadelphia © 1997.

24

A Review of the Neoadjuvant and Adjuvant Treatment of Prostate Cancer

Frederick R. Ahmann

PROSTATE CANCER SIGNIFICANCE

Physicians and patients sometimes summarize the significance of prostate cancer in misleading short phrases: "If you live long enough, you will get it." "Most men with prostate cancer die of something else." While there are isolated facts supporting both of these statements, a more global perspective would lead one to associate the adjective "unpredictable" with this type of cancer.

In autopsy studies, a majority of men do have microscopic foci of prostate cancer after the age of 70 (1). However, such incidental cancers will comprise few of the projected 317,000 new cases that will be clinically diagnosed in 1996 and none of the projected 41,400 deaths (2). The number of prostate cancer-related deaths has been increasing steadily for 25 years and makes prostate cancer the leading cause of cancer-related deaths in men over the age of 60 years (2).

Hence, most men develop a malignant transformation in the prostate that does not progress to clinically significant tumor volumes, and a majority of men clinically diagnosed with prostate cancer will indeed, either with or without treatment, not have their survivals shortened by the disease. Yet 41,000 deaths this year means that almost as many men will die of prostate cancer as women will die of breast cancer (2). Identifying which men are at risk of developing significant prostate cancer and identifying among those already known to harbor prostate cancer which have biologically aggressive disease are the most important unsolved problems in this disease.

NEOADJUVANT AND ADJUVANT THERAPY TENETS

A summary of neoadjuvant and adjuvant therapy trial results in a specific tumor must start with a brief reminder that there are some basic tenets that must be met before such therapeutic approaches should even be tested in a specific tumor (see Table 24-1) (3). For prostate cancer, tenet number one is easily met. There is no question that prostate cancer causes significant morbidity and mortality (2).

As for tenet number two, in men with clinically localized prostate cancer, long-term studies have shown that two local interventions are capable of rendering men free of disease for at least 10 years: radical prostatectomy and radiotherapy (4). Until recently, only actuarial 10- and 15-year overall results could be used to evaluate

TABLE 24-1. Tenets Which Support the Initiation of Neoadjuvant or Adjuvant or Adjuvant Therapy Trials in a Specific Tumor (3)

1. The tumor should be associated with a significant mortality.
2. Potentially curative therapies should be available.
3. Prognostic factors correlating with local therapy failures should be recognized.
4. Effective systemic therapies for advanced disease should be known.

curability. However, the advent of serum PSA levels and the recognition that persistent/rising PSA levels after surgery and rising PSA levels after radiotherapy are highly correlative with treatment failure, has allowed a much more reliable means of assessing potentially curative therapy results (4).

There are least five series with long-term follow-up after radical prostatectomy reporting failure based on serum PSA measurements (4). At 10 years, the freedom from PSA failure ranges between 50 and 70% for prostate cancer found pathologically to be confined to the prostate. Such pathologic staging is not available from radiotherapy trials, but 10-year biochemical failure data have been reported by the Radiation Oncology group at Massachusetts General (5). At that institution, 504 men with clinical stage T1 and T2 lesions were treated with external beam radiotherapy and 20–50% of them were free from PSA progression 10 years later. While it is not possible to compare the overall efficacy of surgery versus radiotherapy, it can be concluded that both interventions are potentially curative.

While these studies would seen to satisfy the second tenet for adjuvant or neoadjuvant therapy trials, one must still ask the question of whether or not death from prostate cancer is a real possibility in most men diagnosed with the disease. Who cares what a man's post-treatment PSA value is if he is likely to die of something else? A group from Sweden has helped clarify this issue as they have pursued for many years a policy of no treatment with radical prostatectomy or definitive radiotherapy in men diagnosed with localized prostate cancer and good prognosis predictors. Their early results suggested that treatment with radiation or surgery did not help people live longer (6). However, recent, long-term updates indicate that this is true only if a man dies of something else within 5–8 years (7). For men who lived more than 10 years, 62% have thus far died of prostate cancer. Hence, observation should be an option best aimed at men with a relatively short life expectancy.

Regarding the third tenet, physicians are increasingly able to identify subgroups of men with localized prostate cancer that have characteristics that predict a higher likelihood of failing local therapies. Table 24-2 lists several of the factors that are commonly used to identify such patients (8,9). While not perfect, the use of such prognostic factors helps identify which men have more biologically aggressive disease.

The last tenet for adjuvant or neoadjuvant therapy trials in prostate cancer is much more easily met. Androgen-suppressive or ablative therapy has been recognized for 50 years as an effective systemic therapy for metastatic disease (10). Recent studies suggest that 90% of men treated with LHRH plus an anti-androgen will have a significant decline in their pretreatment PSA levels (11).

TABLE 24-2. Characteristics of Identifying Prostate Cancers with Prognosis (8,9)

1. Extent of cancer within the prostate
2. Local or regional spread
3. Histologic grade
4. Tumor DNA ploidy studies
5. Pre-treatment serum PSA levels

NEOADJUVANT AND ADJUVANT APPROACHES

As the basic tenets are met, at least four different adjuvant or neoadjuvant treatment strategies could be tested in prostate cancer. The first and simplest strategy would be to deliver radiation post-radical prostatectomy to the prostate bed and/or pelvis when pathologic findings indicate that local recurrences will be likely. Such pathologic findings would include capsular penetration, a positive surgical margin, seminal vesicle involvement, regional lymph node involvement, or a measurable postoperative serum PSA level (8,9).

A second strategy would be to initiate hormonal therapy after a radical prostatectomy when the pathologic findings would predict that the surgery was not highly likely to have cured the disease. In this circumstance, the pathologic findings would include those mentioned above for local recurrence plus bilateral prostate involvement, high tumor histologic grades, preoperative serum PSA levels above 10 ng/ml, and/or DNA studies indicating a nondiploid tumor DNA content (8,9).

The last two strategies involve neoadjuvant hormonal therapy prior to a radical prostatectomy or radiotherapy. Patients would be candidates for such therapeutic studies if their clinical staging indicated bilateral disease, a nondiploid tumor DNA content on biopsy, suspected extracapsular extension, and/or a pretreatment serum PSA level which is greater than 10 ng/ml (8,9).

POST-RADICAL PROSTATECTOMY ADJUVANT RADIOTHERAPY

Several tumor characteristics do predict for local recurrences after a radical prostatectomy. Men with evidence of extracapsular disease (T3) have a known local recurrence rate of between 30 and 60% (12). While no definitive controlled, randomized trials have been completed, there is little doubt that postoperative adjuvant radiotherapy significantly reduces this local recurrence rate. Displayed in Table 24-3 are four representative nonrandomized trials of postoperative adjuvant radiation therapy in such patients. The local recurrence rate is reduced to less than 10%.

Does this reduced local recurrence rate result in an improved survival? Again, there are no randomized controlled trials to definitively answer this question, but three of the four series displayed in Table 24-3 compared their own institutions' surgery alone results with their adjuvant radiation outcomes and could find no suggestion that the lower local recurrence rate resulted in a superior overall survival. This probably should not be surprising as capsular penetration or involvement of

TABLE 24-3. Representative Nonrandomized Trials of Postoperative Radiotherapy after Radical Prostatectomy in Pathologic Stage C Prostate Cancer

Study	Number Enrolled	Median F/U (years)	Local Failure Rate	Survival Effect
Eisbruch (24)	34	5	0%	None
Petrovich (25)	95	6	4%	Not reported
Gibbons (26)	64	9	Reduced	None
Anscher (27)	46	10	8%	None

the seminal vesicles are markers for invasion and are associated with a high risk of micrometastatic disease. Local radiation would seem to have little prospect of reducing micrometastases.

Other studies have demonstrated that post-radical prostatectomy adjuvant radiotherapy when delivered to patients either having a persistent or subsequently rising serum PSA level can reduce the serum PSA levels in a majority of patients (12). However, such serum PSA reductions are usually short-lived and, again, while there are no randomized control trials, postoperative radiation for persistent or rising PSA levels would not appear to offer a significant chance of improved overall survival.

A recent study, however, may indicate that a subgroup of such patients might have a survival benefit from postoperative radiation therapy based on PSA levels. Coetzee et al. evaluated 45 patients with pathologically determined margin-positivity at radical prostatectomy who then underwent adjuvant radiation within 6 months of the surgery. If the postoperative serum PSA level (before starting the adjuvant radiotherapy) did not fall to the undetectable range, the biochemical PSA failure rate of adjuvant radiation was found to be 80% within a year. However, those patients whose serum PSA level did fall to the undetectable range immediately post-operation who then experienced a subsequent rise in PSA, had a much lower failure rate with adjuvant radiation (13). Further studies will need to be done to determine if postoperative serum PSA levels falling to an undetectable range and subsequently rising identifies men who may benefit from adjuvant radiation.

In summary, postoperative adjuvant radiation has not been definitively studied in controlled randomized trials. Nevertheless, some conclusions are possible. Adjuvant radiation reduces the local recurrence rate in men with pathologic findings associated with a high risk of such failures. This improved local control does not appear to result in an improved overall survival. Early data suggest that postoperative serum PSA levels may identify a subgroup of men who achieve a survival advantage. This concept will require additional testing.

POST-RADICAL PROSTATECTOMY ADJUVANT HORMONAL THERAPY

The cure rate for men undergoing radical prostatectomy varies by prognostic factor, but is less than desired for all but small, well-differentiated diploid tumors confined to the prostate. In a similar situation in breast cancer where high-risk patients can be identified, adjuvant hormonal therapy with the anti-estrogen tamoxifen has been successful in prolonging overall survival, particularly in the highest-risk groups (14). Could immediate adjuvant postoperative hormonal therapy provide similar benefits in prostate cancer? Investigation into this concept has been limited by the toxicity profile of hormonal agents until recently. The toxicity profile of either orchiectomy or medical castration is problematic. Currently, there are large national and international trials investigating newer, less toxic hormonal agents in an adjuvant fashion. There are no preliminary results available from these trials at this time.

However, two older trials should be mentioned. In 1993, the National Prostatic Cancer Project reported the results from two prospectively randomized trials of adjuvant treatment after either radical prostatectomy or definitive radiation (15). All men had undergone pelvic lymph node dissection before radiation or radical prostatectomy and then were randomized to receive either no adjuvant therapy, cytotoxic chemotherapy with cyclophosphamide for 2 years, or estramustine phosphate for 2 years. Forty-nine percent of 437 patients enrolled were node-positive and, hence, at quite high risk for metastatic disease. Adjuvant estramustine prolonged the median time to progression but had no effect on overall survival. Adjuvant cyclophosphamide had no clear benefit.

The other trial is a nonrandomized Mayo Clinic study of adjuvant hormonal therapy after radical prostatectomy in men with regional lymph node involvement (16). Two hundred and ninety-four men received adjuvant bilateral orchiectomy or additive hormonal therapy with diethylstilbestrol (DES) postoperatively. The outcome of these patients was compared to 86 other Mayo Clinic patients with positive regional lymph nodes who received no adjuvant treatment post-radical prostatectomy. The adjuvant hormonal therapy in this nonrandomized comparison, appeared to prolong the time to disease progression. The overall effect on survival was minimal.

In summary, adjuvant hormonal therapy after a radical prostatectomy has been poorly tested primarily because of the lack of a suitable hormonal manipulation for adjuvant treatment. In the few studies carried out, such adjuvant therapy in high risk, primarily node-positive patients increased the time to disease progression. There has been, thus far, no obvious impact on survival. Additional studies are needed in this area.

NEOADJUVANT HORMONAL THERAPY PRIOR TO RADICAL PROSTATECTOMY

The development of luteinizing hormone releasing hormone analogues as effective reversible medical castration in the 1980s has permitted the study of neoadjuvant hormonal therapy prior to radical prostatectomy. The overall curability of clinically localized prostate cancer with poor prognostic characteristics is less than satisfactory. Reducing the prostate and prostate cancer size prior to the performance of a radical prostatectomy has been tested and early results are published.

In men clinically staged as having locally extensive disease, a number of trials have shown that the prostate can be reduced in size by an average of 20–40% by hormonal therapy with a concurrent fall in serum PSA levels frequently to values less than 1 ng/ml (17–21). Such nonrandomized results supported testing the value of this downsizing in a randomized clinical trial.

Table 24-4 displays the early results of five prospectively randomized trial of neoadjuvant hormonal therapy prior to radical prostatectomy. Thus far, there is no consensus as to either the ideal hormonal therapy regimen or the duration of therapy. All studies have utilized sustained release luteinizing hormone releasing hormone compounds and many have added an anti-androgen to the LHRH. The combined therapy frequently is commonly called total androgen ablation. The duration of the hormonal therapy has varied between 2 and 8 months. Maximal prostatic shrinkage appears to be obtained only after 6 or more months of therapy, but the majority of the shrinkage has been accomplished after 2–4 months of treatment.

At the University of Miami and collaborating institutions, Soloway et al. randomized 282 men to undergo either androgen deprivation followed by radical prostatectomy or immediate radical prostatectomy (17). No statistical difference was found between the two groups in terms of easier surgery, amount of blood loss, length of hospital stay, or operating time. There was, however, a 30% reduction in pathologic capsule penetration as well as positive surgical margins. No survival or long-term PSA data are available from this trial.

Labrie et al. in Quebec City, Canada, have carried out a similar study in 161 men (18). Three months of total androgen ablation was given before radical prostatectomy versus going directly surgery. The percentage of men with organ confined disease was 28% higher after 3 months of neoadjuvant total hormone ablation. Negative surgical margins were found 26% more commonly in men who received neoadjuvant total androgen ablation. In this study, there has been no clear survival effect yet reported.

In Belgium, Van Poppel and his associates reported on 130 patients treated immediately with a radical prostatectomy or treated with estramustine for 6 weeks prior to the radical prostatectomy (19). Here also, there was a significant reduction in positive surgical margins and an increase in organ-confined disease. Dr. Fair at Sloan-Kettering has studied 182 men with clinical organ confined disease (20). The

TABLE 24-4. Results of Neoadjuvant Hormonal Therapy Prior to Radical Prostatectomy

Study	Number Enrolled	% Down-Staged	Median F/U	Survival Benefit
Soloway (17)	149	31	N/A	Not reported
Labrie (18)	161	29	N/A	Not reported
Van Poppel (19)	130	11	N/A	Not reported
Fair (20)	182	25	2 years	Not reported
Dalkin (21)	61	0	N/A	Not reported

duration of the neoadjuvant hormonal therapy was 2 months with total androgen ablation being utilized. Twenty-five percent of men were downstaged.

However, not all studies have been positive. Dalkin et al. randomized 61 men (21). The clinical characteristics of this patient group suggested they had smaller volume disease than the other studies noted above. Dalkin noted no significant reduction in pathologic staging.

Overall, the clear trend of results from neoadjuvant hormonal therapy studies shows a probability of downstaging in 20–30% of patients who are in higher risk group categories. Whether such benefit applies to men with clinical T1 and T2 disease is less certain. There does not seem to be a significant effect on surgical morbidity, blood loss, or operating time. The effect on overall survival is unclear. One study from San Francisco does have long enough follow-up to provide some insight into this issue. This study reported on the results of neoadjuvant hormonal therapy with total androgen ablation before radical prostatectomy in 30 men (22). At a mean follow-up of slightly less than 3 years, almost three-quarters of these patients had experienced a PSA progression. Longer follow-up from the randomized trials will be very important in determining the overall benefit of neoadjuvant hormonal therapy prior to radical prostatectomy.

NEOADJUVANT HORMONAL THERAPY PRIOR TO RADIATION THERAPY

Similar to the rationale for studying neoadjuvant hormonal therapy prior to radical prostatectomy, the results of primary radiation for clinically localized prostatic carcinoma indicate that, particularly in high-risk patients, the probability of cure is less than ideal. Hence, a theoretical approach of "shrinking" and "downstaging" prostatic carcinoma before the initiation of radiotherapy has been studied. In addition to less tumor volume to treat, such size reductions prior to radiotherapy would have the additional theoretical advantage of resulting in smaller radiation fields, thus reducing potential toxicity to surrounding normal tissues.

There are no definitive randomized trials testing this concept. There are, however, several series which provide information and conclusions are possible. Displayed in Table 24-5 are the results of three such trials. Zelefsky and associates at Sloan-Kettering treated 22 patients with "bulky" prostate cancer with 3 months of LHRH plus eulexin prior to three-dimensional conformal radiotherapy (23). There was a 25% median reduction of prostate size together with a median reduction of 30% in the amount of rectal wall receiving significant radiation, and a median reduction of 50% of bladder volume receiving significant radiation. A lesser reduction in the volume small bowel receiving potentially toxic doses of radiation was accomplished.

Similar findings were reported by others. Analogous to the early results of studies of neoadjuvant hormonal therapy prior to radical prostatectomy, there are no data to indicate that this neoadjuvant approach will lead to a superior treatment outcome in terms of either progression rate or survival. Such treatment would seem to offer some hope of a method of reducing treatment-related toxicity. Controlled randomized clinical trials are in progress testing these hypotheses.

TABLE 24-5. Results of Neoadjuvant Hormonal Therapy Prior to Radiotherapy

Study	Number Enrolled	Prostate Reduction	Median F/U	Survival Benefit
Zelefsky (23)	22	25%	N/A	Not reported
Forman (28)	20	37%	N/A	Not reported
RTOG (29)	477	Not reported	3 years	Not reported

SUMMARY

The theoretical principles for studying adjuvant and neoadjuvant therapies in prostate cancer can be met. There are at least four adjuvant and neoadjuvant treatment strategies being tested in men with prostate cancer. Among the strategies are adjuvant radiotherapy after radical prostatectomy, adjuvant hormonal therapy after radical prostatectomy, and neoadjuvant hormonal therapy prior to either radical prostatectomy or radiotherapy.

No definitive conclusions that can yet be made regarding the success or failure of any of these treatment strategies. Analysis of the data that do exist permits some preliminary conclusions. Adjuvant radiation after radical prostatectomy reduces local failure rates. No effect on overall survival has yet been documented. Adjuvant hormonal therapy after radical prostatectomy is poorly studied, but in men with involved regional lymph nodes at radical prostatectomy, adjuvant hormonal therapy appears to prolong progression-free survival. There is, as yet, no clear indication that such therapy has a positive effect on overall survival.

Neoadjuvant hormonal therapy prior to either radiotherapy or radical prostatectomy reduces prostate and prostate cancer volumes, downstaging some patients. There is no consensus as to which hormonal agent or agents to use or how long to treat neoadjuvantly before the initiation of the radiation or undergoing a radical prostatectomy. Neoadjuvant therapy does not appear to result in easier surgery, less blood loss, or fewer complications. None of the studies with either approach has yet demonstrated a clear effect on progression-free or overall survival. Such neoadjuvant hormonal therapy has mild toxicity but is associated with a significant financial cost.

Randomized controlled clinical trials are currently under way further evaluating all of these treatment strategies. In the next 5–10 years, more definitive conclusions should be available regarding the benefits and risks of such therapies in prostate cancer.

REFERENCES

1. Tulinius H. Latent malignancies at autopsy: A little used source of information in cancer biology. IARC Sci Publ 1991;253.
2. Parker SL, Tong T, Bolden S, Wingo PA. Cancer statistics, 1996. CA 1996;65:5.
3. Jones S, Salmon SE, eds. Adjuvant therapy of cancer II. New York: Grune & Stratton, 1979.
4. Stock RG. Locoregional therapies for early-stage prostate cancer. Oncology 1995;9:803.
5. Zietman AL, Coen JJ, Dallow KC, Shipley WU. The treatment of prostate cancer by conventional radiation therapy: An analysis of long-term outcome. Int J Radiat Oncol Biol Phys 1995;32:287.

6. Johansson JE, Andersson WO, Adam HO, Bergstrom R, Krusemo UB, Kraaz W. Natural history of localised prostatic cancer. Lancet 1989;799.
7. Aus G, Hugosson J, Norln L. Long-term survival and mortality in prostate cancer treated with non-curative intent. J Urol 1995;154:460.
8. Raghavan D. Adjuvant systemic therapy of prostate cancer. Semin Oncol 1995;22:633.
9. Partin AW, Mohler JL, Piantadosi S, et al. Selection of men at high risk for disease recurrence for experimental adjuvant therapy following radical prostatectomy. Urology 1995;45:831.
10. Huggins C, Hodges CV. The effect of castration, of estrogen, and of androgen injections on serum phosphatases in metastatic carcinoma of the prostate: Studies in prostate cancer. Cancer Res 1941;1:293.
11. Schellhammer P, Patterson AL, Sharifi R, et al. A controlled trial of bicalutamide versus flutamide, each in combination with LHRH in patients with advanced prostate cancer. Urology 1995;45:745.
12. Lee WR, Hanks GE. Radiation therapy following radical prostatectomy. Cancer 1995;75(Suppl):1909.
13. Coetzee LJ, Hars V, Paulson DF. Postoperative prostate-specific antigen as a prognostic indicator in patients with margin-positive prostate cancer, undergoing adjuvant radiotherapy after radical prostatectomy. Urology 1996;47(2):232.
14. Zincke H. Combined surgery and immediate adjuvant hormonal treatment for stage D1 adenocarcinoma of the prostate: Mayo Clinic experience. Semin Urol 1990;8(3):175.
15. Schmidt JD, Gibbons RP, Murphy GP, Bartolucci A. Adjuvant therapy for localized prostate cancer. Cancer 1993;71:1005.
16. Fisher B, Brown A, Wolmark N. Prolonging tamoxifen therapy for primary breast cancer: Findings of NSABP clinical trial. Ann Intern Med 1987;106:694.
17. Soloway MS, Sharifi R, Wajsman Z, McLeod D, Wood DP, Puras-Baez A, for the Lupron Depot Neoadjuvant Prostate Cancer Study Group. Randomized prospective study comparing radical prostatectomy alone versus radical prostatectomy preceded by androgen blockade in clinical stage B2 (T2b,Nx,M0) prostate cancer. J Urol 1995;154:424.
18. Labrie F, Cusan L, Gomez JL, et al. Downstaging by combination therapy with flutamide and an LHRH agonist before radical prostatectomy. Cancer Surv 1995;23:149.
19. Van Poppel H, De Ridder D, Elgamal AA, Van De Voorde W, Webrouck P, Ackaert K, Oyen R, Pittomvils G, Baert L, and members of the Belgian Uro-Oncological Study Group. Neoadjuvant hormonal therapy before radical prostatectomy decreases the number of positive surgical margins in stage T2 prostate cancer: Interim results of a prospective randomized trial. J Urol 1995;154:429.
20. Fair WR, Wang Y, Cohen D, et al. Neoadjuvant androgen deprivation therapy (ADT) in patients with clinically localized prostate cancer—Effect on (+) margins and post-operative PSA. J Urol 1995;153:313A.
21. Dalkin BL, Ahmann FR, Nagle R, Calley C. Randomized study of neoadjuvant androgen ablation therapy prior to radical prostatectomy in men with clinically localized prostate cancer. J Urol 1996;155:1357.
22. Cher ML, Shinohara K, Breslin S, Vapnek J, Carroll PR. High failure rate associated with long-term follow-up of neoadjuvant androgen deprivation followed by radical prostatectomy for stage C prostatic cancer. Br J Urol 1995;75:771.
23. Zelefsky MJ, Leibel SA, Burman CM, et al. Neoadjuvant hormonal therapy improves the therapeutic ratio in patients with bulky prostatic cancer treated with three-dimensional conformal radiation therapy. Int J Radiat Oncol Biol Phys 1994;29(4):755.
24. Eisbruch A, Perez CA, Roessler EH, Lockett MA. Adjuvant irradiation after prostatectomy for carcinoma of the prostate with positive surgical margins. Cancer 1994;73:384.
25. Petrovich Z, Lieskovsky G, Freeman J, et al. Surgery with adjuvant irradiation in patients with pathologic stage C adenocarcinoma of the prostate. Cancer 1995;76:1621.
26. Gibbons RP, Jonsson E. Adjuvant radiation therapy following radical prostatectomy for pathologic stage C prostate cancer. Eur Urol 1995;27(Suppl 2):24.
27. Anscher MS, Robertson CN, Prosnitz LR. Adjuvant radiotherapy for pathologic stage T3/4 adenocarcinoma of the prostate: Ten-year update. Int J Radiat Oncol Biol Phys 1995;33(1):37.
28. Forman JD, Kumar R, Haas G, Montie J, Porter AT, Mesina CF. Neoadjuvant hormonal downsizing of localized carcinoma of the prostate: Effects on the volume of normal tissue irradiation. Cancer Invest 1995;13(1):8.
29. Radiation Therapy Oncology Group. Phase III trial of androgen suppression before and during radiation therapy for locally advanced prostatic cancer: Abstract report of RTOG 8610. The prostate supplement, vol 5. New York: Wiley-Liss, Inc., 1994. p 2.

Adjuvant Therapy of Cancer VIII, edited by Sydney E. Salmon. Lippincott–Raven Publishers, Philadelphia © 1997.

25

Adjuvant Trials in Bladder Cancer: Scientific Background, Review, and New Directions

R. T. D. Oliver and C. Boshoff

Although many of the early breakthroughs in understanding the molecular biology and cytogenetics of clonal evolution of cancer came from studying colon tumors (1), developments in our knowledge of the situation in bladder cancer have been rapid recently (2) and are giving hope that it may not be long before it will be possible to use genetic probes to ascertain degrees of evolution for a particular tumor. Already studies of mutated p53 (3), β human choriogonadotrophin expression (4), and granulocyte colony stimulating factor expression (5) by these tumors are giving improved insight into tumor development and identifying potential targets for new therapeutic approaches. In addition, studies of HLA antigen loss as a mechanism for escape from immune surveillance (6) have identified a possible approach for developing the use of gene therapy in this tumor (7).

It is the aim of this review to consider the contribution that randomized trials have made to practice in treatment of bladder cancer and then to focus on possible new directions for future trials.

PATHOLOGY AND EPIDEMIOLOGY

There are two extremes of clinical behavior in bladder tumors: superficial disease which often requires repeated endoscopic treatments and invasive tumors which require radical therapy. Although the large majority of early bladder tumors at the intraepithelial (or *in situ* stage) show some evidence of papillary morphology, i.e., so-called pTa tumors which is also seen when they become invasive, there is a minority of tumors with flat *in situ* intraepithelial morphology which may be precursors for the solid invasive tumors (8). This suggests that there may be two separate paths of clonal evolution. Support for this view comes from cytogenetic studies that show a majority of tumors have 9q loss of heterozygosity as an early event, while there is a minority who do not (9).

The predominance of a papillary morphology raises the question as to whether there is a papilloma virus involved. There have been anecdotal reports of papilloma virus detection using different HPV DNA probes (10), particularly in situations of immunosuppression and by using them at very low stringency (11), the general consensus from most experienced labs working on HPV in cervical cancer is that there is no consistant association. Given that there are in excess of 60 known human papilloma viruses, some of which produce flattened areas of malignancy in the skin, and two or possibly more, morphological variants of intra-epithelial bladder cancer, it is possible that further research needs to be attempted in this field, given the long-term potential of developing a vaccine approach as is currently being used in cervix cancer (12).

In his landmark studies on papilloma-induced tumors in rabbits, Shope demonstrated two mechanisms whereby a benign papillary tumor became malignant. The first was via specific genetic resistance; in this he showed that there were rabbit strains which showed lesser or greater degrees of resistance, some only having benign papillary tumors and others advanced life-threatening invasive tumors after injection with the same viral preparation. The second mechanism he demonstrated was the impact of carcinogens. He demonstrated that it was possible to convert a benign papilloma in a resistant strain of rabbit by repeated painting of the tumor with carcinogen. This latter observation has considerable relevence to bladder cancer as it has long been known to be associated with ingestion of carcinogens such as analine dyes in industry, though also strongly associated with cigarette smoking. The risk of this is reduced by the duration of time off smoking. Less well known is that smoking may play a role in the progression to resistance to immunotherapy (Table 25-1) and in development of invasive disease (13).

CURRENT PRACTICE IN MANAGEMENT OF TRANSITIONAL CELL CARCINOMA OF THE BLADDER

Predominantly patients present with painless hematuria that proves to come from a tumor at cystoscopy. Occasionally a patient is discovered through investigation of cystitis symptoms (most frequently seen in respect of the so-called malignant cystitis associated with carcinoma *in situ*) or even more rarely investigation of uremia due to ureteric obstruction or unexplained metastases.

Conventionally, because it is so difficult to be sure there is not minor degrees of muscle invasion, all new patients are subjected to radical transurethral resection of tumor, examining the exophytic and muscle wall parts separately.

In the setting of unselected tumors, about 60% will prove to be superficial and 40% muscle invasive. For the superficial tumors no further treatment will be required in about 40%, while on occasion, if other health reasons preclude treatment about

TABLE 25-1 Influence of Cigarette Smoking on Durability of Complete Response After Intravesical BCG in Superficial Bladder Cancer (Oliver, unpublished)

	Number of Cases	Continued Complete Response at 12/12
Nonsmokers	18	83%
Smokers	9	22%

P < .004 Fishers exact test.

TABLE 25-2 Natural History of Superficial and Intensive Bladder Cancer

	Superficial	Invasive
Proportion of total cured by primary TURT	40%	5%
Intermittent relapsing pattern controlled by TURT	25%	2%
Relapsing patients needing intravesical chemo + cystectomy	20%	—
Early invasive	5%	25%
Late invasive +/– metastatic	10%	58%

40% of early muscle invasive tumors, i.e., 5% of all invasive tumors, will also remain tumor-free for 5 or more years. Table 25-2 summarizes the other aspects of management which will be discussed in more detail under the section dealing with the randomized trials which have provided the justification for the policy indicated.

INTRAVESICAL TREATMENT OF RECURRENT SUPERFICIAL TUMORS

About 20% of patients with superficial tumors (more than half those with flat carcinoma *in situ*, CIS) are considered at such risk for progression to invasive cancer that they are candidates for radical cystectomy. Because of the deterioration in quality of life such a procedure produces, many different treatments, ranging from chemotherapy through silver nitrate, radioisotopes, physical pressure, or heat have been used in an attempt to suppress recurrence. Today 6- to 12-weekly intravesical treatments with BCG, the attenuated mycobacterium used for tb prophylaxis has become standard in the United States because of the superior results in randomized trials against adriamycin and thiotepa (14,15) which had been the previous standard (Table 25-3). Supplements of vitamin A, possibly because of their known ability to improve immune resistance, have been proven to increase the duration of disease control in BCG recipients (16).

In Europe there is still a degree of dispute about the primacy of BCG as four of six trials against mitomycin failed to show significant benefit (17) and BCG can produce severe problems of toxicity including cystitis, shrunken bladder and even death from BCGosis (18). As there are several different strains of BCG with differing degrees of antigenic strength, the failure to show a difference between mitomycin and BCG in these trials could be unrelated to its anticancer effect. BCG is the only intravesical treatment so far that has 10-year follow-up studies proving that it produces a significant reduction of invasive or metastatic recurrences (19,20).

Because there is animal experimental evidence that surgical trauma in the bladder can induce tumor cell implantation, and data from sites of recurrence after TURT

TABLE 25-3. Progression-free Survival in Recurrent pT1/pT1S Bladder Cancer Randomized Trials (Ref. 17)

	BCG	Adriamycin	Thiotepa	Mitomycin
Lamm et al 1991 (*n* = 131)	70%	34%	—	—
Martinez Pinero et al 1990 (*n* = 171)	82%	52%	54%	—
Janhiamen et al 1990 (*n* = 92)	93%	—	—	62%
de Bruyne et al 1992 (*n* = 338)	58%	—	—	64%

in man that support the view that this could be happening in humans (21), there have been two large-scale randomized trials using single instillations of chemotherapy immediately after the first transurethral resection of tumor (22,23). Both trials had the same standard design, i.e., three-way randomization between control versus intravesical treatment ×1 only versus intravesical treatment ×1 at each 3-monthly check cystoscopy for 1 year (i.e., ×5). Mitomycin ×5 with 64% recurrence-free at 5 years compared to 54% after mitomycin ×1 and 39% in control, has established a significant advantage in this setting (23), although since the trial was reported it has not been widely adopted by urologists as standard practice.

FUTURE DIRECTIONS IN MANAGEMENT OF SUPERFICIAL BLADDER CANCER

Regular check cystoscopies, even when done with a flexible instrument without the need for anaesthesia, for 10 or more years, to say nothing of the indignity of weekly intravesical treatments, is not something that would be voluntarily accepted if alternative, less invasive, approaches were possible. Today the advent of oral drugs such as bropiramine which causes complete regression of established tumors in BCG failures in association with α interferon is offering the first alternative that does not involve bladder instrumentation (24). Because it requires interferon induction, and at present has to be taken for 3 days per week for 12 months, it is far from free of side effects. At the present time what data are available suggests that the results are as good as those from use of BCG, but the results of ongoing large scale randomized trials, currently only being done in CIS patients, are eagerly awaited.

Trials from use of human papilloma virus E7 antigen have begun in carcinoma of the cervix and have already produced evidence of response in patients with advanced disease (12). More work is needed to resolve the continued ongoing debate on whether HPV plays any role in bladder cancer. Given the immunoresponsiveness of superficial bladder cancer, a vaccine could be a very effective approach. With crude

TABLE 25-4. Randomized Trials of Radiation vs Cystectomy as Primary Model of Therapy for Bladder Cancer (Refs. 43, 44, 45)

	Single modality	Combination	χ^2	*P*
Radiation vs radiation + Cystectomy (*n* = 372)	27%	35%	3.0	NS
Cystectomy vs cystectomy + Radiation (*n* = 608)	36%	44%	4.0	.05

tumor cell vaccines being increasingly used in melanoma, and evidence from use of crude papillomavirus-induced tumor cell vaccines in cattle, it is possible that a case could be made to begin studies on crude tumor cell vaccines, perhaps combined with BCG, while awaiting the outcome of more intensive virology studies.

With intralesional studies in melanoma using liposomal preparations of HLA B7 having already demonstrated the ability of gene therapy to induce bystander immunity (25), the wide frequency of HLA loss demonstrable in bladder cancer and the considerable deterioration of quality of life following cystectomy, provides an excellent opportunity to justify treating such cases with HLA liposomal gene therapy.

RANDOMIZED TRIALS IN INVASIVE CANCER

Until recently the principal dispute in bladder cancer was between those who saw cystectomy as the standard and promoted trials to see if any improvement was possible by adding radiation and those who saw radiation as the standard and investigated the gain from adding cystectomy (Table 25-4). Neither approach produced major and statistically significant gain in terms of improved long-term cure. As published results seem to suggest that those treated by primarily surgical approaches were doing better, most recent studies have considered cystectomy as the standard. However this viewpoint has not taken into consideration the considerable degree of case selection that occurs in considering someone fit enough for radical cystectomy. The impact of this is most dramatically demonstrated when the results from Norwegian experience (based on cystectomy after radiation for the fitter, younger group and radiation for the rest) is compared with those from the Royal London Hospital who used radiation as the primary modality for all cases, with cystectomy only being offered as a salvage procedure if the patient failed to respond totally or recurred (26–29). There is a 34% difference in 5-year survival between the primary cystectomy and the primary radiation group in Norway, although when the results are pooled there is no difference from those reported by the Royal London Hospital using radiation as primary management for all cases (Table 25-5).

The most important observation to emerge from all these studies was the influence of tumor down staging by radiation with those patients achieving complete remission post-treatment having a 5-year survival in excess of 60% versus less than

TABLE 25-5 Comparison of Southern Norwegian and Royal London Hospital Experience of Radical Treatment for Invasive Bladder Cancer (Refs. 26, 29)

	No. of Cases	5-Year Survival
Norwegian Preop Radiation and Cystectomy (1980–90)	227	58%
Norwegian Primary Radical Radiotherapy (1980–90)	308	24%
Norwegian Total Radical Experience (1980–90 estimated)	535	38%
Royal London Hospital Primary Radiotherapy (1965–74)	352	34%
Royal London Hospital Primary Radical Radiotherapy (1974–85)	182	40%

30% in the nonresponders or partial responders (26–29). This has become a surrogate end point that is being widely used to assess new approaches to introducing chemotherapy into early management of invasive disease, as there is now increasing support for the view that control of primary disease may be important in determining long-term outcome.

Chemotherapy in Combination with Radical Cystectomy

American centers were the first to develop combination chemotherapy which produced durable complete remission in a minority of patients with established metastatic disease, and subsequently proved in a randomized trial that there was significantly better survival than with single agent (Table 25-6), albeit also demonstrating the big difference case selection to specialist centers produces. As these centers favored surgical approaches, this has been the first approach tried. As yet the major trial involving M-VAC after cystectomy has not fully recruited. Three other smaller trials have reported (Table 25-7). Only in a prematurely terminated trial using M-VAC after cystectomy has there been significant advantage (for review, see ref. 30).

Trials of Radiation versus Neoadjuvant or Synchronous Chemotherapy

No advantage could be demonstrated from combining neoadjuvant cisplatin (31) or methotrexate (32) as single agents before radiation in large-scale randomized trials, although in one trial comparing adriamycin with cisplatin as neoadjuvant before 2000 cGy in 5 days followed by cystectomy there was a statistically better survival (Table 25-7). A small trial comparing cisplatin given synchronously with radiation, stopped prematurely because of lack of interest in single agents when a random-

TABLE 25-6. Comparison of Memorial Hospital vs Intergroup Randomized Trial of M-Vac vs Cisplatin (Ref. 46)

	No of Patients	Response (CR + PR)	Median Survival (Months)
MSKCC cisplatin	38	37%	NA
Intergroup cisplatin alone	133	12%	8.3
M-VAC	121	72%	NA
Intergroup M-VAC	133	33%	13.5

ized trial using neoadjuvant CMV was set up, has shown some suggestion of benefit, albeit because of small numbers statistical significance was only demonstrated in terms of improved pelvic control. The large scale neoadjuvant CMV preconventional treatment trial, coordinated through the MRC in the United Kingdom (33) has now closed with 975 patients recruited. At first analysis, no signficant advantage has been observed, although as only 37% of the patients have died, this can only be considered as a provisional result

Future Directions in Invasive Tumors

Two areas of further interest have emerged from these randomized trials and more specifically from use of the surrogate end point of tumor downstaging. First is the

TABLE 25-7. Neoadjuvant and Adjuvant Chemotherapy in Cystectomy + Radiation-Based Randomized Trials (Ref. 30)

	Control	Trial Arm	*P*
A. Cystectomy-Based Trials			
Adjuvant CISCA ($n = 91$)	37%	44%	NS
Neoadjuvant cisplatin ($n = 122$)	52%	58%	NS
Adjuvant M-VAC ($n = 49$)	35%	73%	.01
B. Radiation-Based Trials			
Adjuvant adria/5FU after radiation ($n = 124$)	37%	35%	NS
Neoadjuvant and adjuvant MTX + irradiation ($n = 376$)	40%	40%	NS
Neoadjuvant cisplatin plus radiation ($n = 255$)	39%	39%	NS
Synchronous radiation + cisplatin ($n = 99$)	43%	61%	.06

TABLE 25-8. Non Randomized Studies of Primary Treatment of Invasive Bladder Cancer (Refs. 30, 42)

	No of Cases	Clinical TO
Cisplatin Combination Chemotherapy + TURT	225	51%
Cisplatin combination chemotherapy alone	300	27%
Radiation +TURT	182	52%
Radiation alone	352	43%
Radiation + concurrent Cisplatin + TURT	145	72%
Radiation + concurrent MOP_q 10+ TURB	11	82%

role of radical transurethral resection of the tumor which in one study when combined with single agent methotrexate produced 53% 3-year survival (34). An overview of chemotherapy and radiotherapy studies (Table 25-8) demonstrates that when radical TURT is done there is a 10–15% higher initial clinical complete remission rate in the bladder. However, given the animal data showing that trauma to urethelium can increase risk of implantation (35), taken with the risks from immunosuppression induced by prolonged anesthesia (36) and transfusion (37) and evidence from studies of prostate cancer demonstrating that pelvic surgery can increase the incidence of blood-borne tumor cells detectable by PCR (38), there has been increasing debate about possible benefits from neoadjuvant medical treatment before radical surgery (39) which is equally relevant to use of radical TURT. There is a strong case for a trial comparing its use as primary treatment with it's use after initial downstaging by chemotherapy (Fig. 25-1).

The second issue arises out of the observation that radiation in terms of initial tumor downstaging is better than any single chemotherapy agent and is at least equal or somewhat better than the best combination chemotherapy (30). Given that long experience with development of combination chemotherapy regimens demonstrates that synchronous use of multiple drugs with differing side effects is the best way to improve the therapeutic ratio, could there be benefit from incorporating radiation as a single agent into synchronous combination with chemotherapy? The data on the comparative effectiveness of single agent cisplatin used in the neoadjuvant compared to the synchronous mode (40) would suggest that there might be advantages, though the degree of toxicity of most combination chemotherapy regimens makes such an approach difficult to contemplate. Recently adapting some of the findings from dose intensification studies in testis cancer to metastatic bladder can-

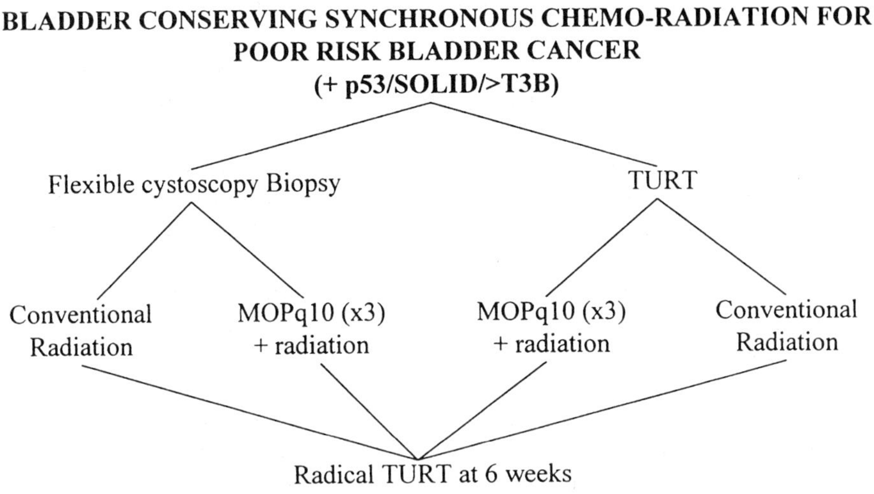

Figure 25-1. Overall survival is compared for 117 patients having resected intermediate or high-grade histologies of non-Hodgkin's lymphoma. Three cycles of CHOP followed by involved-field radiotherapy is superior to 8 cycles of CHOP alone ($P = 0.01$).

cer, our unit has developed a regimen that gives methotrexate vincristine and cisplatin every 10 days (41). Because the frequency of cisplatin in most other regimens is every 21–28 days we were able to demonstrate that the dose intensity of platinum was increased without increased toxicity, and that response was at least equal to that achievable by dose escalation of M-VAC using GCSF (Table 25-9). More recently we have completed a phase I assessment of how to give this regimen synchronously with radiation (42). After preliminary toxicity problems from using large field radiation, our most recently treated cohort of 11 patients receiving this chemotherapy three times during a 4-week course of 5500 cGy has reported 82% complete response (Table 25-8) which justifies further exploration of this approach in the setting of a formal phase II study to prove safety.

TABLE 25-9. Cisplatin Dose Intensification Studies in Bladder Cancer (Ref. 41)

	E-M VAC (ECOG)	E-M VAC (MSKCC)	MOPq10 (RLH)
No of patients	35	16	30
CR + PR	60%	69%	63%
CR	14%	25%	17%
Cisplatin dose intensity (mg/m²/week)	19.6	19.6	27

SUMMARY AND CONCLUSIONS

1. Superficial (both pTa + pTIS) bladder cancer is the most immunotherapeutically sensitive cancer in humans with an excess of 60% of patients becoming long-term relapse-free compared to 40% after adriamycin.
2. In one trial mitomycin equals BCG possibly because it used a more attenuated strain or because mitomycin C has a side effect of contact sensitivity causing allergic response. This might also explain why mitomycin has significant benefit from limited use after TURT.
3. With increasing knowledge of cytogenetic and molecular changes involved in tumor progression, new targets for gene therapy and molecular pharmacology are emerging, although a randomized trial of the effect of stopping smoking on tumor progression would be a more effective priority for the immediate future.
4. There is no demonstrable superiority in randomized trials of cystectomy over radiation in management of invasive bladder cancer. The apparent superiority in literature overviews is a product of case selection.
5. No neoadjuvant/adjuvant chemotherapy strategy has been proven superior to conventional treatment in randomized trial, though in one prematurely curtailed trial there is an indication that synchronous chemotherapy and radiation particularly using combination therapy is worth further study.
6. There is a need for a randomized trial to prove benefits/risks of radical TURT as first line strategy in management of invasive cancer.

REFERENCES

1. Vogelstein B, Fearon ER, Hamilton SR, et al. Genetic alterations during colorectal-tumor development. N Engl J Med 1988;319:527.
2. Dalbagni G, Presti G, Reuter J, Fair W, Cordon-Cardo C. Genetic alterations in bladder cancer. Lancet 1993;342:469.
3. Sarkis A, Bajorin D, Reuter V, et al. Prognostic value of p53 nuclear overexpression in patients with invasive bladder cancer treated with neoadjuvant M-Vac. J Clin Oncol 1995;13:1384.
4. Oliver RTD, Nouri AME, Crosby D, et al. Biological significance of beta hCG, HLA and other membrane antigen expression on bladder tumors and their relationship to tumor infiltrating lymphocytes (TIL). J Immunogenet 1989;16:381.
5. Daruwalla P, Oliver R, Heath E, et al. Granulocytosis and lymphopenia as prognostic factors in transitional carcinoma. B J Urol (submitted 1996).
6. Oliver RTD, Nouri AME. T cell immune response to cancer in humans and its relevance for immunodiagnosis and therapy. Cancer Surv 1991;13:173.
7. Nouri AME, Hussain FR, Oliver RTD. The frequency of major histocompatibility complex antigen abnormalities in urological tumors and their correction by gene transfection or cytokine stimulation. Cancer Gene Ther 1994;1:119.
8. Pugh R. The pathology of cancer of the bladder: An editorial over-view. Cancer 1973;32:1267.
9. Tyrkus M, Powell I, Fakr W. Cytogenetic studies of carcinoma *in situ* of the bladder: Prognostic implications. J Urol 1992;148:44.
10. Rovere GQD, Oliver RTD, McCance DJ, Castro JE. Development of bladder tumor containing HPV type 11 DNA after renal transplantation. Br J Urol 1988;62:36.
11. Sinclair AL, Nouri AME, Oliver RTD, Sexton C, Dalgleish AG. Bladder and prostate cancer screening for human papilloma virus by polymerase chain reaction: Conflicting results using different annealing temperatures. Br J Biol Sci 1993;50:350.
12. Fiander A, Nimako M, Adams M, et al. Immunotherapy in cervical cancer patients. Eur J Cancer 1995;31a(Suppl 581). [Abstr.]
13. England H, Paris A, Paris J. The correlation of T1 bladder tumor history with prognosis and follow-up requirements. Br J Urol 1981;53:593.

14. Lamm D, Blumenstein B, Crawford E, et al. A randomized trial of intravesical doxorubicin and immunotherapy with bacillus Calmette-Guerin for transitional-cell carcinoma of the bladder. N Engl J Med 1991;325:1205.
15. Martinez-Pineiro J, Leon JJ, Martinez-Pineiro, et al. Bacillus Calmette-Guerin versus doxorubicin versus thiotepa: A randomized prospective study in 202 patients with superficial bladder cancer. J Urol 1990;143:502.
16. Lamm D, Riggs D, Shriver J, et al. Megadose vitamins in bladder cancer—A double-blind clinical-trial. J Urol 1994;151:21.
17. Lamm D. BCG in perspective—Advances in the treatment of superficial bladder cancer. Eur Urol 1995;27:2.
18. Lamm D, Vandermeijden A, Morales A, et al. Indicence and treatment of complications of bacillus-Calmette-Guerin intravesical therapy in superficial bladder cancer. J Urol 1992;147:596.
19. Lamm D, Riggs D, Taynelis C, Nseyo U. Apparent failure of current intravesical chemotherapy prophylaxis to influence the long-term course of superficial transitional-cell carcinoma of the bladder. J Urol 1995;153:1444.
20. Herr H, Schwalb D, Zhang Z-F, et al. Intravesical bacillus Calmette-Guerin therapy prevents tumor progression and death from superficial bladder cancer: Ten-year follow-up of a prospective randomized trial. J Clin Oncol 1995;13:1404.
21. Oliver RTD. Monoclonality of multiple bladder cancers. N Engl J Med 1992;327(6):433.
22. MRC Working Party on Urological Cancer. The effect of intravesical thiotepa on the recurrence rate of newly diagnosed superficial bladder cancer. Br J Urol 1985;57:680.
23. Tolley D, Hargreave T, Smith P, et al. Effect of intravesical mitomycin C on recurrence of newly diagnosed superficial bladder cancer: Interim report from the Medical Research Council subgroup on superficial bladder cancer (urological cancer working party). B Med J 1988;296:1759.
24. Nabel G, Chang A, Hersh E, et al. Combined experience from phase 1 studies with allovectin-7, a direct gene transfer immunotherapeutic, in patients with metastatic solid tumors. Proc Am Soc Clin Oncol 1995;14. [Abstr. 582.]
25. Sarosdy M, Lowe B, Schellhammer P, et al. Bropiramine immunotherapy of bladder CIS: Positive phase II results of an oral interferon inducer. Proc Am Soc Clin Oncol 1994;13. [Abstr. 719.]
26. Waehre H, Ous S, Klevmark B, et al. A bladder cancer multi-institutional experience with total cystectomy for muscle-invasive bladder cancer. Cancer 1993;72:3044.
27. Fossa S, Waehre H, Aass N, et al. Bladder cancer definitive radiation therapy of muscle-invasive bladder cancer. A retrospective analysis of 317 patients. Cancer 1993;72:3036.
28. Blandy JP, England HR, Evans SJW, et al. T3 bladder cancer—The case for salvage cystectomy. Br J Urol 1980;52:506.
29. Jenkins BJ, Caulfield MJ, Fowler CC, et al. Reappraisal of the role of radical radiotherapy and salvage cystectomy in the treatment of invasive (T2/T3) bladder cancer. Br J Urol 1988;62:343.
30. Zietman A, Shipley W, Kaufman D. The combination of cisplatin based chemotherapy and radiation in the treatment of muscle-invading transitional cell cancer of the bladder. Int J Radiat Oncol Biol Phys 1993;27:161.
31. Wallace D, Raghaven D, Kelly K, et al. Neo-adjuvant (pre-emptive) cisplatin therapy in invasive transitional cell carcinoma of the bladder. Br J Urol 1991;67:608.
32. Shearer R, Chilvers C, Bloom H, et al. Adjuvant chemotherapy in T3 carcinoma of the bladder. A prospective trial: Preliminary report. Br J Urol 1988;62:558.
33. Hall RR. Neo-adjuvant CMV chemotherapy and cystectomy or radiotherapy in muscle invasive bladder cancer. First analysis of MRC/EORTC intercontinental trial. Proc Amer Soc Clin Oncol 1996; 15:Abstr. 612:214.
34. Hall R, Newling D, Ramsden P, et al. Treatment of invasive bladder cancer by local resection and high dose methotrexate. Br J Urol 1984;56:668.
35. Alexander P, Murphy P, Skipper D. Preferential growth of blood borne cancer cells at site of trauma: A growth promoting role of macrophages. Adv Exp Med Biol 1988;33:245.
36. Oliver RTD, Riddle P, Blandy JP. Operative factors & tumor membrane antigen changes in escape from immune surveillance of bladder cancer. In: EORTC Genitourinary Group monograph 10—Urological oncology: Reconstructive surgery, organ conservation, and restoration of function. New York, 1991;161.
37. Heiss M, Mempel W, Delanoff C, et al. Blood transfusion-modulated tumor recurrence: First results of a randomized study of autologous versus allogeneic blood transfusion in colorectal cancer surgery. J Clin Oncol 1994;12:1859.
38. Eschwege P, Dumas F, Blanchet P, et al. Haematogenous dissemination of prostatic epithelial cells during radical prostatectomy. Lancet 1995;346:1528.
39. Oliver R. Does surgery disseminate or accelerate cancer? Lancet 1995;346:1506.

40. Ghersi D, Stewart L, Parmar M, et al. Does neoadjuvant cisplatin-based chemotherapy improve the survival of patients with locally advanced bladder cancer: A meta-analysis of individual patient data from randomized clinical trials. Br J Urol 1995;75:206.
41. Boshoff C, Oliver R, Gallagher C, Ong J. Accelerated cisplatin-based chemotherapy for advanced bladder cancer. Eur J Cancer 1995;31A:1633.
42. Boshoff C, Gallagher CJ, Oliver RTD, et al. A pilot study of combination chemotherapy with concurrent radiotherapy in patients with locally advanced bladder cancer. Proc Am Soc Clin Oncol 1995;14:249,Abstr. 670.
43. Lerner P, Skinner G. Radical cystectomy for bladder cancer. In: Vogelzang N, ed. Comprehensive textbook in genito urinary oncology. Baltimore: Williams & Wilkins, 1996. p 442.
44. Bloom H, Hendry W, Wallace D, Skeet R. Treatment of T3 bladder cancer: Controlled trial of preoperative radiotherapy and radical cystectomy versus radical radiotherapy. Br J Urol 1982;54:136.
45. Sell A, Jakobsen A, Nerstrom B, et al. Treatment of advanced bladder cancer category T2 T3 and T4a. Scand J Urol Nephrol Suppl 1991;138:193.

Adjuvant Therapy of Cancer VIII, edited
by Sydney E. Salmon. Lippincott–Raven
Publishers, Philadelphia © 1997.

26
Adjuvant Concepts in Testicular Cancer

Lawrence H. Einhorn

Testis cancer has become a model for a curable neoplasm (1). Overall, 80% of patients with metastatic testis cancer will be cured with modern chemotherapy strategies. The volume of metastatic disease and the multiplicity of anatomic sites at the initiation of chemotherapy are important determinants of chemocurability (2).

CLASSICAL ADJUVANT CHEMOTHERAPY

Retroperitoneal lymph node dissection (RPLND) is frequently employed, following orchiectomy, in patients with early stage nonseminomatous germ cell tumors (NSGCT). At Indiana University, most patients with clinical stage I and clinical stage II NSGCT with less than 3 cm maximal transverse diameter of retroperitoneal mass will undergo a nerve-sparing RPLND (3). Over 95% of such patients will have antegrade ejaculation.

Adjuvant cisplatin combination chemotherapy is attractive in patients with pathologic stage II disease (with no gross disease left behind and normal post-RPLND serum tumor markers). In other cancers, the prevention of a postoperative relapse will increase the overall survival, as cure is rare in other solid tumors. However, testis cancer is unique in this setting. Patients not cured by RPLND will usually relapse in the first postoperative year, and occasionally (about 10%) in the second postoperative year, and rarely are relapses seen beyond 2 years. Relapses are manifested as either pulmonary metastases, supraclavicular nodes, or elevated serum alphafetoprotein (AFP) or human chorionic gonadotropin (HCG). Retroperitoneal relapse is uncommon in patients who have an adequate RPLND. Patients can thusly be followed postoperatively once a month the first year, every 2 months the second year, and every 6–12 months subsequently. This should guarantee that if a relapse occurs, it will present as favorable (minimal or moderate) extent disease and have >90% probability of cure with three courses of cisplatin, etoposide, and bleomycin (4).

A phase II intergroup study was initiated in 1979 and completed in 1985 for patients with pathologic stage II disease. Patients were randomized to close observation as detailed above versus two courses of cisplatin combination chemotherapy at 4-week intervals. One hundred and ninety-three patients were evaluable. Of the 97 observed patients, 47 (48%) have recurred, compared to 1 of 96 patients with adjuvant chemotherapy. However, the follow-up schedule was effective in detecting small volume relapse, and virtually all relapses were cured with subsequent cisplatin combination chemotherapy. Thus, there was no difference in overall survival (5). This large intergroup study has confirmed the excellent results with either of the two strategies. The probability of recurrence can be predicted by the size and number of positive retroperitoneal nodes. Two courses of adjuvant chemotherapy will obviate any serious concern about relapse, and such patients are followed just every 3 months for the first postoperative year, every 6 months the second year, and then annually. However, it is equally attractive to delay chemotherapy until relapse, at which time three courses of cisplatin + etoposide + bleomycin will cure virtually all patients.

"ADJUVANT" ORCHIECTOMY

The testis is a relative sanctuary site. Occasionally, chemotherapy for metastatic disease is started before orchiectomy is performed (massive metastatic disease or occult testis primary). We have recently reviewed the results of orchiectomy after induction chemotherapy (6). This retrospective review of delayed orchiectomy with concomitant RPLND was analyzed in 160 patients. The orchiectomy specimen contained only necrosis in 70 (44%), teratoma in 50 (31%), and germ cell cancer in 40 (25%). Of the 40 with cancer in the orchiectomy specimen, 17 (42%) had necrosis and 16 (40%) teratoma in the RPLND, with no cancer in the larger retroperitoneal metastases remaining postchemotherapy. Thus, orchiectomy is necessary in this patient population.

CLINICAL STAGE I DISEASE

Clinical stage I disease implies that postorchiectomy there is no clinical evidence of testis cancer. Physical examination, serum HCG and AFP, and abdominal and chest CT scans are all normal. There are three potential therapeutic options: namely, nerve-sparing (NS) RPLND, surveillance, or chemotherapy. Risk factors for failure to cure with orchiectomy alone include vascular or lymphatic invasion in the orchiectomy specimen, predominance of embryonal carcinoma (and presumably choriocarcinoma), and absence of yolk sac tumor. The overall probability of relapse with surveillance is 30%. At Indiana University, our preferred strategy is NS RPLND. However, there are some patients who have very favorable prognostic and histologic characteristics, and in this setting, surveillance is equally attractive. I personally do not favor primary chemotherapy for poor-risk clinical stage I NSGCT. Although most, if not all, patients are cured with two courses of cisplatin combination chemotherapy, this significantly increases the morbidity of therapy, including infertility due to impaired spermatogenesis. Also, clinical stage I patients should have a cure rate that approaches 100%. Occasional stage I patients who receive two courses of cisplatin combination chemotherapy may indeed harbor occult grossly positive retroperitoneal nodes, and two courses may be insufficient to routinely cure all of these patients.

There is no controversy concerning the management of pathologic stage I NSGCT. These patients will have an 8–10% probability of relapse and do not need any form of adjuvant therapy. Virtually all relapses should be cured with chemotherapy, assuming appropriate follow-up is done post-RPLND.

Standard therapy in the United States for clinical stage I seminoma is adjuvant abdominal radiotherapy. There have been several published series evaluating surveillance in this patient population in Canada and Europe. A nationwide Danish surveillance study entered 261 patients with clinical stage I seminoma. The median follow-up was 48 months (range 6–67 months). Forty-nine (19%) patients relapsed, with most recurrences in the retroperitoneal nodes. Thirty-seven (76%) of 49 relapses were treated with radiotherapy, 33 of 37 (89%) are continuously disease-free (NED), and 36 of 37 are currently NED. The other 12 patients initially received chemotherapy and there were no subsequent relapses, but there were two deaths from sepsis. The size of the testis tumor was significant. The 4-year relapse-free survival with orchiectomy alone was 94%, 82%, and 62% for tumors <3, 3–6, and >6 cm (7). Similar data (80% cure rate with orchiectomy alone) were reported by investigators at Princess Margaret Hospital in Toronto. However, I personally feel the standard approach should remain adjuvant radiotherapy, except perhaps for patients with small (<3 cm) tumors.

RADIOGRAPHIC STAGE I NSGCT WITH ELEVATED MARKERS

Most patients with NSGCT and normal chest and abdominal CT scans will also have normal postorchiectomy markers (clinical stage I disease). However, a special clinical situation is seen in patients with normal physical exam, and normal CT scans, but persistently elevated HCG and/or AFP. Data from both Memorial Sloan-Kettering Cancer Center and Indiana University suggest that chemotherapy, rather than an RPLND, is the optimal postorchiectomy strategy for this group of patients. Davis et al. examined 11 such patients who were treated with RPLND postorchiectomy. All 11 patients had persistent marker elevation following RPLND and required chemotherapy (8). Saxman et al. retrospectively reviewed 30 similar patients, also treated with RPLND postorchiectomy. Of six patients with elevated AFP, five (83%) had relapse and required chemotherapy, as did six of 24 (25%) with HCG elevation.

REFERENCES

1. Einhorn LH. Treatment of testicular cancer: A new and improved model. J Clin Oncol 1990;8:1777.
2. Birch R, Williams SD, Cone A, Einhorn LH, et al. Prognostic factors for favorable outcome in disseminated germ cell tumors. J Clin Oncol 1986;4:400.
3. Donohue JP, Thornhill JA, Foster RS, Rowland RG, Bihrle R. Retroperitoneal lymphadenectomy for clinical stage A testis cancer: Modification of technique and impact on ejaculation. J Urol 1993;149:237.
4. Einhorn LH, Williams SD, Loehrer PJ, et al. Evaluation of optimal duration of chemotherapy in favorable prognosis disseminated germ cell tumors: An SECSG protocol. J Clin Oncol 1989;7:387.
5. Williams SD, Stablein DM, Einhorn LH, et al. Pathologic stage II testis cancer: Immediate adjuvant chemotherapy versus observation with treatment at relapse. N Engl J Med 1987;3178:1433.
6. Leibovitch I, Little JS, Foster RS, Rowland RG, Bihrle R, Donohue JP: Delayed orchiectomy after chemotherapy for metastatic nonseminomatous germ cell tumors. J Urol 1996;155:952.
7. von der Maase H, Specht L, Jacobsen GK, et al. Surveillance following orchiectomy for stage I seminoma of the testis. Eur J Cancer 1993;29A:1931.
8. Davis BE, Herr HW, Fair WR, Bosl GJ. The management of patients with nonseminomatous germ cell tumors of the testis with serologic disease only after orchiectomy. J Urol 1994;152:111.
9. Saxman SB, Nichols CR, Foster RS, Messemer JE, Donohue JP, Einhorn LH: The management of patients with clinical stage I nonseminomatous testicular tumors and persistently elevated serologic markers. J Urol 1996;155:587.

VI

Lymphoma, Melanoma, and Sarcoma

Adjuvant Therapy of Cancer VIII, edited
by Sydney E. Salmon. Lippincott–Raven
Publishers, Philadelphia © 1997.

27

CHOP Plus Radiotherapy Is Superior to CHOP Alone for Adjuvant Therapy of Resected Localized Unfavorable Non-Hodgkin's Lymphoma: A Southwest Oncology Group Study

Thomas P. Miller, Steve Dahlberg, James R. Cassady, David J. Adelstein, Catherine M. Spier, Thomas M. Grogan, Susan Carlin, Ellen Chase, Michael LeBlanc, and Richard I. Fisher

Treatment of intermediate and high-grade histologies of non-Hodgkin's lymphoma (NHL) provides a paradigm for adjuvant therapy of cancer. Approximately 20% of patients with aggressive histologic subtypes of NHL have limited disease (stage I or II) and excisional biopsies (lumpectomy) often remove all visible or palpable disease. Without additional therapy, however, such patients invariably relapse and recurrent disease frequently involves distant sites. Localized NHL has been treated with regional radiotherapy with mixed results (1–4). Carefully selected patients following aggressive staging techniques (even laparotomy on occasion) can be cured with regional radiotherapy. However, results are not optimal because lymphomas are generally systemic diseases and hematogeneous spread occurs early in the disease course.

Advanced stages of NHL can be successfully treated with doxorubicin-containing combination chemotherapy and at least 30% of such patients are cured (5). Thus, the expectation is that systemic chemotherapy can eliminate microscopic metasatic disease. In 1979, Miller and Jones first published results using doxorubicin-containing chemotherapy as initial therapy in 23 patients with apparent localized forms of NHL (6). Some of these patients received consolidative involved field radiotherapy following chemotherapy. The survival estimate at 5 years exceeded 90% and the results seemed dramatically improved compared to historical series using radiotherapy alone. Subsequent single institution experiences confirmed that impression and have been reviewed in detail (7–9). Most of the series are relatively small and do not distinguish patients having resected disease from those patients having residual palpable or visible lymphoma. In the current study, 117 patients who had all disease resected at the time of initial biopsy were treated with adjuvant doxorubicin-containing combination chemotherapy (CHOP). The study was designed to determine whether three cycles of CHOP chemotherapy followed by involved field radiotherapy was superior to chemotherapy alone using eight cycles of CHOP (Figure 27-1).

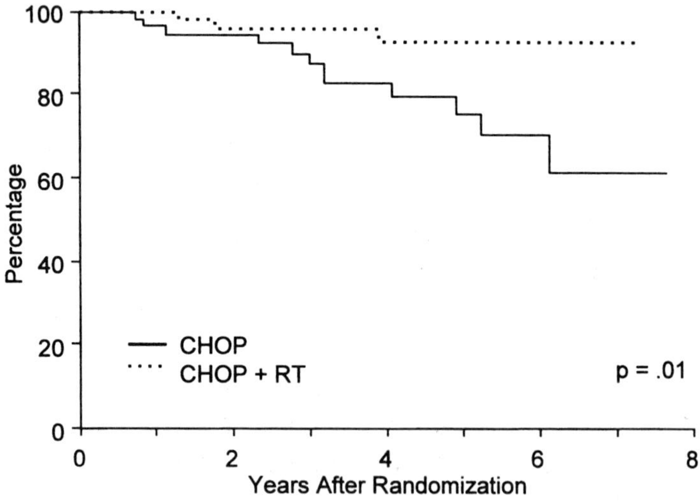

Figure 27-1. Localized lymphoma—SWOG 8736. Overall survival is compared for 117 patients having resected intermediate or high-grade histologies of non-Hodgkin's lymphoma. Three cycles of CHOP followed by involved-field radiotherapy is superior to 8 cycles of CHOP alone ($P = 0.01$).

METHODS

Between 1987 and 1995, 404 eligible patients were entered onto Southwest Oncology Group study 8736 (SWOG 8736) which was a therapeutic trial designed to compare two treatment programs for patients with visually localized (stage I or II) aggressive histologies of non-Hodgkin's lymphoma. Patients were eligible for entry who had biopsy-proven intermediate or high-grade histologies of non-Hodgkin's lymphoma (except lymphoblastic subtype) according to the Working Formulation. Stage I and IE and nonbulky II and IIE were included. The final stage designation was determined using extent of disease measurements made prior to lymph node excisional biopsy. All patients were ambulatory and included SWOG performance status of 0, 1, or 2. Patients were excluded who had a history of congestive heart failure, symptoms or findings of central nervous system disease, or any prior treatment for lymphoma. Clinical staging procedures were used to determine the extent of disease prior to registration and included peripheral blood counts, serum chemistries, a chest radiograph, a CT scan of the abdomen and pelvis, and a bone marrow biopsy.

Eligible patients were stratified at the time of registration on the basis of age (65 years or older versus less than 65 years), stage (I versus II), histology (diffuse large cell versus all other subtypes), location of disease involvement (gastrointestinal sites involved versus all other sites), and whether or not disease had been resected (complete resection versus residual disease).

This report describes 117 patients who had all disease resected at the time of diagnosis and prior to randomization. These patients were randomized to receive eight cycles of CHOP chemotherapy versus three cycles of CHOP chemotherapy followed by involved field radiotherapy. CHOP chemotherapy included cyclophosphamide, 750 mg/m^2, IV on day 1; doxorubicin, 50 mg/m^2, IV on day 1; vincristine, 1.4 mg/m^2 (maximum of 2.0 mg), IV on day 1; and prednisone, 100 mg, PO on days 1–5. The radiotherapy was delivered to all involved sites of disease determined prior to biopsy. The minimum dose was 4000 cGy. A maximum dose of 5500 cGy was given and the exact total dose was at the discretion of the treating radiotherapist. In general, higher doses were given if, in the opinion of the treating radiotherapist, residual overt disease persisted after the patient had received 4000 cGy. The daily dose varied between 180 and 200 cGy.

RESULTS

Of 404 patients entered in SWOG 8736, 117 patients had all visible and evaluable disease resected at the time of initial biopsy. Most of these 117 patients had stage I or IE disease at the time of diagnosis (109 patients). Although the study was not designed to test the effect of surgical resection of disease, patients having had all disease resected had a better overall survival than those patients with residual disease (287 patients). The 5-year survival estimate for patients having disease resected was 89%, whereas the 5-year estimate for patients with residual disease was 78% ($P = 0.01$). The difference in progression-free survival was even greater comparing patients with all disease resected to those patients with residual visible or palpable disease ($P = 0.001$). As a comparison of patients with all disease resected to patients with residual disease is confounded by stage (primarily comparison of stage I versus stage II), we considered only patients with stage I and compared patients having all disease resected to patients with residual disease for survival ($P = 0.07$) and progression-free survival ($P = 0.03$).

The primary objective of the study was to compare eight cycles of CHOP to three cycles of CHOP followed by involved field radiotherapy. For 117 patients having all disease resected, three cycles of CHOP plus radiotherapy was superior to eight cycles of CHOP with regard to survival ($P = 0.01$) and progression-free survival ($P = 0.03$) (see Figure 27-1). The 5-year estimate of survival for patients treated with CHOP alone was 76% and for patients treated with CHOP plus radiotherapy was 93%. Comparisons of additional subsets of patients are limited by patient numbers and generally lack power to detect differences. Nevertheless, the treatment of gastrointestinal lymphoma has been discussed in numerous retrospective series and we took the opportunity to look at 40 patients prospectively registered who had gastrointestinal involvement with aggressive histologies of NHL. These data show no difference in overall survival comparing 16 patients having had all disease resected prior to treatment to 24 patients treated with chemotherapy or chemotherapy plus radiotherapy and having residual disease ($P = 0.58$). Further, overall survival curves were superimposable when comparing 20 patients with gastrointestinal disease treated with eight cycles of CHOP to 20 patients treated with CHOP plus radiotherapy

($P = 0.86$). Survival curves were also superimposable for patients treated with CHOP compared to patients treated with CHOP plus radiotherapy whether there was residual disease ($P = 0.90$) or whether all disease was resected ($P = 0.70$).

DISCUSSION

The results of SWOG 8736 indicate that three cycles of CHOP plus RT is superior to eight cycles of CHOP for adjuvant treatment of resected NHL. Further, the 5-year survival estimate of 93% following treatment with CHOP plus RT indicates that microscopic metastatic lymphoma can be successfully eliminated with as few as three cycles of chemotherapy. We can only surmise that the apparent beneficial effects of involved field RT result from elimination of residual disease at the resection site that was not apparent to the treating physician following surgical resection. The study was not designed to test the efficacy of surgical resection, and thus, there was no effort directed to wide excision or regional lymphadenectomy. Similar results have been reported following lumpectomy in breast cancer wherein lumpectomy plus adjuvant chemotherapy is inferior to lumpectomy followed by mastectomy or RT with adjuvant chemotherapy.

The best sequence of treatment for localized NHL has been previously investigated. Patients with clinically localized NHL have been aggressively staged including a laparotomy, and 10–28% are reported to have occult abdominal disease (3,10–13). Inasmuch as laparotomy represents a limited sampling of possible involved sites of disease, we presume the incidence of occult microscopic metastases is much higher. Further, several retrospective reviews of patient outcome following treatment with RT alone consistently note that 10–20% of clinically staged patients progress (usually in distant sites) during the time required to complete treatment with RT (4,14,15). Thus, there is evidence to suggest that the optimal sequence for adjuvant treatment of resected NHL begin with chemotherapy of proven curative potential. In the current study all patients received doxorubicin-containing chemotherapy as initial adjuvant therapy for resected disease.

Treatment of aggressive histologies of NHL involving the gastrointestinal tract has been reviewed in detail (16). Controversy exists over the roles of surgery, radiotherapy, and chemotherapy (17,18). The current study was not designed to specifically investigate the best management of gastrointestinal NHL and lacks the power to reach firm conclusions. Nevertheless, 40 patients having gastrointestinal disease were prospectively registered, eliminating some of the selection bias of past retrospective reviews. In this "pilot" setting, we see no support for the concept that gastrointestinal disease must be resected based on overall survival or complications of treatment (only one patient treated with residual NHL in the stomach required surgical intervention following treatment with chemotherapy). We also observed no leads as to whether CHOP alone or CHOP plus RT might be a superior treatment strategy for this particular site of disease involvement.

In conclusion, (a) three cycles of CHOP followed by involved-field RT was superior to eight cycles of CHOP alone as adjuvant therapy of resected aggressive histologies of NHL, (b) resecting localized NHL may improve survival, and (c) more patients with localized gastrointestinal lymphoma must be studied to determine the relative utility of surgery, radiotherapy, or chemotherapy.

ACKNOWLEDGMENTS

This investigation was supported in part by the following PHS Cooperative Agreement grant numbers awarded by the National Cancer Institute, DHHS: CA38926, CA32102, CA13612, CA46282, CA04919, CA22433, CA20319, CA12644, CA04920, CA46441, CA27057, CA42777, CA46113, CA35281, CA42028, CA28862, CA35261, CA58861, CA45377, CA37981, CA58686, CA35431, CA45807, CA58416, CA35090, CA45807, CA32734, CA46136, CA35128, CA35119, CA35176, CA52772, CA58348, CA12213, CA45560, CA45466, CA58882, CA45450, CA35178, CA16385, CA52654, CA58415, CA35192, CA46368, CA35262, CA58723, CA52771, CA63850, CA52654.

REFERENCES

1. Miller TP. Therapy of localized non-Hodgkin's lymphomas. In: DeVita VT Jr, Hellman S, Rosenberg SA, eds. Cancer: Principles and practice of oncology updates III (6). Philadelphia: J. B. Lippincott, 1989.
2. Miller TP, Grogan TM. Patients with localized non-Hodgkin's lymphomas provide opportunities for future research. Oncology 1991;5:127–131.
3. Sweet DL, Kinxie J, Gacke ME, et al. Survival of patients with localized diffuse histiocytic lymphoma. Blood 1981;58:1218.
4. Hudson BV, Hudson GV, MacLennan KA, et al. Clinical stage I non-Hodgkin's lymphoma: Long term follow-up of patients treated by the British National Lymphoma Investigation with radiotherapy alone as initial therapy. Br J Cancer 1994;69:1088–1093.
5. Fisher RI, Gaynor ER, Dahlberg S, et al. Phase III comparison of CHOP vs. m-BACOD vs. ProMACE-CytaBOM vs. MACOP-B in patients with intermediate or high-grade non-Hodgkin's lymphoma: Results of SWOG-8516 (Intergroup 0067), the national high priority lymphoma study. N Engl J Med 1993;328:1002–1006.
6. Miller TP, Jones SE. Chemotherapy of localized histiocytic lymphoma. Lancet 1979;8:358–360.
7. Jones SE, Miller TP, Connors JM. Long term follow-up and analysis for prognostic factors for patients with limited stage diffuse large cell lymphoma treated with initial chemotherapy with or without adjuvant radiotherapy. J Clin Oncol 1989;7:1186–1191.
8. Cabanillas F. Chemotherapy as definitive treatment of stages I–II large cell and diffuse mixed lymphomas. Hematol Oncol 1981;3:25.
9. Connors JM, Klimo P, Fairey RN, et al. Brief chemotherapy and involved field radiation therapy for limited-stage histologically aggressive lymphoma. Ann Intern Med 1987;107:25.
10. Veronesi U, Musumeci R, Pizzatti F, et al. The value of staging laparotomy in non-Hodgkin's lymphomas. Cancer 1974;33:446–459.
11. Lester JN, Fuller LM, Conrad FG, et al. The roles of staging laparotomy, chemotherapy, and radiotherapy in the management of localized diffuse large cell lymphoma: A study of 75 patients. Cancer 1982;49:1746–1753.
12. Goffinet DR, Warnke R, Dunnick NR, et al. Clinical and surgical (laparotomy) evaluation of patients with non-Hodgkin's lymphomas. Cancer Treat Rep 1977;61:981–992.
13. Chabner BA, Johnson RE, DeVita VT, et al. Sequential staging in non-Hodgkin's lymphoma. Cancer Treat Rep 1977;61:993–997.
14. Landberg TG, Hakanssan LG, Moller TR, et al. CVP-remission-maintenance in stage I or II non-Hodgkin's lymphomas: Preliminary results of a randomized study. Cancer 1979;44:831.
15. Bajetta E, Buzzoni R, Bonadonna G, et al. Combined radiotherapy-chemotherapy (CVP versus bACOP) in stage I–II diffuse non-Hodgkin's lymphomas. In: Salmon SE, Jones SE, eds. Adjuvant therapy of cancer III. New York: Grune & Stratton, 1981.
16. List AF, Hande KR. Lymphomas of the gastrointestinal tract. In: MacDonald JS, ed. Gastrointestinal oncology: Basic and clinical aspects. Boston: Martinus Nijhoff Publishers, 1987.

17. Flemming ID, Mitchell S, Dilawari RA. The role of surgery in the management of gastric lymphoma. Cancer 1982;49:135.
18. Rosenfelt F, Rosenberg SA. Diffuse histiocytic lymphoma presenting with gastrointestinal tract lesions. Cancer 1980;45:2188.

Adjuvant Therapy of Cancer VIII, edited by Sydney E. Salmon. Lippincott–Raven Publishers, Philadelphia © 1997.

28

Adjuvant Therapy of High-Risk Melanoma: The Role of High-Dose Interferon α-2b

John M. Kirkwood, Myla Hunt Strawderman, Marc S. Ernstoff, Thomas Smith, Ernest Borden, and Ronald Blum

Skin cancers are the most prevalent of all neoplasms, with nearly a million new cases developing each year in the United States. The vast majority of these are basal cell or squamous neoplasms, related to cumulative sun exposure and readily cured by local excision. Melanoma is the most lethal of the cancers that arise in the skin, and while the surgical cure rate for melanoma is >80% overall, more than 7,000 deaths each year are attributable to metastatic melanoma in the more than 34,000 new cases observed each year. The rate of incidence of this disease continues to rise at ~4% per year, more rapidly than other solid tumors, and the rising death rate demands new therapies.

Melanoma has been the subject of an extensive immunological literature, as a consequence of the well-documented responsiveness of this tumor to a variety of immunological interventions ranging from microbial immunostimulants and vaccines to cytokines including the interferons (IFNs). This discussion will be limited to the effects of interferons upon melanoma.

The interferons derived from buffy-coat leukocytes, lymphoblastoid cell lines, and recombinant DNA technology have each shown evidence of antitumor activity in melanoma. Interferons of type I, and specifically the recombinant DNA-produced IFN α-2 subspecies (IFN α-2a, b, and c produced by Hoffman LaRoche, Schering-Plough, and Boehringer-Ingelheim) have been studied in large enough clinical trials to demonstrate reproducible evidence of antitumor activity, which is as great as that of any single systemic antitumor modality for patients with metastatic melanoma (1).

The clinical evidence of antitumor activity of interferons that have been reported in patients with metastatic disease served as the impetus for a series of adjuvant trials of the interferons which commenced in the early 1980s in the United States and abroad. The criteria of risk for melanoma recurrence and death that served to define eligibility for these trials varied considerably, ranging from regional nodal metastasis (constituting the highest risk determinant) to primary tumor depth of greater than 1.5 mm (T3), or 4.0 mm (T4), which constitute determinants of intermediate risk apart from nodal metastasis.

The first-reported adjuvant trials of interferon in melanoma were nonrandomized and generally employed nonrecombinant interferons of buffy-coat leukocyte origin. These trials are difficult to interpret, although they have been viewed as positive in reference to historic experience; the trial of Kokoshka (2) utilized low dosages of interferon given for 6 months, and raised the possibility that treatment diminished the frequency of relapses for patients during the interval of their therapy—with subsequent loss of any effect after the discontinuation of therapy.

The industrial production of recombinant IFN α-2 afforded clinical investigators more plentiful, pure, and consistent preparations of interferon and spurred the initiation of multicenter cooperative groups in the United States and Europe. These diverse trials of IFN α-2 administered by IM, IV, and/or SC routes for 3 months, 12 months, 24 months, or 36 months have recently begun to yield the first evidence of effective therapy for melanoma in the literature. The entry criteria, treatment regimens, and summary outcomes of these trials and the cooperative groups that performed them are summarized in Table 28-1.

The trials of the Eastern Cooperative Oncology Group (ECOG) and North Central Cancer Treatment Group (NCCTG) commenced in 1983–1984 and are the most mature, having recently been reported at maturity (3–5).

The ECOG trial E1684 has revealed the first significant impact of adjuvant therapy upon relapse and survival. This trial employed maximal tolerable dosages of IFN α-2b administered daily × 5 per week for the first 4 weeks by the IV route, and three times weekly for the next 48 weeks by the SC route. IFN α-2b was shown to be tolerable at dosages of up to 20 μ/m^2/day by the IV route, and 10 μ/m^2/day by the SC route, in early trials conducted at our center (6–8). On the basis of these phase I studies of IFN α-2b, and early phase II trials which in aggregate suggested that clinical antitumor response to IFN α-2b was most frequent when the agent was administered at the maximal tolerable dosages, an adjuvant trial was proposed to test the potential benefit of dosages of IFN α-2b, 20 μ/m^2/day administered IV daily × 5 for 4 weeks, then 10 μ/m^2/day thrice weekly for the next 48 weeks. This regimen of high-dose IFN α-2b administered for one year was compared with observation in a randomized multicenter setting in a trial designated E1684, which was open for accrual from 1984 to 1990.

Patients with resected histologically proven cutaneous melanoma who had a high risk for recurrence were eligible for this trial if they had no prior systemic adjuvant therapy or evidence of distant metastases. Four groups of patients were stratified at entry according to stage: (i) patients with deep primary lesions of > 4 mm Breslow depth, but without metastatic disease identified on elective regional lymphadenectomy; (ii) patients with any depth of primary, and clinically inapparent regional lymphadenopathy, who revealed microscopic involvement of regional nodes at elective lymphadenectomy; (iii) patients with synchronous primary melanomas of any depth and palpable regional lymphadenopathy; and (iv) patients with a prior primary melanoma who developed regional recurrence at the first lymph node station. Candidates in groups (i–iii) were eligible within 56 days of primary biopsy, while candidates in group (iv) were eligible within 42 days of lymphadenectomy. Treatment was administered until relapse or the occurrence of dose-limiting toxicity; all patients were monitored similarly on both arms for relapse occurrence, and the cause and date of death.

TABLE 28-1 Controlled Trials of Postoperative Adjuvant Therapy with Adjuvant IFN in α-2 and γ

Cooperative Group/PI	Agent	Eligible Subjects	No. of Subjects	Investigational Treatment	Study Status
ECOG 1684/ Kirkwood	IFN-α2b	T_4*, N_{1-2}**	287	Intensive-dose IV × 1 mo followed by SC TIW regimen × 11 mos	Significant disease-free and overall survival benefit at 7yrs
NCCTG/ Creagan	IFN-α2a	T_{3-4}, N_{1-2}	262	Moderate dose limited duration IM regimen × 3 mos	Stage III trend to benefit
SWOG/ Meyskins	IFN-γ	T_{3-4}, N_{1-2}	284	Immunologically active 0.2 mg/d dose SC TIW × 1 yr	Closed, negative
EORTC/ Kleeberg	IFNγ vs. IFN-α	T_{3-4},***, N_{1-2}	800	Low-dose IFNα vs. immunology action 0.2 mg/d IFNγ × 1 yr	Closed, under analysis
WHO #16/ Cascinelli	IFN-α2a	N_{1-2}***	444	Low-dose prolonged SC TIW regimen x 2 yrs	No disease-free or relapse benefit at 3 yrs
ECOG 1690/ INT-2055/ Kirkwood	IFN-α2b	T_4*, N_{1-2}	642	Intensive-dose IV x 1 mo + SC x 11 mos (total 1 yr) vs. low-dose prolonged SC TIW (2 mos + yr) regimen	Closed, under analysis

ECOG, Eastern Cooperative Oncology Group; WHO, World Health Organization Melanoma Programme; NCCTG, North Central Cancer Treatment Group; SWOG, Southwestern Oncology Group; EORTC, European Organization for Research and Treatment of Cancer.

* Deep primary >4 mm, without satellites.

** Regional node involvement without extracapsular soft tissue extension.

*** Regional nodal involvement including extracapsular extension.

**** Deep primary >3 mm.

Of the 287 patients enrolled in this study, 286 were included in an intent-to-treat analysis, and 280 noncancelled with both relapse endpoint and toxicity information were included in an efficacy sample analysis (9). Patients were distributed evenly between treatment (n = 143) and observation (n =137) arms in terms of all analyzed prognostic factors, including stage, microstage (Breslow depth and Clark level), tumor ulceration and site, age, and sex among others. In the small node-negative stratification group (i) with T4 pN0 tumors, however, analysis reveals a treatment-stage interaction, and for this stratum taken alone, there exists an imbalance in the distribution of cases with ulceration that favored the observation group. The numbers of patients in this stratum (15–16 per group) unfortunately preclude further analysis.

The toxicities associated with treatment in this trial were significant: all treated patients experienced some toxicities, but these were generally those of the well-recognized flu-like syndrome associated with a range of biologicals (e.g., fatigue in 96%, fever, chills). Dose-limiting grade 3 or worse toxicity was observed in approximately one-third of patients in the first 4 weeks of IV therapy, and in approximately one-third of patients during the balance of the year of SC therapy subsequently. Apart from the constitutional and flu-like manifestations expected of IFN α-2, neutropenic or thrombocytopenic toxicity and abnormal liver functions were not uncommon. Two patients who entered this trial early and were not monitored or treated according to protocol experienced lethal hepatotoxicity. With subsequent attention to the criteria for dose modification, no further instances of such toxicity have been encountered. Anorexia, nausea and vomiting, headaches, and depression were also notable. Despite toxicity however, three-fourths of patients who entered the trial and did not relapse were able to complete the 1 year of therapy.

The analysis of this trial at a median interval of more than 6.9 years for the 109 survivors reveals an overall treatment impact upon relapse-free survival that is highly significant, and consistent throughout the planned group sequential monitoring evaluations of this trial's outcome ($P_2 < .005$). The trial revealed an impact upon overall survival that was significant at final intention-to-treat analysis ($P_2 = .047$), as well as significant in Cox multivariate analysis (9).

Cox multivariate analysis of the factors that are associated with relapse-free survival and overall survival of melanoma in this trial revealed that postoperative treatment with high-dose IFN α-2b therapy as administered in E1684 was among the most significant predictors of continuous relapse-free survival as well as overall survival ($P = .001$) and associated with an improvement of RFS amounting to approximately by 50% over observation in this trial. Only freedom from nodal involvement and time from diagnosis or recurrence to treatment were of similar prognostic import (Table 28-2).

Interferon α-2b therapy at high dosage as administered in this trial prolonged overall survival by 12 months (from 33.4 to 45.8 months) and median relapse-free survival 9 months, from 11.8 to 20.6 months. The comparison of 5-year relapse-free survival among treated patients and those observed reveals an increment of 42% (from 26% to 37%), while 5-year overall survival was increased 24% (from 37% to 46%).

TABLE 28-2. The Factors Identified as Significant Predictors of Favorable Outcome in E1684

Stage of disease (pathologic absence of lymph node metastasis)
Time from diagnosis or recurrence to randomization > 30 days
Treatment with IFN α-2b
Lack of ulceration of the primary lesion
Age younger than 50 years

The analysis of this trial in terms of the individual stratification groups reveals no benefit for those patients in the small node-negative group for which the (unbalanced) presence of ulceration is a confounding factor.

The several groups of node-positive patients exhibit a highly consistent and favorable impact of IFN α-2b therapy at high dosage, which was analyzed separately at the request of the FDA ODAC 7/25/95. The results of this analysis are depicted in terms of relapse-free and overall survival of the combined node-positive strata (ii, iii, and iv) at 6.9 years of median follow-up (Figure 28-1). Among node-positive patients, the increment in 5-year relapse-free survival is highly significant, both in terms of relapse-free (P_2 = .0006) and overall survival (P_2 = .006). The continuous relapse-free survival of this group of patients, which comprised the majority of entrants to E1684, is improved by approximately 80% (from 21% for observation to 38% for treatment at 5 years) with IFN α-2b therapy.

The temporal pattern of benefit from IFN α-2b therapy has been analyzed in terms of the hazard function for relapse and death, revealing a disproportionate early impact of therapy, at the time when the liability to relapse is greatest in patients with resected stage IIB and III melanoma. This may indicate the critical nature of the initial month of IV therapy employed in E1684, although this has yet to be tested in any cooperative group trial.

CONCLUSION

The results of E1684 are the first to demonstrate significant relapse-free and overall survival prolongation in a mature multicenter randomized controlled trial. The benefit of high-dose IFN α-2b therapy given for the first month by the IV route, and for the next 11 months by the SC route, includes the improvement of continuous relapse-free survival by 42% at 5 years.

An analysis of the impact of high-dose IFN α-2b therapy upon node-positive participants in E1684, performed at the request of the FDA ODAC, reveals an even larger 80% increment in the continuous relapse-free benefit associated with therapy. The stable continuous relapse-free survival advantage observed with IFN α-2b as administered in E1684 suggests a curative potential. The subsequent Intergroup E1690 trial, which is testing the same dose and schedule of IFN α-2b for 1 year, as

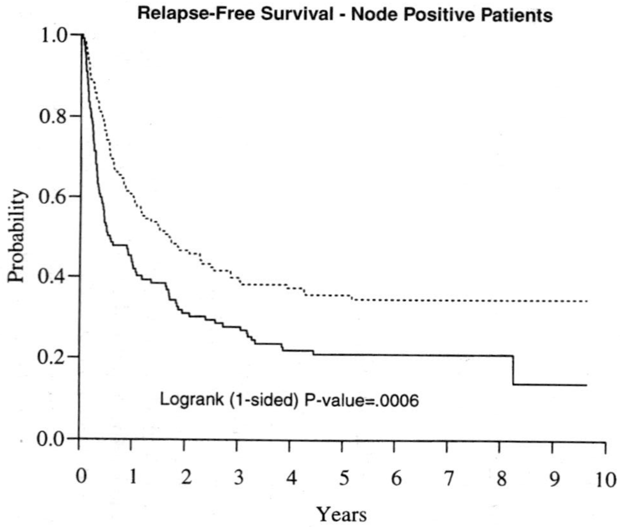

Group	0-2	2-4	4-6	6-8	8-10
——— OBS	84/122	11/37	1/26	0/15	1/4
········ IFN	68/127	11/58	3/45	0/32	0/13

Time Interval (# events/# at risk)

A

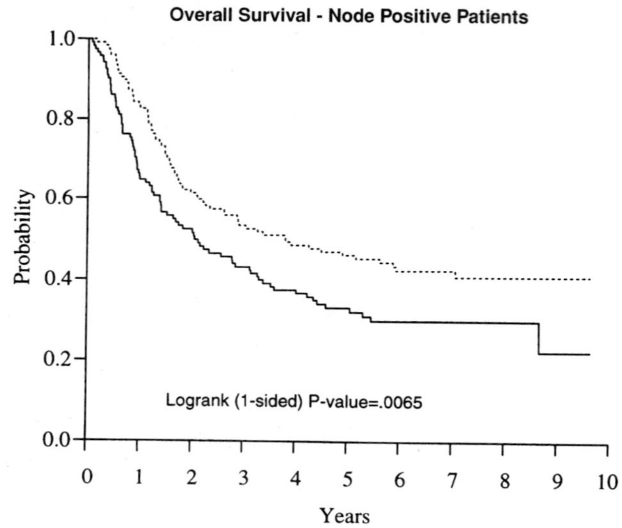

Group	0-2	2-4	4-6	6-8	8-10
——— OBS	58/122	18/63	8/44	0/24	1/7
········ IFN	49/127	16/78	7/61	1/41	0/16

Time Interval (# events/# at risk)

B

Figure 28-1. Relapse-free (A) and overall survival (B) of node-positive patients on high-dose IFN α-2b therapy, at 6.9 years median follow-up.

well as a lower dose of IFN α-2b given SC TIW for 2 years, has also been analyzed in terms of immunological and in vitro antitumor mechanisms of IFN α-2. This may permit a more rational selection of patients who are most likely to benefit from this new therapy in the future.

The toxicity of IFN α-2b as administered in E1684 was significant, but manageable, using the supportive measures that have been effective for symptomatic toxicity of a variety of biologicals. These, together with the dose modification criteria employed in the protocol E1684 and adopted by the FDA, permit the safe administration of adjuvant therapy of high-risk stage IIB or III melanoma.

REFERENCES

1. Kirkwood JM: Melanoma, in Anonymous Biologic Therapy of Cancer: Principles and Practice 1994. pp 388–411.
2. Kokoschka EM, Trautinger F, Knobler RM, Pohl-Markl H, Micksche M: Long-term adjuvant therapy of high-risk malignant melanoma with interferon α-2b. J Invest Dermatol 1990; 95(6): 193S–197S.
3. Creagan ET, Dalton RJ, Ahmann DL, Jung S, Morton RF, Langdon RM, Jr., Kugler J, Rodriguez LJ: Randomized, surgical adjuvant clinical trial of recombinant interferon α-2a in selected patients with malignant melanoma. J Clin Oncol 1995;13:2776–2783.
4. Cascinelli N: Evaluation of efficacy of adjuvant rIFN, α-2a in melanoma patients with regional node metastases. Proc ASCO 1995;14:A1296.
5. Kirkwood JM, Sosman J, Ernstoff M, Ross M, Gerstner C, Bryant J, Whiteside T, Johnson C:E2690: a study of the mechanism of IFN α-2b in high risk melanoma in the ECOG/intergroup trial E1690. Proc Am Assoc Cancer Res 1995;36:641.
6. Miotti S, Mantovani LT, Pupa SM, Bellosta P, Colnaghi MI: Characterization of two anti-idiotypic monoclonal antibodies raised against anti-tumor monoclonal antibody MOv18. J Immunol Res 1989;1(2):59–65.
7. Kirkwood JM, Ernstoff M, Davis CA, Reiss M, Ferraresi R, Rudnick SA: Comparison of intramuscular and intravenous recombinant α-2 interferon in melanoma and other cancers. Ann Intern Med 1985;103(1):32–36.
8. Sertoli MR, Bernengo MG, Ardizzoni A, Brunetti I, Falcone A, Vidili MG, Cusimano MP, Appino A, Doveil G, Fortini C, et al: Phase II trial of recombinant α-2b interferon in the treatment of metastatic skin melanoma. Oncology 1989;46(2):96–98.
9. Kirkwood J, Hunt M, Smith T, et al: A randomized controlled trial of high-dose IFN α-2b for high-risk melanoma: the ECOG trial EST-1684. Proc Am Soc Clin Oncol 1993;12:390.

Adjuvant Therapy of Cancer VIII, edited by Sydney E. Salmon. Lippincott–Raven Publishers, Philadelphia © 1997.

29

Is Interferon-γ Detrimental? Results of a Southwest Oncology Group Randomized Trial of Adjuvant Interferon-γ versus Observation in Melanoma

Vernon K. Sondak, Kenneth J. Kopecky, John W. Smith II, Evan M. Hersh, Robert D. Noyes, Ralph J. Tuthill, Thomas P. Miller, Lynn G. Feun, James H. Doroshow, Lawrence E. Flaherty, and Frank L. Meyskens, Jr., for the Southwest Oncology Group

Cutaneous malignant melanoma has an excellent prognosis after surgical excision if the lesion is diagnosed and treated at an early stage of development. However, as the tumor invades more deeply and/or spreads to regional lymph nodes, prognosis worsens considerably (1–3). Patients with AJCC stage II and III disease are therefore appropriate candidates for postsurgical adjuvant therapy aimed at decreasing the likelihood of regional and systemic metastases. Since many of these patients can be cured with surgical excision alone, however, any adjuvant therapy must not only be effective but reasonably well tolerated and free of long-term adverse effects.

A variety of observations suggest an important role for immunologic mechanisms in controlling the spread or proliferation of melanoma cells: the occasional presence of a vigorous immune response in the primary lesion and regional nodes, the presence of tumor-specific or tumor-associated antigens, documented "spontaneous" remission of advanced disease, and demonstration of altered histocompatibility antigen repertoire with disease progression (4,5). At the time of planning of this trial, previous adjuvant studies had used a nonspecific immunologic approach, principally bacillus Calmette-Guerin (BCG). Early positive reports in the adjuvant setting as well as activity against advanced disease precipitated a multitude of randomized trials with BCG (6,7). Utilizing BCG alone or in combination with chemotherapy, all these randomized adjuvant trials have been negative (8). Likewise, adjuvant studies using other nonspecific immunostimulants (*Corynebacterium parvum*, levamisole, and transfer factor) also produced disappointing results (8–11). More efficacious immunomodulatory approaches were clearly needed.

Interferons are a group of proteins and glycoproteins produced by cells in response to virus, double-stranded RNA, antigen, or mitogen (12). A wide range of biological activities have been identified for these proteins including antiviral and antiproliferative activity and the ability to modulate surface antigens and various cells of the immune system (12,13). Interferons have been classified into three major classes based on various biochemical properties (14). Interferon-γ (IFN-γ) is an acid-labile interferon produced primarily by T-lymphocytes in response to mitogen or antigen exposure (14). This interferon has a variety of immunomodulatory effects including stimulation of natural killer cell-mediated cytotoxicity, macrophage activation, and enhancement of HLA Class II antigen expression and shedding, which is related to cytotoxic lymphocyte function (12,15–17). Short-term phase I studies showed that the molecule was well tolerated and that immune parameters could be favorably modulated (18–21). Although it was recognized at the time of the design of this trial, and confirmed subsequently (22), that IFN-γ was not active against advanced melanoma, its favorable immunologic profile and low toxicity argued for consideration of its use in the adjuvant setting (23). Therefore, a randomized, controlled phase III trial of subcutaneous IFN-γ following definitive local surgery for AJCC stage II and stage III melanoma patients was undertaken (SWOG-8642).

PATIENTS AND METHODS

Patient Eligibility

Patients with stage II (primary thickness >1.5 mm, N0M0) or III (regional nodal and/or in transit or satellite metastases) cutaneous malignant melanoma were eligible. Patients with stage II melanoma were required to have a primary lesion with a Breslow's thickness >1.5 mm; complete local excision with at least 1-cm margins within 4 weeks of entry; and clinically negative lymph nodes or, if clinically positive, pathologically negative nodes demonstrated by excision and histologic examination. Patients with stage III disease had resection of the primary lesion (if present) and of the regional lymph nodes and any in transit or satellite metastases within 4 weeks of registration. Strict criteria for surgical excision and lymph node dissection were defined and review of the adequacy of surgery was done by a single surgeon (R.D.N.). Initial protocol entry was based on pathologic examination conducted by the local pathologist(s); the slides of all patients were subsequently reviewed by one central pathologist (R.J.T.) to determine final eligibility.

Staging procedures were required to assure that patients were free of detectable residual disease. For stage II patients, a CT scan of the regional lymph nodes was required if they were not visualized on a chest or abdominal scan. Patients under age 18, with performance status worse than 0–1 by SWOG criteria, with any prior treatment for melanoma other than surgery, or with prior therapy with interferon of any type were not eligible.

Randomization and Treatment Schedules

Patients who gave written informed consent in accordance with local institutional guidelines were randomly assigned to receive either recombinant human IFN-γ (rIFN-γ; 0.2 mg daily by subcutaneous injection for 1 year or until relapse) or no treatment. The rIFN-γ was provided by Genentech, Inc. (South San Francisco, California). This randomization was stratified by stage (II versus III).

The results of phase I and single-dose pharmacokinetic studies of rIFN-γ in cancer patients were known at the start of the current trial and significant biologic activity on immune parameters was evident (19–21). The dosage and schedule of rIFN-γ in SWOG-8642 were based on results of trials conducted by the Biological Response Modifiers Program of the National Cancer Institute (21). The immunomodulatory effects of IFN-γ were documented in patients with a high risk of recurrence after surgical excision of a primary melanoma lesion (i.e., the same patient population under study here) and included improved macrophage activation, increased NK cell-mediated cytotoxicity, and enhancement of Fc receptor and HLA class II expression on monocyte cells. Optimal enhancement was demonstrated at a dose of 0.1 mg/m^2/day administered intramuscularly on a daily schedule; subsequent studies with a subcutaneous route showed comparable benefit. For practical reasons, a dose of 0.2 mg/day rIFN-γ was chosen for the present study; body surface area was calculated to allow correlation between outcome and relative dose expressed as mg/m^2.

All patients were to be seen every 6 months for the duration of the trial and underwent a history and physical examination as well as screening hematologic parameters and chemistries and chest x-rays at each visit. Patients were free to withdraw from treatment at any time after enrollment on the study. The investigational treatment was discontinued if the patient experienced a recurrence of melanoma. The protocol was approved by the Human Subjects Review Board of each of the participating institutions.

Toxicity

Toxicities were graded according to standard guidelines. Reductions of interferon dosage were made in the event of side effects (fever, chills, night sweats, fatigue, anorexia, myalgia, and headache).

Statistical Analysis

The objectives of this randomized phase III trial were to compare the two treatment arms with respect to disease-free survival (DFS) and overall survival, and to estimate the rates of toxicities associated with rIFN-γ therapy. DFS was measured from date of randomization until recurrence of melanoma or death from any cause, censored at the date of last contact for patients not known to have relapsed or died. Overall survival was measured from date of randomization until death from any cause, censored at the date of last contact for patients not known to have died. The study design called for 230 eligible patients registered over a period of 2.5 years, followed by an additional follow-up period of 1.5 years. Based on formulae of Lachin for comparison of exponential distributions (24), this would provide a one-sided test at critical level $\alpha = 0.05$ with statistical power of 0.80 to detect an increase in DFS at 2.5 years from 60% to 75%. One-sided tests were considered appropriate for analysis of treatment effects since interest lay in the alternative hypothesis of improved outcomes with rIFN-γ. Distributions of DFS and overall survival were estimated for graphical purposes by the method of Kaplan and Meier (25) and compared between treatment groups using the log rank test (26). Multivariate analyses of DFS and overall survival in relation to stage, treatment and other factors were based on the proportional hazards regression model of Cox (27). The primary comparisons between treatment groups were done using one-sided tests against alternative hypotheses of superior outcome in the rIFN-γ arm; statistical significance of results was therefore expressed using one-sided *P*-values (P_1). Two-sided *P*-values (P_2) were used for certain other tests as appropriate. In accordance with the study monitoring policy of SWOG in effect at the time, results of treatment comparisons were presented only to the study's Data Monitoring Committee until that committee approved disclosure of the study's findings. The analysis in the current report is based on data available as of August 2, 1994, and expands upon previously published results (28,29).

RESULTS

A total of 284 patients were registered between October 1987 and November 1989. Eighty-two (29%) were deemed ineligible, the reasons being: (a) pre-study tests either not done or not done within the specified time frame, or pathology reviews not able to be completed (48 patients); or (b) inadequate surgery (14 patients), stage I disease (Breslow's thickness ≤1.5 mm, 6 patients), stage IV (metastatic) disease (5 patients), pretreatment surgery outside required time frame (4 patients), central pathology review diagnosis not melanoma (2 patients), inadequate cardiac function (1 patient), Parkinson's disease (1 patient), and registration after treatment start (1 patient).

A planned interim analysis in August 1989 suggested that rIFN-γ was unlikely to have a beneficial effect. Consequently, the study's Data Monitoring Committee initiated an accelerated schedule of interim analysis which, 8 months later, effectively ruled out the possibility that rIFN-γ could produce a statistically significant improvement in disease-free survival, despite having fewer than the planned number of eligible patients. Therefore, in June 1990, the Monitoring Committee decided against enrolling any additional patients to this study. In addition, physicians with patients still on rIFN-γ were notified of the study's and allowed to decide with their patients whether to discontinue interferon therapy. A total of six eligible patients randomized to rIFN-γ discontinued therapy after 8–10 months, instead of the 12 months specified by the protocol. These patients were included in all analyses of outcome and toxicity. Since the number of eligible patients (202) fell short of the planned number (230), and the results of the interim analyses precluded reopening the study to accrue additional eligible patients, two secondary analyses were performed in addition to the primary analysis of fully eligible patients. One secondary analysis included the 48 ineligible patients in group (a) above along with the 202 fully eligible patients, and the second was based on strict intention to treat, i.e., included all 284 randomized patients regardless of eligibility. However the conclusions reached were not altered in any fashion as a result of these additional analyses, hence only the results of the primary analysis are detailed here.

TABLE 29-1. Characteristics of Fully Eligible Patients

Characteristic	rIFN-γ ($n = 97$)	Observation ($n = 105$)
Median age (range)	45 (21–79)	46 (21–74)
Gender		
Males	72 (74%)	67 (64%)
Females	25 (26%)	38 (36%)
Race		
White	97 (100%)	105 (100%)
Stage		
Stage II	39 (40%)	35 (33%)
Stage III	58 (60%)	70 (67%)
Primary Site		
Trunk	46 (47%)	47 (45%)
Extremity	29 (30%)	30 (29%)
Head/neck	16 (16%)	17 (16%)
Other/unknown	6 (6%)	11 (10%)

Disease-Free and Overall Survival

The demographic characteristics of the 202 fully eligible patients are shown in Table 29-1. The two arms were well-balanced for age, stage, and primary site, although the proportion of women was somewhat lower in the rIFN-γ group. One hundred of the 202 patients have died, and the median duration of follow-up for the remaining 102 patients is 58 months (range 34–76 months). Results are shown by stage and treatment arm in Table 29-2 and Figures 29-1 and 29-2. DFS was not significantly better in the rIFN-γ arm compared to the observation arm ($P_1 = 0.81$ for log rank test stratified by stage). Estimated DFS at 2.5 years among patients with stage II disease was 64% in the rIFN-γ arm (95% confidence interval 49–79%) and 66% in the observation arm (95% CI 50–81%). The corresponding DFS estimates for patients with stage III disease were 31% with rIFN-γ (95% CI 19–43%) and 41% with observation (95% CI 30–53%). Estimated DFS at 5 years among patients with stage II disease was 56% in the rIFN-γ arm (95% CI 40–71%) and 56% in the observation arm (95% CI 40–73%). The corresponding 5-year DFS estimates for patients with stage III disease were 29% with rIFN-γ (95% CI 18–41%) and 29% with observation (95% CI 17–41%). The estimated relative risk of relapse or death among rIFN-γ patients was 1.18 (95% CI 0.82–1.68). A relative risk of 1.0 indicates no difference between treatments, and a risk >1.0 indicates a poorer outcome with rIFN-γ. Multivariate proportional hazards regression analyses (stratified by stage) were performed to assess whether adjustment for the small imbalances of the treatment arms with respect to the factors in Table 29-1 might modify the estimated treatment effect.

Text continues on page 266

TABLE 29–2. Endpoint Analysis of All Fully Eligible Patients

	Stage II		Stage III	
	rIFN-γ	**Observation**	**rIFN-γ**	**Observation**
No. of Patients	39	35	58	70
Alive in remission (%)	21 (54%)	20 (57%)	17 (29%)	22 (31%)
Dead without relapse (%)	2 (5%)	0 (0%)	0 (0%)	3 (4%)
Relapsed: alive (%)	2 (5%)	4 (11%)	5 (9%)	11 (16%)
Relapsed: dead (%)	14 (36%)	11 (31%)	36 (62%)	34 (49%)
Median DFS	Not reached	Not reached	10 months	19 months
%Disease-free at 2.5 yrs (95% CI)	64% (49–79%)	66% (50–81%)	31% (19–43%)	41% (30–53%)
%Disease-free at 5 yrs (95% CI)	56% (40–71%)	56% (40–73%)	29% (18–41%)	29% (17–41%)
Median survival	Not reached	Not reached	25 months	57 months
% Alive at 2.5 yrs (95% CI)	79% (67–92%)	89% (78–99%)	47% (34–59%)	57% (46–69%)
% Alive at 5 yrs (95% CI)	62% (47–78%)	67% (51–83%)	38% (25–50%)	47% (34–60%)

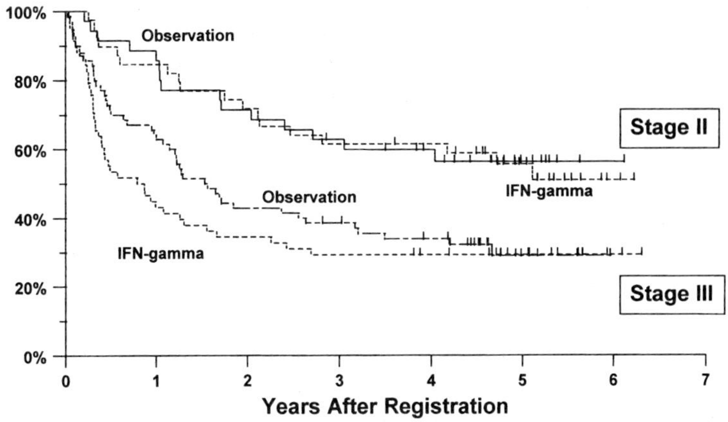

No. at Risk		0	2	4	6
	II, Obs	35	25	17	1
	II, IFN	39	28	23	2
	III, Obs	70	30	21	0
	III, IFN	58	20	15	2

Figure 29-1. Disease-free Survival by Stage and Treatment Arm. (From Meyskens FL Jr, Kopecky KJ, Taylor CW, et al. Randomized trial of adjuvant human interferon gamma versus observation in high-risk cutaneous melanoma. J Natl Cancer Inst 1995;87:1710. Used with permission.)

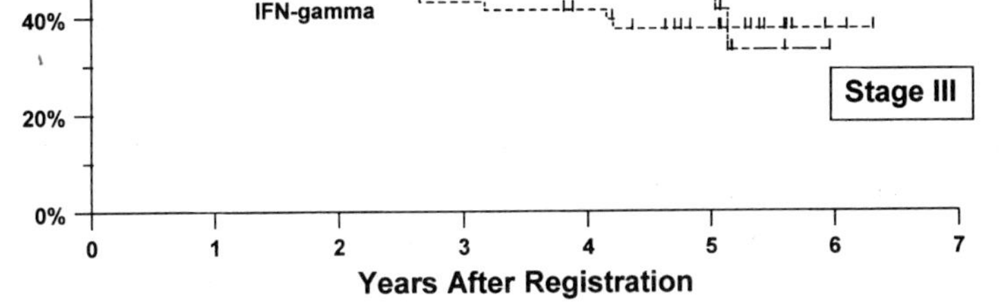

No. at Risk		0	2	4	6
	II, Obs	35	31	20	1
	II, IFN	39	33	26	2
	III, Obs	70	43	33	0
	III, IFN	58	30	22	2

Figure 29-2. Overall Survival by Stage and Treatment Arm. (From Meyskens FL Jr, Kopecky KJ, Taylor CW, et al. Randomized trial of adjuvant human interferon gamma versus observation in high-risk cutaneous melanoma. J Natl Cancer Inst 1995; 87:1710. Used with permission.)

This adjustment did not change the lack of apparent treatment effect (P_1 = 0.74). In addition there was no evidence of significant interaction between the effects of treatment and stage (P_2 = 0.82), gender (P_2 = 0.34), age (treated as a continuous variable, P_2 = 0.96), or primary site (extremity vs. trunk vs. all others, P_2 = 0.17).

There was also no significant effect of rIFN-γ treatment on overall survival (Figure 29-2, P_1 = 0.81). Estimated probability of survival at 2.5 years among patients with stage II disease was 79% in the rIFN-γ arm (95% CI 67–92%) and 89% in the observation arm (95% CI 78–99%). The corresponding survival estimates for patients with stage III disease were 47% with rIFN-γ (95% CI 34–59%) and 57% with observation (95% CI 46–69%). Estimated probability of survival at 5 years among patients with stage II disease was 62% in the rIFN-γ arm (95% CI 47–78%) and 67% in the observation arm (95% CI 51–83%). The corresponding survival estimates for patients with stage III disease were 38% with rIFN-γ (95% CI 25–50%) and 47% with observation (95% CI 34–60%). The estimated relative risk of death among rIFN-γ patients was 1.31 (95% CI 0.88–1.95). The effect of treatment remained nonsignificant (P_1 = 0.88) after adjusting for the effects of gender, age, and primary site in multivariate proportional hazards regression analysis stratified by stage. In addition there was no evidence of interaction between the effects of treatment and stage (P_2 = 0.94), gender (P_2 = 0.60), age (P_2 = 0.82), or primary site (P_2 = 0.21). These results suggest that there were no subgroups of patients in which rIFN-γ had a significant effect on DFS or survival.

The study was designed to have adequate power to detect an increase in DFS at 2.5 years from 60% with no postsurgical treatment to 75% with rIFN-γ. For exponentially distributed DFS, this can be expressed as an alternative hypothesis that the relative risk of relapse or death for rIFN-γ patients relative to observation patients is 0.56. Based on proportional hazards regression analysis stratified for stage, the possibility that the true relative risk is 0.56 was convincingly rejected (P_1 = 0.0001). In fact the even more stringent alternative hypothesis that the relative risk is 0.75 (a 25% improvement with rIFN-γ, corresponding to an increase of 2.5-year DFS from 60% to 68%) was also rejected (P_1 = 0.007). Therefore the results of this study provide strong evidence for lack of any clinically meaningful beneficial effect of rIFN-γ, even though the trial had fewer than the planned number of fully eligible patients.

Some studies have suggested that the immunomodulatory effect of IFN-γ was very dose-dependent with a bell-shaped curve evident (23). Since the patients in the current trial were administered a fixed dose of rIFN-γ, we examined whether the treatment effect varied accordingly to body surface area (BSA) or weight. In particular, for the group whose BSA was 1.90–2.09 (for whom the dose of rIFN-γ was closest to the "optimal" dose of 0.1 mg/m^2/day), there was no suggestion of a beneficial effect of treatment. The estimated relative risks for rIFN-γ versus observation in this group of patients were 1.09 in the analysis of DFS (95% CI 0.63–1.89) and 1.31 for overall survival (95% CI 0.72–2.39), which indicate slightly though not significantly poorer outcomes with rIFN-γ. Proportional hazards regression analysis based on the fully eligible patients and stratified by stage suggested the possibility of a trend in the effect of rIFN-γ over the range of BSA, with the dele-

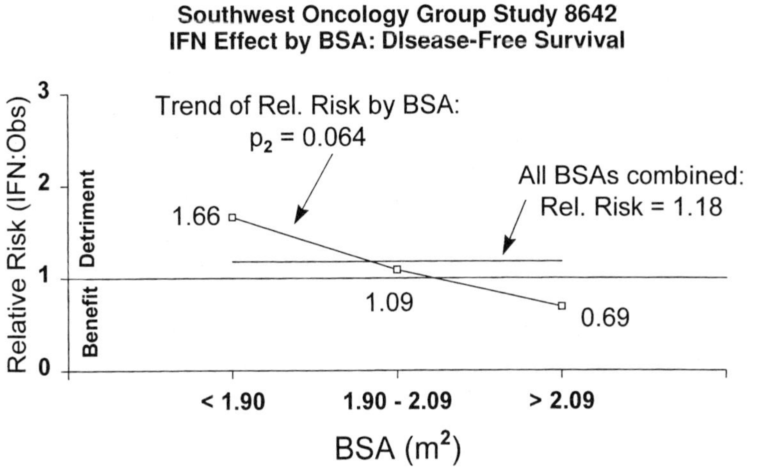

Figure 29-3. Interferon Effect on Disease-free Survival by Body Surface Area (BSA).

terious effect seen with rIFN-γ increasing with decreasing BSA (Figures 29-3 and 29-4). This trend, which was marginally significant ($P_2 = 0.064$) for DFS but not significant for survival ($P_2 = 0.17$) suggests that the highest relative doses of rIFN-γ may have been most detrimental. Similar results were obtained in analyses based on weight rather than BSA.

Possible Detrimental Effect of rIFN-γ

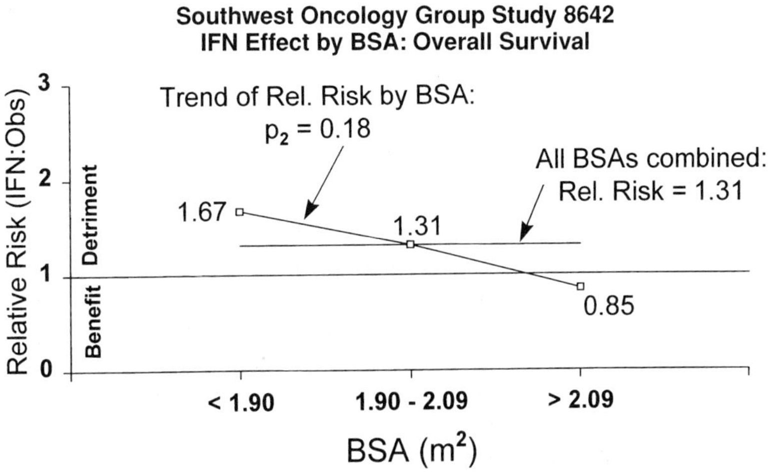

Figure 29-4. Interferon Effect on Survival by Body Surface Area (BSA).

This study was not designed to address the possibility that treatment with rIFN-γ might be detrimental in terms of either DFS or overall survival. Nonetheless, the treatment group actually had a poorer outcome (relative risk for DFS 1.18 and for overall survival 1.31) than the observation arm. As indicated above, there was a trend for patients receiving the highest relative doses of rIFN-γ (by virtue of having the smallest body surface area) to have the poorest DFS. In order to address this unexpected possibility, we conducted a *post hoc* two-sided analysis of our data. This analysis revealed no evidence of a statistically significant beneficial or detrimental effect of rIFN-γ on DFS ($P_2 = 0.38$) or overall survival ($P_2 = 0.17$). This study, however, had comparatively little power for these unanticipated, *post hoc* tests of possible detrimental effects. Thus, while this study did not find significant evidence of a detrimental effect of rIFN-γ, it also cannot rule out the possibility that rIFN-γ increases the risk of relapse or death by even as much as 50% (i.e., that the relative risk is 1.50).

Toxicity

A total of 133 patients who were randomized to the rIFN-γ arm were evaluated for toxicity (Table 29-3). This included all but four patients who were randomized to rIFN-γ, whether eligible or not. The four patients randomized to rIFN-γ but not evaluated for toxicity included two who received no rIFN-γ, one who received only one injection, and one for whom data were inadequate to assess toxicities. There were no grade 4 or 5 (fatal) toxicities. Twenty-four patients (18%) had grade 3 toxicities. Three of these were neurological toxicities: confusion, confusion and insomnia, and personality change. Four patients had grade 3 granulocytopenia or leukopenia. Other grade 3 toxicities included depression, migraine, elevated liver enzymes, pruritus, and flu-like symptoms (fatigue, headache, chills, fever, myalgia, loss of appetite, and diarrhea). Toxicities notable for their frequency included chills and fever (94 patients, 71%), headache (85 patients, 64%), and nausea and anorexia (46 patients, 35%). Sixteen patients (12%) had grade 1 neurologic toxicities, almost entirely consisting of mild confusion.

DISCUSSION

The results of this trial indicate that an immunomodulatory dose of recombinant human IFN-γ given daily by subcutaneous injection did not significantly improve the natural history of resected cutaneous melanoma of AJCC stage II or III. Neither disease-free survival nor overall survival was significantly longer among the patients treated with IFN. The results of our study argue strongly against the possibility that IFN-γ, in this biologically active dose and schedule, exerts any clinically meaningful beneficial effect in the adjuvant therapy of melanoma. Although an interim analysis raised concern about the possibility of an adverse effect of rIFN-γ (28), this could not be substantiated in the present analysis.

It remains difficult to conceive how IFN-γ therapy could exert an adverse effect upon survival given its known biologic activities. It is possible that the dose of

TABLE 29-3. Number of Treated Patients with a Given Type and Degree of Toxicity (Eligible and Ineligible Patients Included)

	rIFN-γ (n=133) Grade					
Toxicity	**0**	**1**	**2**	**3**	**4**	**5**
Allergy/rash/epidermitis	127	5	0	1	0	0
Cardiac-other	131	2	0	0	0	0
Chills/fever	39	82	7	5	0	0
Depression	129	3	0	1	0	0
Diarrhea	102	26	4	1	0	0
Dizziness/hot flashes	107	25	1	0	0	0
General neurologic	114	16	0	3	0	0
Granulocytopenia	102	17	11	3	0	0
GI other	130	3	0	0	0	0
Headache	48	56	25	4	0	0
Hepatic-enzyme	118	10	4	1	0	0
Hepatic-other	128	5	0	0	0	0
Ileus/constipation	132	1	0	0	0	0
Leukopenia	117	9	6	1	0	0
Mucositis/stomatitis/ulcers	131	1	1	0	0	0
Nausea/vomiting/anorexia	87	38	6	2	0	0
Paresthesia	132	0	1	0	0	0
Peripheral neuropathy	132	1	0	0	0	0
Somnolence/coma	132	1	0	0	0	0
Miscellaneous—other*	25	75	25	8	0	0
Maximum Grade Any Toxicity						
Number	9	55	45	24	0	0

*The majority of Miscellaneous—other toxicities reported were fatigue and myalgia.

rIFN-γ chosen was outside the immunomodulatory range. At least one study published subsequent to the design of our trial, however, suggested that a dose of 0.1 mg/m^2/day administered subcutaneously represented the "optimal" immunomodulatory dose for patients with metastatic melanoma, and that a higher dose was no better (30). In our study, a fixed dose of 0.2 mg/day was utilized, rather than an adjusted dose based on body surface area. Nonetheless, those patients whose BSA was such that they received 0.1 mg/m^2/day or more did not fare better, and in fact may have fared worse than those treated with a lower dose of rIFN-γ or none at all.

The possibility that melanoma patients might form neutralizing antibodies following subcutaneous injections of rIFN-γ has been investigated, and no evidence of such antibodies has been detected (31). Finally, it is possible that the rIFN-γ patients had more frequent medical encounters while on treatment than observation patients, resulting in a lead-time bias whereby relapses were detected earlier in the rIFN-γ patients. This would not necessarily explain, however, why the detrimental effect of rIFN-γ was seen most prominently in patients with the smallest BSA. It is noteworthy that at least two other randomized, controlled trials of adjuvant therapy with rIFN-γ at a dose of 0.2 mg/day administered subcutaneously conducted in other tumor types were similar to our own in finding a worse but not significantly worse outcome for patients treated with rIFN-γ (32,33). In both these trials, concomitant immunologic studies verified that the rIFN-γ treatment led to a statistically significant upregulation of HLA-DR and Fc receptors on monocytes (32,34).

In marked contrast to the results of adjuvant rIFN-γ therapy stands the results of a trial using high-dose interferon-α2b for the adjuvant treatment of patients with cutaneous melanoma of AJCC stages IIB and III (35). If subsequent trials confirm a benefit for adjuvant IFN-α, we would be wise to examine the clinical and biological differences between these two similar molecules for the lessons that might apply to the design of future adjuvant trials in melanoma and other malignancies. Perhaps the important difference between the two interferons is that the α-form is more active in patients with advanced melanoma (approximately 16% objective response rate) (36) than the γ-form (0 to 5% objective response rate) (21,37,38). However, high doses of rIFN-α are much more toxic than rIFN-γ, and treatment-related deaths have occurred in the adjuvant setting (35). It is also clear that IFN-γ is the ligand for a different receptor than IFN-α (39), and that monocytes and macrophages represent primary immunologic targets of IFN-γ, as opposed to T lymphocytes (15,21).

The current trial was based on a careful (although short-term) assessment of the immunomodulatory effects of rIFN-γ in patients with resected cutaneous melanoma (21,22). Why then should the current trial show no benefit of adjuvant rIFN-γ in a similar group of patients? The outcome of this trial should give investigators considerable pause in using the results of short-term nontherapeutic end points (e.g., immune modulation) in the design of long-term therapeutic trials for melanoma. Whether we should demand that an agent being considered for adjuvant therapy for melanoma must have activity against advanced disease is a concept that should be revisited for intense discussion. In view of the negative results from the current study and other studies of rIFN-γ (32,33), as well as the negative results of randomized trials using levamisole (9,10), transfer factor (11), and vitamin A (40), we should question whether agents with favorable immunologic and biologic properties, but which lack therapeutic efficacy against measurable disease, are indeed appropriate for adjuvant therapy trials. If immunologic studies are to be used to select candidate biologic response modifiers for adjuvant studies, it will be important to refine our understanding of which immune cells (e.g., monocytes versus T cells) should be targeted for modulation.

ACKNOWLEDGMENTS

This investigation was supported in part by the following PHS Cooperative Agreement grants awarded by the National Cancer Institute, DHHS: CA13612, CA46368, CA42028, CA20319, CA45377, CA46282, CA45560, CA35128, CA58861, CA12644, CA46113, CA35192, CA04919, CA35261, CA35090, CA35431, CA45807, CA35176, CA22433, CA35117, CA42777, CA46441, CA46136, CA58686, CA35283, CA35119, CA37981, CA35084, CA35200, CA35262, CA27057, CA16385, CA35281, CA58882, CA35178, CA58416, CA04920, CA03389, CA35429, CA12213, CA38926, CA32102.

REFERENCES

1. Breslow A, Cascinelli N, Van der Esch EP, Morabito A. Stage I melanoma of the limbs: Assessment of prognosis by levels of invasion and maximum thickness. Tumori 1978;64:273.
2. Meyskens FL Jr, Berdeaux DH, Parks B, Tong T, Loescher L, Moon TE. Cutaneous malignant melanoma (Arizona Cancer Center Experience): I. The natural history and prognostic factors influencing survival in patients with stage I disease. Cancer 1988;62:1207.
3. Berdeaux, DH, Meyskens FL Jr, Parks B, Tong T, Loescher L, Moon TE. Cutaneous malignant melanoma: II. The natural history and prognostic factors influencing the development of stage II disease. Cancer 1989;63:1430.
4. Shiku H, Takahaski T, Resnick LA, Oettgen HF, Old LJ. Cell surface antigens of human malignant melanoma. III. Recognition of autoantibodies with unusual characteristics. J Exp Med 1977;145:784.
5. Houghton AN, Eisinger M, Albino AP, Cairncross JG, Old LJ. Surface antigens of melanocytes and melanomas. Markers of melanocyte differentiation and melanoma subsets. J Exp Med 1989;156:1755.
6. Morton DL, Eilber FR, Joseph WL, Wood WC, Trahan E, Ketcham AS. Immunological factors in human sarcomas and melanomas: A rational basis for immunotherapy. Ann Surg 1970;172:740.
7. Gutterman JU, Marligit G, McBride C, Frei E 3d, Freireich EJ, Hersh EM. Active immunotherapy with B.C.G. for recurrent malignant melanoma. Lancet 1973;1(814):1208.
8. Barth A, Morton DL. The role of adjuvant therapy in melanoma management. Cancer 1995;75:726.
9. Spitler LE, Sagebiel R. A randomized trial of levamisole versus placebo as adjuvant therapy in malignant melanoma. N Engl J Med 1980;303:1143.
10. Lipton A, Harvey HA, Balch CM, Antle CE, Heckard R, Bartolucci AA. *Corynebacterium parvum* versus bacille Calmette-Guerin adjuvant immunotherapy of stage II malignant melanoma. J Clin Oncol 1991;9:1151.
11. Blume MR, Rosenbaum EH, Cohen RJ, Gershow J, Glassberg AB, Shepley E. Adjuvant immunotherapy of high risk stage I melanoma with transfer factor. Cancer 1981;47:882.
12. Stewart WE II. The interferon system. New York: Springer-Verlag, 1981.
13. Rubin BY, Gupta SL. Differential efficacies of human type I and type II interferons as antiviral and antiproliferative agents. Proc Natl Acad Sci USA 1980;77:5928.
14. Cabana V, Teodorescu M, Dray S. Interferon nomenclature [letter to the editor]. J Immunol 1980;125:2353.
15. Nathan CF, Horowitz CR, de la Harpe J, et al. Administration of recombinant interferon-γ to cancer patients enhances monocyte secretion of hydrogen peroxide. Proc Natl Acad Sci USA 1985;82:8686.
16. Herlyn M, Guerry D, Koprowski H. Recombinant γ-interferon induces changes in expression and shedding of antigens associated with normal human melanocytes, nevus cells, and primary and metastatic melanoma cells. J Immunol 1985;134:4226.
17. Houghton AN, Thomson TM, Gross D, Oettgen HF, Old LJ. Surface antigens of melanoma and melanocytes: Specificity of induction of Ia antigens by human γ interferon. J Exp Med 1984;160:255.
18. Foon KA, Sherwin SA, Abrams PG, et al. A phase I trial of recombinant gamma interferon in patients with cancer. Cancer Immunol Immunother 1985;20:193.
19. Kurzrock R, Rosenblum MG, Sherwin SA, et al. Pharmacokinetics, single-dose tolerance and biological activity of recombinant γ interferon in cancer patients. Cancer Res 1985;45:2866.

20. Kleinerman ES, Kurzrock R, Wyatt D, Quesada JR, Gutterman JU, Fidler IJ. Activation or suppression of the tumoricidal properties of monocytes from cancer patients following treatment with human recombinant γ-interferon. Cancer Res 1986;46:5401.
21. Maluish AE, Urba WJ, Longo DL, et al. The determination of an immunologically active dose of interferon-gamma in patients with melanoma. J Clin Oncol 1988;6:434.
22. Schiller JH, Pugh M, Kirkwood JM, Karp D, Larson M, Borden E. Eastern Cooperative Group trial of interferon gamma in metastatic melanoma: An innovative study design. Clin Cancer Res 1996;2:29.
23. Jaffe HS, Herberman RB. Rationale for recombinant human interferon-gamma adjuvant immunotherapy for cancer. J Natl Cancer Inst 1988;80:616.
24. Lachin JM. Introduction to sample size determination and power analysis for clinical trials. Controlled Clin Trials 1981;2:93.
25. Kaplan EL, Meier P. Nonparametric estimation from incomplete observations. J Am Stat Assoc 1958;53:457.
26. Mantel N. Evaluation of survival data and two new rank order statistics arising in its consideration. Cancer Chemother Rep 1966;50:163.
27. Cox DR. Regression models and life tables. J R Stat Soc B 1972;34:187.
28. Meyskens FL Jr, Kopecky K, Samson S, et al. Recombinant human interferon gamma: Adverse effects in high-risk stage I and II cutaneous malignant melanoma [letter]. J Natl Cancer Inst 1990;82:1071.
29. Meyskens FL Jr, Kopecky KJ, Taylor CW, et al. Randomized trial of adjuvant human interferon gamma versus observation in high-risk cutaneous melanoma. J Natl Cancer Inst 1995;87:1710.
30. Kopp WC, Smith JW II, Ewel CH, et al. Immunomodulatory effects of interferon-gamma in patients with metastatic malignant melanoma. J Immunother 1993;13:181.
31. Dummer R, Muller W, Nestle F, et al. Formation of neutralizing antibodies against natural interferon-beta, but not against recombinant interferon-gamma during adjuvant therapy for high-risk malignant melanoma patients. Cancer 1991;67:2300.
32. Wiesenfeld M, O'Connell MJ, Wieand HS, et al. Controlled clinical trial of interferon-γ as postoperative surgical adjuvant therapy for colon cancer. J Clin Oncol 1995;13:2324.
33. Jett JR, Maksymiuk AW, Su JQ, et al. Phase III trial of recombinant interferon gamma in complete responders with small-cell lung cancer. J Clin Oncol 1994;12:2321.
34. Pujol JL, Gibney DJ, Su JQ, Maksymiuk AW, Jett JR. Immune response induced in small-cell lung cancer by maintenance therapy with interferon gamma. J Natl Cancer Inst 1993;85:1844.
35. Kirkwood JM, Strawderman MH, Ernstoff MS, Smith TJ, Borden ED, Blum RH. Interferon α-2b adjuvant therapy of high-risk resected cutaneous melanoma: The Eastern Cooperative Oncology Group trial EST 1684. J Clin Oncol 1996;14:7.
36. Balch CM, Houghton AN, Peters LJ. Cutaneous melanoma. In: De Vita VT Jr, Hellman S, Rosenberg SA, eds. Cancer: Principles and practice of oncology, 4th ed. Philadelphia: J. B. Lippincott, 1993. p 1612.
37. Creagan ET, Ahmann DI, Long HJ, Frytak S, Sherwin SA, Chang MN. Phase II study of recombinant interferon-gamma in patients with disseminated malignant melanoma. Cancer Treat Rep 1987;71:843–844.
38. Ernstoff MS, Trautman T, Davis C, et al. A randomized phase I/II study of cutaneous versus intermittent intravenous interferon gamma in patients with metastatic melanoma. J Clin Oncol 1987;5:1804.
39. Zoon KC, Arnheiter H. Studies of the interferon receptor. Pharmacol Ther 1984;24:259.
40. Meyskens FL Jr, Liu PY, Tuthill RJ, et al. A randomized trial of vitamin A versus observation as adjuvant therapy in high risk primary malignant melanoma: A Southwest Oncology Group Study. J Clin Oncol 1994;12:2060.

Adjuvant Therapy of Cancer VIII, edited
by Sydney E. Salmon. Lippincott–Raven
Publishers, Philadelphia © 1997.

30

The Recent Experience at the Rizzoli Institute in the Treatment of Osteosarcoma

P. Picci, G. Bacci, S. Ferrari, A. Brach del Prever, A. Tienghi, A. Comandone, A. M. Mancini, H. Zmerly, G. Rulli, and M. Mercuri

Most malignant neoplasms of bone benefit from primary (neoadjuvant) chemotherapy. For osteosarcoma, this strategy has dramatically changed treatment options and has led to longer survival and better quality of life (1). When osteosarcoma was treated with surgery alone the cure rate was very low (10% in the Rizzoli experience) and most patients were surgically treated with amputation (95% in the Rizzoli experience) (2–5). Using five slightly different protocols, adjuvant chemotherapy was employed from 1973 to 1982 in 238 patients (2). The results obtained (about 44% DFS) are similar to those reported by other institutions (3–9). In this period a 2% severe cardiotoxicity due to the use of doxorubicin (DOX) was also observed.

Primary chemotherapy was adopted at the Rizzoli Institute in March 1983. The aim of this first study was to ameliorate the patients' quality of life, try to increase the percentage of limb salvage procedures, and attempt to diminish the treatment toxicity of chemotherapy, by reducing or avoiding the use of DOX. Preoperative treatment consisted of two cycles of intravenous methotrexate (MTX) (given at the dose of 750 mg/m^2 versus 7.5 g/m^2, after randomization) and of 120 mg/m^2 intraarterial cisplatinum (CDP). Postoperatively, chemotherapy was chosen according to the amount of necrosis observed on the resected specimen. Patients with necrosis greater than 90% continued with the same two drugs used preoperatively (MTX and CDP for two cycles). In patients with an intermediate necrosis (between 60 and 90%), four cycles of 90 mg/m^2 of DOX were added to three cycles of MTX and CDP. Patients with a lesser degree of necrosis were switched to an alternative treatment which consisted of five cycles of DOX and bleomycin-cyclophosphamide-dactinomycin (BCD) (10,11). Because we observed early relapses in patients with necrosis greater than 90% who were treated postoperatively without DOX, after January 1994, the same postoperative treatment was used in these patients as was the case for patients whose tumor specimens had 60–90% necrosis. This study, which was closed in August 1986, included 127 treated patients, did not significantly modify the overall DFS (45% at 9 years of minimum follow-up), but nonetheless gave important results. The number of amputations decreased from 82% in the previous years to 26%, without an increase of local recurrences (6/127, 5%). Sixty-six patients (52%) had a good necrosis and a significantly better DFS (60%) compared to those 60 patients with a lower extent of necrosis (DFS 32%). This study also gave important indications: (a) It was not possible to avoid the use of DOX (DFS was 27% in the 15 patients treated without DOX, in comparison to 47% for the 112 patients treated with DOX). (b) High-dose MTX gave better results than low-dose MTX (good necrosis 60% versus 41%). (c) The attempt to salvage those patients with very low necrosis by completely changing the postoperative treatment with DOX and BCD failed. Severe cardiotoxicity was not observed in this study.

Based on these results, in September 1986 a second neoadjuvant study was started. The aims were to intensify preoperative treatment to increase the number of patients with good necrosis and try to salvage patients with a poor necrosis not by changing postoperative treatment but by adding other drugs to those used preoperatively. Therefore, preoperatively, DOX was added to MTX and CDP. Postoperatively, patients with necrosis >90% continued with the same three drugs, while for patients with a lower extent of necrosis, we added ifosfamide (IFO) (10 g/m^2 over 5 days) and etoposide (VP16) (120 mg/m^2/day for 3 days administered along with CDP) (12). This study accrued 144 patients and was closed in December 1989. The percentage of patients with good necrosis increased from 52% in the first study to 78% in this study. The percentage of amputations continued to decrease, from 26% in the first study to 8% in this study, with only four (3%) local recurrences. The overall disease-free survival (DFS), at a minimum follow-up of 72 months, is 69%. Analyzing these data in terms of necrosis, there are no differences in DFS between patients with good necrosis (70%) and patients with poor necrosis (66%).

This study revealed two other important factors: the role of MTX Cmax (the peak of MTX serum concentration at the end of infusion), and the role of dose/intensity. Disease-free survival was strictly correlated to MTX Cmax. Those patients with a Cmax > 700 μmol/liter had a DFS of 86%, compared to 61% for those patients with a lower Cmax (13). Regarding dose/intensity, DFS decreased from 84% for values >90% to 50% for a dose/intensity lower than 70% (14,15). Despite these good results, the total dose of DOX (480 mg/m^2) resulted in severe cardiotoxicity in six patients. Therefore, in an effort to reduce cardiac toxicity, in the subsequent protocol we reduced the total dose of DOX.

The third study was activated in January 1990. It included a preoperative treatment similar to the previous one (however the MTX dose was increased to 10 g/m^2). A substudy was included to evaluate intra-arterial versus intravenous infusion of CDP during preoperative treatment. Accordingly, 36% of the patients entered on this protocol received CDP intravenously rather than intra-arterially. The first postoperative dose of DOX was administered at 90 mg/m^2, while subsequent doses of DOX were administered at 60 mg/m^2 along with CDP. Patients with necrosis lower than 90% also received three cycles of IFO. Inasmuch as we were administering DOX along with CDP, use of VP16 discontinued. In comparison to the second study, while the total dose of DOX in this protocol was reduced to 390 mg/m^2, the total length of treatment was also decreased; therefore, the dose/intensity for all single drugs was increased. The study enrolled 98 patients and was closed in September 1991. Eleven amputations, 9 rotation plasties, and 78 limb salvage procedures were performed. Six patients suffered local relapse. While 55% of all treated patients had greater than 90% tumor necrosis, 62% of those receiving intra-arterial CDP and 42% of those receiving intravenous CDP had such extensive necrosis (16).

After a minimum follow-up of 50 months, 54% of the patients from the third study are continuously disease-free. There is no statistical difference between patients with necrosis greater than 90% or lower, although a trend is present (61% versus 48%). This study confirmed the importance of dose/intensity and the importance of serum MTX concentration at the end of the infusion. Cardiotoxicity was not observed.

The fourth study, which included 60 patients, was opened in October 1991 and closed in December 1992. This study was performed with the German group COSS. Due to the very good results obtained in the previous studies using IFO, this drug (at the dose of 6 g/m^2 over 3 days in combination with CDP and DOX) was included preoperatively in one arm of this study and was compared to the previously used three-drug arm. In the four-drug arm, CDP was given intravenously, while in the three-drug arm it was given intra-arterially. Postoperatively, all the patients were treated with the four drugs for three cycles, without differences due to chemotherapy-induced necrosis. Greater than 90% necrosis was observed in 48 patients (80%), with no differences between the patients treated with the four-drug arm (13/17, 76%) and those treated with the three-drug arm (35/43, 81%). Regarding surgery, only 3 patients underwent amputation, 5 had a rotation plasty, and the remaining 52 had a limb salvage procedure. One patient relapsed locally. After a minimum follow-up of 36 months, 39 patients (65%) remain continuously disease-free, with no difference between the two treatment arms.

Evaluation of the data from previous studies revealed the importance of total (100%) tumor necrosis. We observed that in the second study the DFS for these patients was 90% compared to 70% for patients with residual viable tumor. The same observation, which was confirmed in the third study (72% versus 56%), was considered in the design of the fifth study.

The fifth study was opened in January 1993 and closed in July 1995, with 121 evaluable cases. IFO was used preoperatively in all the patients and the dose of MTX (12 g/m^2) was escalated if the MTX Cmax did not reach 700 μmol/liter at the end of the infusion. Postoperatively, the same four drugs were given for three cycles. Patients with total necrosis received only two cycles. One patient underwent amputation and two underwent rotation plasties. The remaining 118 patients were treated with limb-salvage procedures. Necrosis was greater than 90% in 73.5% of the cases, with total necrosis observed in 31.4%.

At a median follow-up of 18 months (6–30 months), 99 patients (82%) remain continuously disease-free, 3 died of acute toxicity, 2 died of unrelated causes, and 17 relapsed (12 with distant metastases and 5 with local recurrences). While still preliminary, the results seem better than those in prior studies with respect to MTX Cmax, good and total necrosis, and in reduction in extent of surgery.

CONCLUSIONS

Our "step by step" experience in the neoadjuvant treatment of osteosarcoma suggest the following:

1. Despite its cardiac toxicity, use of doxorubicin is essential in osteosarcoma.
2. To obtain maximal effects of methotrexate, dosing must be individually tailored to achieve an optimal serum concentration.

3. When used with DOX and MTX, intra-arterial cisplatinum has greater efficacy. Moreover, when IFO is added preoperatively to this combination, intravenous rather than intra-arterial CDP appears sufficient, with comparable results.
4. Ifosfamide is a first-line drug and has to be employed from the beginning of the preoperative treatment.
5. Dose intensity must be maintained at the highest possible rate, and unnecessary delay or drug dose reduction must be avoided.
6. There are no pretreatment prognostic factors that we believe justify the use of less than all of the most effective drugs (DOX, CDP, MTX, IFO), from the beginning of treatment.
7. Total (100%) necrosis might be a prognostic factor which might justify reduction in the aggressiveness of postoperative treatment.

The major objective of future osteosarcoma protocols will be to identify reliable biologic prognostic factors which permit individualizing treatment from the outset, thereby sparing toxicities to patients with the best prognosis, and limiting very aggressive and toxic regimens to just those patients with a poor prognosis.

REFERENCES

1. Picci P, Ferrari S, Bacci G, Gherlinzoni F. Treatment recommendations for osteosarcoma and adult soft tissue sarcomas. [editorial]. Drugs 1994;47:82.
2. Campanacci M, Bacci G, Bertoni F, et al. The treatment of osteosarcoma of the extremities: Twenty year experience at the Istituto Ortopedico Rizzoli. Cancer 1981;48:1569.
3. Jaffe N, Frei E III, Watts H, et al. High-dose methotrexate in osteogenic sarcoma: A 5 year experience. Cancer Treat Rep 1978;62:259.
4. Rosen G, Suwansirikul S, Kuon C, et al. High-dose methotrexate with citrovorum factor rescue and adriamycin in childhood osteogenic sarcoma. Cancer 1974;33:1151.
5. Sutow WW, Gehan EA Vietti TJ, et al. Multidrug chemotherapy in primary treatment of osteosarcoma. J Bone Joint Surg 1976;58A:629.
6. Goorin AM, Perez-Atayde A, Gebhardt M, et al. Weekly high-dose methotrexate and doxorubicin for osteosarcoma: The Dana-Farber Cancer Institute/The Children Hospital—Study III. J Clin Oncol 1987;5:1178.
7. Krailo M, Ertel L, Makley J, et al. A randomized study comparing high-dose methotrexate with moderate dose methotrexate as components of adjuvant chemotherapy in childhood non-metastatic osteosarcoma. A report from the Children's Cancer Study Group. Med Ped Oncol 1987;15:69.
8. Link MP, Goorin AM, Miser AW, et al. The effect of adjuvant chemotherapy on relapse free survival in patients with osteosarcoma of the extremity. N Engl J Med 1986;314:1600.
9. Winkler K, Beron G, Kotz R, et al. Neoadjuvant chemotherapy for osteogenic sarcoma: Results of a cooperative German/Austrian study. J Clin Oncol 1984;2:617.
10. Bacci G, Picci P, Ruggieri P, et al. Primary chemotherapy and delayed surgery (neoadjuvant chemotherapy) for osteosarcoma of the extremities. The Rizzoli's experience in 127 patients treated preoperatively with methotrexate i.v. (high vs moderate dose) and cisplatinum i.a. Cancer 1990;65:2539.
11. Bacci G, Picci P, Pignatti G, et al. Neoadjuvant chemotherapy for non metastatic osteosarcoma of the extremities: The experience at the Rizzoli Institute. Clin Orthoped Relat Res 1991;270:87.
12. Bacci G, Picci P, Ferrari S, et al. Primary chemotherapy and delayed surgery for non-metastatic osteosarcoma of the extremities. Results in 164 patients preoperatively treated with high dose of methotrexate (iv) followed by cisplatinum (ia) and adriamycin (iv). Cancer 1993;72:3227.
13. Ferrari S, Sassoli V, Orlandi M, et al. Serum methotrexate concentrations and prognosis in patients with osteosarcoma of the extremities treated with a multidrug neoadjuvant regimen. J Chemother 1993;5:135.

14. Bacci G, Picci P, Avella M, et al. The importance of dose-intensity in neoadjuvant chemotherapy of osteosarcoma. A retrospective analysis of a study in which high dose methotrexate, cisplatinum, and adriamycin were used preoperatively. J Chemother 1990;2:127.
15. Prasad R, Bacci G, Picci P, et al. Neoadjuvant chemotherapy of high grade osteosarcoma and prognostic significance of percentage tumor necrosis and drug dose intensity. In: Salmon SE, ed. Adjuvant therapy of cancer VI. Philadelphia: W. B. Saunders, 1990. p 574.
16. Bacci G, Picci P, Avella M, et al. Effect of intra-arterial versus intra-venous cisplatin in addition to systemic adriamycin and high-dose methotrexate on histologic tumor response of osteosarcoma of the extremities. J Chemother 1992;4:185.

Adjuvant Therapy of Cancer VIII, edited by Sydney E. Salmon. Lippincott–Raven Publishers, Philadelphia © 1997.

31

Adjuvant Therapy of Sarcomas of Bone and Soft Tissue

Karen H. Antman

Bone and soft tissue sarcomas currently represent 1% of adult malignancies and 15% of pediatric malignancies. Adjuvant chemotherapy is currently established in the treatment of rhabdomyosarcomas, osteosarcomas, and Ewing's sarcomas but remains controversial in other adult soft tissue sarcomas.

RANDOMIZED ADJUVANT TRIALS IN BONE SARCOMAS

Osteosarcoma

Based on a consistent 20% 5-year disease-free survival of surgically treated patients, early adjuvant chemotherapy trials documented significantly improved disease-free survivals of 50–80% compared to historical controls. However, Mayo Clinic data from 1963 to 1974 demonstrated an improved disease-free survival for sequential cohorts of patients treated with surgery only, from 13% for patients treated 1963 to 1968, to 42% for 1972 to 1974, prompting the design of randomized trials (1).

Three small randomized trials have subsequently compared observation to two-, five-, and six-drug drug chemotherapy regimens (Table 31-1). In the Mayo Clinic study, postoperative high-dose methotrexate and vincristine did not significantly improve disease-free survival when compared to observation alone (2). In contrast, investigators for the Pediatric Oncology Group (POG) (3,4) and at UCLA

TABLE 31-1. Randomized Adjuvant Chemotherapy Trials in Osteosarcoma with an Observation Control Arm

		Observation			Chemotherapy			
Institution	**Regimen**	**No.**	**%DFS**	**%S**	**No.**	**%DFS**	**%S**	***P***
Mayo Clinic	MVA	18	44	62	20	40	80	NS
POG	MABCDP	18	11	NA	18	61	NA	<0.001
UCLA	MABCD	28	39	65	27	59	86	0.005

AM, high-dose methotrexate; P, cisplatin; V, vincristine; A, doxorubicin; C, cyclophosphamide; B, bleomycin; D, actinomycin D; DFS, disease-free survival; S, survival (2–5 years); NS not significant; POG, Pediatric Oncology Group; UCLA, University of California at Los Angeles, NA not available

TABLE 31-2. Randomized Adjuvant Chemotherapy Trials in Osteosarcoma Assessing the Role of High Dose Methotrexate

Institution	No	Drugs 1	Drugs 2	% DFS 1	% DFS 2	%S 1	%S 2
EORTC	198	DPM	DP	41	57	64	50
Ontario	120	DM	D, M	49	53	NA	NA
CCSG	166	DM	Dm	40	40	NA	NA
Bologna	127	PM	Pm	66	42	NA	NA
CALGB	89	DM	D	40	52	57	82
Mayo Clinics	38	VM	observation	40	43	52	55

NA, Not available; P, Cisplatin; m, Methotrexate moderate dose; D, Doxorubicin; M, Methotrexate, high dose

(5) reported a significantly improved disease-free survival after five- and six-drug adjuvant regimens, respectively, and the UCLA study also demonstrated a significantly prolonged survival. Based on these randomized trials, doxorubicin- and cisplatin-based adjuvant chemotherapy is now accepted as standard treatment.

The optimal combination of agents and schedule is not yet established, however. While five trials show no advantage for high-dose methotrexate (Table 31-2), one randomized trial demonstrated an advantage for high-dose over standard-dose methotrexate (6,7). Two trials demonstrate a significant advantage for the group that received no methotrexate (8,9) Three other studies show no difference between the high-dose methotrexate arm and either low-dose (10) or no methotrexate (2) or delayed high-dose methotrexate (11). Because most studies varied more than one variable, it is not possible to draw definitive conclusions from these data. Cyclophosphamide, bleomycin, and actinomycin D used in earlier studies have been largely abandoned.

Ewing's Sarcoma

Current multimodality treatment results in cure of about 70% of children under 10 years of age with localized disease and about a third of children with metastases. Patients older than 16 years of age have a significantly worse prognosis despite treatment on the same protocols as younger children.

Primary treatment consists of combination chemotherapy with doxorubicin, vincristine, and cyclophosphamide or ifosfamide prior to and concurrent with radiotherapy to the involved bone. Although dose schedules of other combinations vary, the Intergroup Ewing Sarcoma Study used 1.5 mg/m^2 vincristine per weeks 1–6 and 8–13; actinomycin D, 0.015 mg/kg daily, days 1–5 every 12 weeks; cyclophosphamide, 600 mg/m^2/week; and doxorubicin, 30 mg/m^2 daily, days 1–3 every 3 weeks. Doxorubicin has significantly improved survival in randomized trials. Adjuvant surgery is controversial but is often considered for resection of expendable bones or if tumor remains after chemotherapy and radiation.

Mesna, adriamycin, ifosfamide, and dacarbazine (MAID) resulted in a 77% response rate for 13 adults with unresectable or metastatic Ewing's sarcoma in a SWOG trial (manuscript submitted). There were two complete and eight partial responses. At 5 years, three patients have not progressed.

RANDOMIZED ADJUVANT CHEMOTHERAPY TRIALS FOR SOFT TISSUE SARCOMA

Adjuvant chemotherapy is currently established in the treatment of rhabdomyosarcomas. Combination chemotherapy regimens usually include cyclophosphamide, actinomycin, and vincristine. In randomized trials the addition of doxorubicin did not improve survival. Mesna, adriamycin, ifosfamide, and dacarbazine (MAID) resulted in a 64% response rate for 25 adults with unresectable or metastatic rhabdomyosarcoma sarcoma in a SWOG trial (manuscript submitted). There were seven complete and nine partial responses. At 5 years, three patients have not progressed.

Adjuvant chemotherapy in other adult soft tissue sarcomas remains controversial although there is general agreement on several principles. The risks of adjuvant chemotherapy are not currently warranted in patients with low-grade lesions, given their low probability of metastatic spread. There is no study which shows a survival or metastasis-free survival advantage for nonextremity lesions or in uterine sarcomas.

Initial pilot studies in adult soft tissue sarcomas evaluating patients receiving adjuvant chemotherapy versus historical controls were promising, with large statistically significant differences observed. However, the survival of the control arms in subsequent randomized studies has usually been significantly superior to that of historical controls. Thus only randomized studies with nontreatment control arms appear to be reliable (Table 31-3). Because surgical salvage of pulmonary metastases or recurrent local disease is possible in some patients, survival may be a more meaningful end point than disease-free survival.

Of the 12 reported adjuvant studies, only two studies (one from the Rizzoli Center in Bologna (12) and the other from the Foundation Bergonie in Bordeaux) show a significant overall survival advantage for chemotherapy. One study (EORTC) demonstrated a significant improvement in local control for adjuvant chemotherapy, but no overall survival benefit (13). Subset analyses in two additional studies from M. D. Anderson Hospital (14,15) and the National Cancer Institute (16) currently indicate a significant disease-free survival advantage for adjuvant chemotherapy in extremity lesions but no significant improvement in survival. [While the NCI reported a significant prolonged survival for the subset of chemotherapy-treated extremity primaries on initial reports (17–22), survival is no longer significantly different, due to late relapses (16).] In the subset analysis of the same NCI study for retroperitoneal sarcomas, the survival of the control group is superior to the treatment group. Of the 14 randomized trials, the survival of the observation arm exceeds that of the chemotherapy arm in three studies (Mayo Clinic, ECOG, Scandinavian study). Doxorubicin-associated cardiotoxicity has occurred in about 10% of treated patients, occasionally contributing to treatment-related deaths.

Text continues on page 284

TABLE 31-3. Randomized Adjuvant Trials in High Grade Soft Tissue Sarcomas

Institute	Drugs	N	%DFS			%S		
			–	+	*P*	–	+	*P*
EORTC (13)	ACVD	468	43	56	.007	56	63	NS
Extremities		233	64	64	NS	55	42	NS
Bordeaux (25)	ACVD	59	16	57	<.01*	53	87	<.01
Extremities		36	NA	NA	NA	NA	NA	NA
Mayo Clinic (26)	AVDAd	61	68	65	NS	70	70	NS
Extremities		48	67	88	.08	83	63	NS
MD Anderson (14, 15)	ACVAd	47	83	76	NS	NA	NA	NS
Extremities		43	35	54	<.05	46	65	NS
NCI (16, 27-29)	ACM							
Non ext/non retroperitoneal		31	49	77	.075	58	68	NS
Trunk		22	47	92	<.01	61	82	NS
Retroperitoneal		15	NA	NA	NA	100	47	.06**
Extremities		67	28	54	<.05	60	54	NS

Scandinavia (30)	A	181	56	62	NS	70	75	NS
Extremities		155	NS	NS	NS	NS	NS	NS
Pooled DFCI/MGH, ISSG, ECOG (31)	A	168	53	66	NS	65	68	NS
Extremities		72	64	79	NS	70	79	NS
GOG (32)	A	156	47	59	NS	52	60	NS
UCLA (33)								
Extremities	A	119	54	56	NS	74	78	NS
Rizzoli (12)								
Extremities	A	77	45	73	<.05	70	91	<.05

DFS, disease-free survival; S, survival; – , without chemotherapy; +, with chemotherapy; EORTC, European Organization for the Research and Treatment of Cancer; DFCI/MGH, Dana Farber Cancer Institute/Massachusetts General Hospital; ISSG, Intergroup Sarcoma Study Group; ECOG, Eastern Cooperative Oncology Group; GOG, Gynecologic Oncology Group; UCLA, University of California at Los Angeles; NCI, National Cancer Institute; A, doxorubicin (doxorubicin); V, vincristine; Ad, Actinomycin D; C, cyclophosphamide; D, dacarbazine; NA, not available; NS, not significant

* Authors reported metastatic-free survival.

** 2 year survival inferior in chemotherapy arm.

Modified with permission from Mazanet R, Antman KH. Sarcomas of soft tissue and bone. Cancer 1991:68:463–73.

Studies of Schedule or Mode of Chemotherapy Administration

There have been two randomized trials of two different preoperative or adjuvant chemotherapy schedules. One from UCLA studied intraarterial versus intravenous doxorubicin. End points were feasibility of limb salvage (98% versus 100%, respectively), local recurrence (7% versus 8%), incidence of complications (18% versus 10%), and median tumor necrosis (70% versus 60%) (23). The authors concluded that intravenous doxorubicin had at least equivalent efficacy with less toxicity.

In the second study, 87 adults with extremity sarcomas treated at Memorial Sloan-Kettering Cancer Center in New York City received continuous infusion versus bolus doxorubicin. While fewer patients receiving continuous infusion had a >10% decrease in ejection fraction (42% versus 61% for bolus infusion), survival status was superior for those receiving bolus doxorubicin (24).

PENDING META-ANALYSIS

A meta-analysis of adjuvant data in soft tissue sarcomas will be reported by the Medical Research Council Cancer Trials Office, United Kingdom, on behalf of the Sarcoma Meta-Analysis Collaboration. Three meta-analyses of published data have been reported to be positive. Such analyses from publications are problematic and less reliable than meta-analyses of individual patient data. Published data are subject to publication bias and may only include positive subsets of patients. All randomized trials published and unpublished must be included for a valid study.

FUTURE STUDIES

Future randomized trials should include patients at high risk for metastases (large, high-grade lesions) with a reasonable likelihood of local control (radical resection or resection with uninvolved margins and radiotherapy). Totally resected low-grade sarcomas are currently cured in 80% of cases, and thus should not be included in adjuvant trials. Small (<5 cm) high-grade sarcomas may have a better prognosis than large intermediate-grade sarcomas and thus also should not be included. As grades II and III are not reliably distinguished pathologically, some investigators have advocated inclusion both in adjuvant trials. A doxorubicin and ifosfamide adjuvant regimen is being compared to no further treatment by the EORTC.

REFERENCES

1. Taylor W, Ivins J, Dahlin D, Edmonson J, Pritchard D. Trends and variability in survival from osteosarcoma. Mayo Clin Proc 1978;53:695–700.
2. Edmonson J, Green S, Ivins J, et al. A controlled pilot study of high-dose methotrexate as post-surgical adjuvant treatment for primary osteosarcoma. J Clin Oncol 1984;2:152–156.
3. Link M, Goorin A, Miser A, et al. The effect of adjuvant chemotherapy on relapse-free survival in patients with osteosarcoma of the extremity. N Engl J Med 1986;314:1600–1606.
4. Link M, Shuster J, Goorin A, et al., eds. Adjuvant chemotherapy in the treatment of osteosarcoma: Results of the multi-institutional osteosarcoma study. In: Ryan JR, Baker LO, eds. Recent concepts in sarcoma treatment. Dordrecht, Netherlands: Kluwer Academic Publishers, 1988. pp 283–290.
5. Eilber F, Guiliano A, Eckardt J, Patterson K, Moseley S, Goodnight J. Adjuvant chemotherapy for osteosarcoma: A randomized prospective trial. J Clin Oncol 1987;5:21–26.

6. Picci P, Bacci G, Campannacci R. Neoadjuvant chemotherapy for localized osteosarcoma of the extremities. Experience related to 103 cases treated between March 83–March 86. In: Salmon S, ed. Adjuvant therapy of cancer V. Orlando, Florida: Grune & Stratton, 1987. pp 711–718.
7. Picci P, Bacci G, Capanna R, et al., eds. Neoadjuvant chemotherapy for osteosarcoma. In: Ryan JR, Baker LO, eds. Recent concepts in sarcoma treatment. Results of a prospective study. Dordrecht, Netherlands: Kluwer Academic Publishers, 1988. pp 291–296.
8. Bramwell V, Burgers M, Sneath R, et al. Preliminary report of the first European osteosarcoma intergroup study. Proc Am Soc Clin Oncol 1988;7:273.
9. Cortes E, Necheles T, Holland J, Carey R. Adjuvant chemotherapy for primary osteosarcoma: A Cancer and Leukemia Group B experience. In: Salmon SE, Jones S, eds. Adjuvant therapy of cancer IV. Orlando, Florida: Grune & Stratton, 1984. pp 201–210.
10. Kraillo M, Ertel I, Makley J. A randomized study comparing high-dose methotrexate with moderate dose methotrexate as components of adjuvant chemotherapy in childhood nonmetastatic osteosarcoma: A report from the Childrens Cancer Study Group. Med Pediatr Oncol 1987;15:69–77.
11. Jenkin R, Biship A, Bourchard H. Osteosarcoma. A preliminary report of a trial of adjuvant chemotherapy. Am Soc Clin Oncol 1981;22:525. [Abstr.]
12. Picci P, Bacci G, Gherlinzoni F, et al. Results of a randomized trial for the treatment of localized soft tissue tumors of the extremities in adult patients. In: Ryan JR, Baker LO, eds. Recent concepts in sarcoma treatment. Dordrecht, Netherlands: Kluwer Academic Publishers, 1988. pp 144–148.
13. Bramwell V, Rouesse J, Steward W, et al. Adjuvant CYVADIC chemotherapy for adult soft tissue sarcoma: Reduced local recurrence but no improvement in survival. J Clin Oncol 1994;12(6):1137–49.
14. Lindberg RD, Murphy WK, Benjamin RS, et al. Adjuvant chemotherapy in the treatment of primary soft tissue sarcomas: Preliminary report. In: van Oosterom AT, van Unnik JAM, Management of bone and soft tissue tumors. Chicago: Year Book Medical Publishers, Inc., 1977. pp 343–352.
15. Benjamin TO, Terjanian TO, Fenoglio CJ, et al. The importance of combination chemotherapy for adjuvant treatment of high-risk patients with soft-tissue sarcomas of the extremities. In: Salmon S, ed. Adjuvant therapy of cancer V. Orlando, Florida: Grune & Stratton, 1987. pp 735–744.
16. Baker AR, Chang AE, Glatstein E, Rosenberg SA. National Cancer Institute experience in the management of high-grade extremity soft tissue sarcomas. In: In: Ryan JR, Baker LO, eds. Recent concepts in sarcoma treatment. Dordrecht, Netherlands: Kluwer Academic Publishers, 1988. pp 123–130.
17. Rosenberg SA, Tepper J, Glatstein E, et al. Prospective randomized evaluation of adjuvant chemotherapy in adults with soft tissue sarcomas of the extremities. Cancer 1983;52:424–434.
18. Rosenberg SA. Prospective randomized trials demonstrating the efficacy of adjuvant chemotherapy in adult patients with soft tissue sarcomas. Cancer Treat Rep 1984;68:1067–1078.
19. Rosenberg SA, Chang AE, Glatstein E. Adjuvant chemotherapy for treatment of extremity soft tissue sarcomas: Review of National Cancer Institute experience. Cancer Treat Symp 1985;3:83–88.
20. Rosenberg SA. Adjuvant chemotherapy of adult patients with soft tissue sarcoma. In: DeVita V, Hellman S, Rosenberg S, eds. Important advances in oncology. Philadelphia: J. B. Lippincott, 1985. pp 273–294.
21. Rosenberg SA, Suit HD, Baker LH. Sarcomas of soft tissue. In: DeVita V, Hellman S, Rosenberg S, eds. Cancer: Principles & practice of oncology, 2nd ed. Philadelphia: J. B. Lippincott, 1985. p 1243.
22. Rosenberg SA, Lotze MT, Muul LM, et al. A progress report on the treatment of 157 patients with advanced cancer using lymphokine-activated killer cells and interleukin-2 or high-dose interleukin-2 alone. N Engl J Med 1987;316:890–897.
23. Eilber FR, Giuliano AE, Huth JF, Weisenburger T, Eckardt J. Intravenous vs. intraarterial adriamycin, 2800 r radiation and surgical excision for extremity soft tissue sarcomas: A randomized prospective trial. Proc Am Soc Clin Oncol 1990;9:309. [Abstr. 1194.]
24. Casper ES, Gaynor JJ, Hajdu SI, et al. A prospective randomized trial of adjuvant chemotherapy with bolus versus continuous infusion of doxorubicin in patients with high-grade extremity soft tissue sarcoma and an analysis of prognostic factors. Cancer 1991;68(6):1221–1229.
25. Ravaud A, Nguyen BB, Coindre JM, et al. Adjuvant chemotherapy with CyVADIC in high-risk soft tissue sarcoma: A randomized prospective trial. In: Salmon SE, ed. Adjuvant therapy of cancer VI. Philadelphia: W. B. Saunders Company, 1990. pp 556–566.
26. Edmonson JH, Fleming TR, Ivins JC, et al. Randomized study of systemic chemotherapy following complete excision of nonosseus sarcomas. J Clin Oncol 1984;2:1390–1396.
27. Chang A, Kinsella T, Glatstein E, et al. Adjuvant chemotherapy for patients with high-grade soft-tissue sarcomas of the extremity. J Clin Oncol 1988;6:1491–1500.
28. Glenn J, Sindelar WF, Kinsella T. Results of multimodality therapy of resectable soft-tissue sarcomas of the retroperitoneum. Surgery 1985;97:316–325.
29. Glenn J, Kinsella T, Glatstein E, et al. A randomized, prospective trial of adjuvant chemotherapy in adults with soft tissue sarcomas of the head and neck, breast, and trunk. Cancer 1985; 55:1206–1214.

30. Alvegard TA, Sigurdsson H, Mouridsen H, et al. Adjuvant chemotherapy with doxorubicinin high grade soft tissue sarcoma: A randomized trial of the Scandinavian Sarcoma Group. J Clin Oncol 1989;7:1504–1513.
31. Antman K, Ryan L, Borden E, et al. Pooled results from three randomized adjuvant studies of doxorubicin versus observation in soft tissue sarcoma: 10-Year results and review of the literature. In: Salmon S, ed. Adjuvant therapy of cancer VI. Philadelphia: W. B. Saunders Company, 1990. pp 529–544.
32. Omura GA, Major FJ, Blessing JA, et al. A randomized clinical trial of adjuvant adriamycin in uterine sarcomas: A Gynecologic Oncology Group study. J Clin Oncol 1985;3:1240–1245.
33. Eilber FR, Giuliano AE, Huth JF, Morton DL. Adjuvant Adriamycin in high-grade extremity soft-tissue sarcomas—A randomized prospective trial. Proc Am Soc Clin Oncol 1986;5:125. [Abstr. C-488.]

VII

Conference Summary

Adjuvant Therapy of Cancer VIII, edited by Sydney E. Salmon. Lippincott–Raven Publishers, Philadelphia © 1997.

32

Adjuvant Therapy of Cancer VIII: Concluding Perspectives

Anne Schott and Laurence H. Baker

The purpose of adjuvant therapy is to prevent cancer recurrence after primary surgical management and is generally the realm of the medical oncologist and radiation oncologist. Whereas radiation therapy is useful in prevention of local recurrence, systemic medical therapy would appear more suited to preventing metastatic disease.

In order to metastasize, cancer cells must first develop biological weaponry which allows uncontrolled proliferation, angiogenesis, and invasiveness. These developments must be accompanied by an ability to evade the host's immune system, to recognize and penetrate other organs conducive to growth, and to establish a new environment suitable for continued growth and further cycles of metastasis. A cell that has metastasized, therefore, has gone through a rigorous selection process and is poised and ready to spread again. In the case of many solid tumors, unfortunately, this selection has rendered the patient incurable by existing therapies. Therefore, the successful treatment of clinically undetectable residual disease after surgery, and the prevention and treatment of micrometastasis would be expected to have a positive impact on patient survival.

SCIENTIFIC OVERVIEW

The Eighth International Conference on the Adjuvant Therapy of Cancer was an opportunity to review the current state of the art in the management of patients with no detectable cancer after surgery. The meeting commenced with the Scientific Overview, opened by Dr. Sydney Salmon, who discussed his vision of the adjuvant treatment of cancer in the 21st century. Dr. Salmon noted that basic scientific efforts are currently focused on developing techniques to eliminate cells with altered genes, to block oncogene expression, to repair damaged tumor suppressor genes, and to convert tumor cells to normal cells with tools such as differentiating agents. Some of these methods would incorporate the use of "gene therapy," which is the term used to describe the introduction of genetic material for the purpose of altering a cell in a desired way. The challenges and pitfalls of gene therapy were further elaborated by Dr. Evan Hersh. Although exciting advances have been made, there are significant obstacles to overcome before gene therapy will realize its full potential in the management of cancer. Although over 100 gene therapy protocols are now funded in the United States, it has been suggested by leading scientists and the NIH that more work be done at the basic science level before further clinical trials are undertaken.

In keeping with the theme of "obstacles and opportunity," Dr. J. J. Grous discussed the use of the bradykinin analog RMP-7 to overcome the blood brain barrier, long an obstacle to the penetration of chemotherapy agents into the central nervous system. RMP-7 was found to increase levels of carboplatin in rat brain gliomas, and the combination of RMP-7 + carboplatin increased survival over carboplatin alone. In humans, RMP-7 was well tolerated and increased glioma permeability as measured by PET scan. No information was presented on human response rates to RMP-7 combined with chemotherapy, but phase II clinical trials are under way. One may envision future uses of such agents in the adjuvant treatment of primary brain tumors, as well as in hematologic malignancies and solid tumors which frequently metastasize to brain and meninges.

Dr. Bailes discussed another obstacle to the improvement of cancer therapy—the managed care system. Clinical trials are essential to the improvement of existing medical therapies, and the growth of managed care has made it increasingly difficult to enroll patients in clinical protocols, due to the refusal of such programs to pay for the care of patients on investigational treatments. Several suggestions were made to improve the participation of managed care patients. For example, simplification of protocols would make them easier to apply in the community, and less costly, thus overcoming the most pressing obstacles to managed care acceptance of clinical trials. Furthermore, discussions with managed care companies to establish guidelines for the use of novel therapies would serve in the interest of both the managed care company and the researchers, and could allow patients options that would otherwise be denied. Overall, Dr. Bailes has observed a trend toward allowing off-label uses of drugs.

Dan Green provided a sobering review of the late effects of adjuvant chemotherapy in children and adolescents. Long-term consequences include the risk of left ventricular failure following doxorubicin, risk of Fanconi's syndrome following ifosfamide therapy, sterilization occurring in males following alkylating agents such as procarbazine, and congenital defects in children sired by a cancer survivor. Long-term screening strategies for these cancer survivors was also emphasized.

AIRWAY TUMORS

Dr. Hong presented compelling biologic data supporting the concepts of multi-step carcinogenesis and field carcinogenesis. In all cases, Chung, Hong, et al. examined primary head and neck cancers and secondary cancers for concordance of p53 expression. There was discordance in all cases, indicating that the development of the second primary tumor occurs as an independent clonal event. Also importantly, it was recently reported by this group that there is a loss of heterozygosity at 9p21 and 3p12 in patients with dysplasia and carcinoma *in situ*. These concepts, as well as the important observation that there is differential expression of nuclear retinoic acid receptors and especially the suppression of retinoic acid receptor-β, all support the concepts of multi-step carcinogenesis and field carcinogenesis. Further, this specific receptor can be upregulated by treatment with retinoids, laying important groundwork for the ongoing chemoprevention trials in these patients. Dr. Hong also provided an update of the completed VA laryngeal trial, again demonstrating that the survival rate is the same whether or not total laryngectomy is part of the treatment plan. The value of avoidance of laryngectomy is obvious.

LeChevalier briefly reviewed the role of adjuvant chemotherapy of non-small cell lung cancer (NSCLC). A meta-analysis of the 14 trials comparing surgery alone versus surgery followed by adjuvant chemotherapy was performed using updated individual data. This analysis suggests that the use of long-term alkylating therapy resulted in a 15% detriment while cisplatin-based regimens produced a 13% reduction in the risk of death and an absolute benefit of chemotherapy of 5%. Similarly, when trials were analyzed comparing surgery and radiotherapy with and without chemotherapy, there was a 6% reduction in death and a 2% absolute benefit. Neoadjuvant approaches have also been studied and the two reported randomized trials of stage IIIA demonstrated significant benefit from chemotherapy. However, both trials were small and the populations heterogeneous. Larger trials are needed to support this approach.

BREAST CANCER

A total of four sessions were devoted to the discussion of the adjuvant treatment of breast cancer. Most lectures were in the form of updates of mature clinical trials and single institution experiences with various treatment regimens. The fourth session was in the form of a roundtable discussion with leading figures in breast cancer fielding questions from the audience participants.

Large-Scale Adjuvant Trials

Dr. Pinuccia Valagussa, substituting for Gianni Bonadonna, gave an update of the Milan experience with cyclophosphamide, methotrexate, and fluorouracil (CMF) in node-positive breast cancer. The encouraging results show continued disease-free (DFS) and overall survival (OS) benefit of CMF at 20 years postenrollment. A subsequent study comparing 6 versus 12 cycles of CMF showed no additional benefit from the longer chemotherapy schedule, at 18 years follow-up. In summary, these results continue to support the use of six cycles of this standard drug regimen in the adjuvant treatment of breast cancer. Studies in high-risk patients (>10 nodes positive) which examined treatment with sequential doxorubicin-CMF versus high-dose sequential chemotherapy indicated a benefit to dose intensity in this group of patients. The most recent Milan trials examined the use of neoadjuvant chemotherapy in patients with locally advanced (>3 cm) breast cancer. In this group of patients, response to primary chemotherapy correlated with patient outcome, suggesting that primary tumor response also predicts the sensitivity of micrometastatic disease. Further trials examining the use of taxol as adjuvant or neoadjuvant therapy are planned. Hopefully, the future will allow us to predict patient response based on tumor genotype and phenotype, and lead to the design of rational therapies which can be tailored to a particular patient's tumor.

Dr. Fisher presented an historical overview of the National Surgical Adjuvant Breast and Bowel Project (NSABP) trials in breast cancer. The Halsteadian approach to breast cancer, now 100 years old, stated that breast cancer spreads in a direct and orderly fashion, and that the way to cure it is to remove the breast and all surrounding tissues. Bernard Fisher and his brother, Ted, suggested an alternate hypothesis—that breast cancer spread is chaotic and that radical surgery would not necessarily improve cure rates. That was the basis of the lumpectomy versus mastectomy trial, NSABP B-06. As a result of that seminal trial, the surgical management of breast cancer has been completely transformed. For example, 20 years ago centers such as the University of Michigan performed mastectomy on 80% of breast cancer patients, but now 80% are treated with lumpectomy followed by radiation therapy. One of the first adjuvant treatment trials was also from the NSABP, comparing cytotoxic therapy using L-phenylalanine mustard (L-PAM) versus no treatment. This study was positive, providing a rational basis for further study of adjuvant chemotherapy in breast cancer. The third major contribution of the NSABP was in the careful examination of endocrine manipulation as breast cancer therapy. NSABP B-14 evaluated the use of tamoxifen versus placebo in node-negative, estrogen receptor-positive (ER+) breast cancers. Whereas a clear benefit was seen with the use of tamoxifen after 5 years, continued use of this medication after 5 years did not supply any additional improvement in overall or disease-free survival. This study establishes the current standard of care to include the discontinuance of tamoxifen after 5 years. It is suggested that this practice be extrapolated to node positive patients as well, until other data are available on this group of patients.

The breast cancer discussion continued with Dr. Buzdar, who reviewed the M. D. Anderson experience with combination chemotherapy utilizing 5-FUra, doxorubicin, and cyclophosphamide (FAC). In this single institution, the 15-year reduction in mortality was comparable to that seen in larger intergroup trials, thus confirming the legitimacy of doxorubicin-containing regiments as adjuvant therapy.

Dr. Boccardo addressed the long-standing theory that the effectiveness of adjuvant chemotherapy in premenopausal women is, in a large part, related to the induction of amenorrhea. If this were true, then more effective pharmacological ovarian ablation may prove beneficial in treating breast cancer, particularly in ER+ patients. In a multi-center Italian trial, six cycles of CMF are being compared with tamoxifen plus gosrelin in pre- and perimenopausal, ER+ patients. The combination of tamoxifen and gosrelin had a 72% incidence of drug-induced amenorrhea, whereas CMF stopped menstrual periods in 68%. At 3-year follow-up of 235 patients, there was no apparent difference in disease-free or overall survival between the two groups. However, there was a suggestion that continued menstruation in the CMF group was an adverse prognostic factor. These results are at present underpowered and preliminary and will need to be examined at a later date.

High-Dose Chemotherapy

Drs. Frei, Viens, and Peters presented information on the use of high-dose chemotherapy in breast cancer patients. Dr. Frei began with an historical review of the STAMP program. This approach, examined in three separate trials, utilized multiple alkylating agents sequentially and in high doses. The premise for this work was the observation that different alkylating agents were non-cross-resistant and that combination therapy is in general more effective than single agent therapy. Perhaps surprisingly, there was a significant difference in results based on the order of use of phenylalanine mustard (PAM), with a disease-free survival of 20% when PAM was given prior to a combination of other alkylating agents, in contrast to a 60% disease-free survival when PAM was given later in the sequence. This observation led to the "one drug–multiple mechanisms" concept; in other words, resistance to a given single agent results from the induction of more than one resistance mechanism. This hypothesis is supported by *in vitro* and *in vivo* studies.

Dr. Peters gave an update on the results of autologous bone marrow transplant (ABMT) as adjuvant therapy in patients with >10 positive lymph nodes. In phase II trials, patients treated with CAF for four cycles followed by ABMT had a DFS at seven years of approximately 60%. In comparison, similar high-risk patients in a recent CALGB study received doxorubicin-containing chemotherapy and had an approximately 40% DFS. We all await results from phase III studies which will more definitively answer the question of whether ABMT should be recommended off-protocol in high-risk patients. In addition to this review, Dr. Peters presented new data from a subset analysis of a randomized study performed at Duke University examining immediate versus delayed transplant in patients with metastatic breast cancer. In this analysis, patients who reached complete remission with AFM (doxorubicin, continuous infusion 5-FUra, and methotrexate) induction chemotherapy were randomized to receive transplant immediately or in early relapse. The intriguing results showed that remission induction followed by observation, with bone marrow transplant after relapse, resulted in a better overall survival when compared to immediate transplant after remission induction. One explanation offered for this result was that a "transient drug resistance" mechanism was activated by induction chemotherapy, a theory which seems similar to the "one drug–multiple mechanisms" concept discussed by Dr. Frei.

Dr. Viens described the use of a high dose intensity chemotherapy regimen in nonmetastatic breast cancer, utilizing growth factor and peripheral blood stem cell support. This regimen, designed to be given in an outpatient setting, required an average of 4 days of hospitalization per cycle, usually for the complication of febrile neutropenia. Disease-free and mortality data were only available at 16-month follow-up and must be compared at a later date to conventional chemotherapy.

Biologic Observation and Potential Clinical Relevance

Dr. Hrushesky reviewed the long-known but often forgotten observation that breast cancers change in response to the menstrual cycle. Many retrospective studies suggest that operation during the luteal phase leads to a decreased recurrence rate. Dr. Hrushesky made an unabashed appeal to the NSABP to test this observation.

Dr. Pollack presented data from the North Central Cancer Treatment Group (NCCTG) on the use of octreotide given concurrently with tamoxifen in metastatic breast cancer. It has been known for many years that insulin, like estrogen, is a required growth factor for breast cancer. Both octreotide and tamoxifen have been shown to suppress serum levels of the IGF-1 mitogen factor in laboratory studies. As part of the NCCTG study, a subset of 18 patients receiving either tamoxifen alone or tamoxifen + octreotide were examined for treatment-related changes in serum IGF-1 levels. Both treatments resulted in decreased IGF-1 levels, and the percent decline at 3–6 weeks after institution of treatment was greater in the combination arm than the tamoxifen alone arm. Whether this biological end point will translate into a survival benefit is as yet unknown.

To conclude this section, Dr. Paterson reported the use of the diphosphonate clodronate in two clinical trials. In one trial, patients with cancer metastatic to bone were examined for skeletal morbidity with placebo versus clodronate. In this group, clodronate reduced the number of hypercalcemic events and reduced the cumulative incidence of skeletal morbidity (increased calcium, vertebral fractures, and radiation for bone pain). In a second study, patients with metastatic cancer but no bone metastases were randomized to receive clodronate or placebo. Again, patients on clodronate had fewer hypercalcemic events, fractures, and radiation for bone pain. In addition, there were fewer bony metastases as a site of first recurrence. As more potent and specific diphosphonates become available, cost-benefit analyses and quality-of-life analyses will be helpful in determining the appropriate clinical use of these agents.

GASTROINTESTINAL CANCER

Dr. David Kelsen reminded the group that, just as our treatments are evolving, the diseases themselves may undergo a change as well. Esophageal cancer, once primarily found to occur in older individuals with a long history of tobacco and ethanol abuse, has shown a significant shift in the United States toward a disease which affects younger, predominantly white, males. In addition to this change in epidemiology, the predominant histologic type now seen is no longer epidermoid cancer, but adenocarcinoma. The environmental and genetic reasons for this alteration is not yet known. While earlier trials showed a survival benefit of chemotherapy and radiation in inoperable esophageal cancer, it is not clear that these data, collected mainly in patients with epidermoid cancer, applies to the current spectrum of esophageal cancer.

Three colorectal adjuvant studies were reported by Wolmark, Pronzato, and Wong. All three trials questioned the role of levamisole in the management of these patients. Wolmark, reporting the NSABP C-05 trial, contrasted 5-FUra and leukovorin (lv) versus 5-FUra and levamisole (lev) versus 5-FUra + lv + lev in 2151 patients. The addition of levamisole provided no benefit. The INTACC (Intergruppo Nationale Terapie Adiuvante Carcinoma Colon) study attempted to assess the addition of high-dose 6-S-leucovorin to 5-FUra and levamisole to prolong survival in 1700 colon cancer patients. While the results are still quite early, there have been 127 relapses and 66 deaths on the 5-FUra/levamisole arm versus 51 deaths and 116 relapses on the leucovorin arm. Wong reported a nonrandomized but prospective comparison of 5-FUra + eucovorin versus 5-FUra/levamisole as adjuvant therapy after resection of stage III colon cancer. Patients with the poorer prognostic features of poorly differentiated histology or tumor perforation of the visceral peritoneum or invasion of contiguous structures were treated with the leucovorin arm while the better prognostic stage III patients received the levamisole arm. The 5-FUra/leucovorin arm had 8 relapses and 3 cancer deaths ($n = 46$) while the patients with the presumed better prognosis treated with 5-FUra and levamisole ($n = 57$) had 17 relapses and 12 cancer deaths.

GYNECOLOGIC AND GENITOURINARY CANCER

The role of adjuvant chemotherapy in ovarian cancer was reviewed by Alberts. Although there are many published studies in early ovarian cancer, almost all show either no significant advantage or are seriously underpowered. The data from these studies led to the European wide ACTION-ICON I trial in patients with stage I disease wherein patients are randomized to treatment at relapse (observation group) or chemotherapy with either cisplatin or carboplatin. This modern trial attempts to provide a definitive answer after decades of conflicting and confusing data. In stage III ovarian cancer, it is important to distinguish patients with optimal disease versus the rest (suboptimal and stage IV) because the results are very different. Such analysis could be performed in four published trials. In one the study of the Southwest Oncology Group, comparing intraperitoneal chemotherapy versus intravenous chemotherapy, the median survival is 49+ months for the IP route versus only 41 months for IV chemotherapy. The Gynecologic Oncology Group is helping define the role of paclitaxel which now should be included in treatment of optimal stage III patients.

Dr. Ahmann provided an overview of the developing investigations of prostate cancer adjuvant treatment. In this area, the importance of developing intermediate markers for therapeutic advantage are clearly needed. The role that PSA may play as a marker was explored. Androgen blockade is being studied as an adjuvant to prostatectomy and in other studies as an adjuvant to radiation therapy. No trials of adjunctive chemotherapy have been undertaken.

Professor Oliver provided an update on adjuvant trials in bladder cancer and stressed important scientific discoveries to serve as background for current and future trials. The studies of mutated p53, HCG expression, and G-CSF expression by bladder tumors is giving new insight into possible approaches for developing gene therapy in this cancer.

In superficial tumors, 6–12 weeks of intravesical BCG therapy has become a standard approach in the United States. Superficial bladder cancer is the most immunotherapeutically sensitive cancer in men, with an excess of 60% of patients becoming long-term relapse-free compared to 40% with doxorubicin. In Europe there is still some controversy when comparing BCG to mitomycin therapy.

The value of adjuvant chemotherapy in invasive bladder cancer is still unclear. One relatively small trial did show benefit of M-VAC chemotherapy as adjunct to cystectomy. No advantage has yet been shown using chemotherapy as adjunctive to radiation therapy. The surrogate endpoint of downstaging as a result of preoperative radiation therapy has emerged.

Dr. Einhorn reviewed the adjuvant concepts of therapy in testicular cancer. The role of adjuvant orchiectomy was introduced. Since the testis is a relative sanctuary from chemotherapy and since occasionally chemotherapy is started before orchiectomy is performed, the role of orchiectomy was reviewed in 160 cases. The orchiectomy specimen contained only necrosis in 44%, teratoma in 31%, and germ cell cancer in 25%. Of the 40 patients with cancer in the orchiectomy specimen, 17 had necrosis and 16 had teratoma in the retroperitoneal lymph node dissection, with no cancer in the larger retroperitoneal metastasis remaining postchemotherapy. Einhorn also summarized his approach to patients with stage I nonseminomatous germ cell tumors in which he anticipates that the cure rate should approach 100% with either of three initial approaches including: (a) observation following orchiectomy, (b) nerve-sparing retroperitoneal lymph node dissection (RPLND), or (c) chemotherapy. The preferred strategy he employs is the lymph node dissection by his expert urologist.

LYMPHOMAS, MELANOMA, AND SARCOMA

Lymphoma

The recently completed Southwest Oncology Group (SWOG 8736) study was the topic of a discussion by Dr. Thomas Miller. This study compared CHOP chemotherapy versus CHOP plus radiotherapy (RT) in localized intermediate- and high-grade non-Hodgkin's lymphoma (NHL). Presented at the conference was a subset analysis of those patients whose lymphoma was completely resected at the time of diagnostic biopsy. In those patients, three cycles of CHOP plus RT was superior to eight cycles of CHOP. In addition, the OS was better in this subset of patients than in those left with residual disease after biopsy. Results of the entire group (resected and unresected) will be presented at this year's ASCO meeting.

Melanoma

The topic of adjuvant treatment of melanoma was addressed in a balanced manner, with the presentation of two trials on the use of interferon in melanoma. Dr. Kirkwood reviewed data from an ECOG trial recently published in the *Journal of Clinical Oncology* examining the use of high-dose interferon-α2β as adjuvant treatment in high-risk melanoma patients. This trial showed a statistically significant benefit of treatment, with an increase in 5-year DFS from 26% in untreated to 37% in treated patients, with an even greater consistency of benefit in node-positive patients. This encouraging result must be weighed against significant toxicity associated with the regimen. In addition, several other trials using interferon-α2β and other interferons in different schedules showed no benefit. Dr. Vernon Sondak presented one such trial from SWOG, using IFN-γ as adjuvant treatment in resected stage II or II melanoma. The dose and schedule used (0.2 mg Q.D. S.Q. for 1 year) was selected because of demonstrated favorable immunomodulatory effects. Unfortunately, this rational approach did not result in improved DFS or OS.

Sarcomas

The impressive progress made in the combined modality treatment of patients with osteosarcoma was reviewed by Dr. Picci in describing consecutive protocols utilized at the Rizzoli Institute in Bologna. These investigators began using adjunctive chemotherapy in 1973. In 1973 and prior to adjunctive use of chemotherapy, 90% of patients diagnosed with osteosarcoma died of that disease and *all patients were surgically treated with an amputation*. The last study based upon a neoadjuvant strategy using ifosfamide reports 82% of 121 patients continuously free of disease (median follow-up of 18 months) and *only one patient was amputated*. Conclusions drawn from these experiences include: (a) doxorubicin is absolutely necessary, (b) doses of methotrexate need to be individualized to maximize benefit, (c) ifosfamide is a first line drug and needs to be employed in the preoperative treatment, and (d) total necrosis (100%) may be a prognostic factor for reduction of postoperative chemotherapy.

Dr. Antman contrasted the effectiveness of adjuvant chemotherapy focusing upon the randomized trials. In osteosarcoma there have been three such trials. The UCLA study showed significant improvement in disease-free and overall survival. The Pediatric Oncology Group reported significant improvement in disease-free survival only, while the Mayo clinic trial showed improvement in neither disease-free nor overall survival. Conversely, of twelve reported adjuvant studies in soft tissue sarcomas, only two studies show a significant overall survival advantage for chemotherapy, while in three studies, the survival of the observation arm patients exceed that of the chemotherapy arm patients. The initial report of a meta-analysis using updated individual patient data will be presented at the 1996 ASCO meeting. Three literature reviews of the randomized prospective trials support the use of adjuvant chemotherapy. Clearly, the benefit of chemotherapy is much more impressive in bone sarcomas than in soft tissue sarcomas.

CONFERENCE SUMMARY

At the conclusion of the *Adjuvant Therapy of Cancer V Conference* (1987), Larry Einhorn summarized the conference by saying, "... adjuvant breast cancer chemotherapy studies remain positive. The role of tamoxifen continues to be emerging." At the *Eighth Conference* 9 years later, we see the continued wisdom of those remarks. At 20 years of follow-up, the Milan breast cancer trial remains positive in every aspect. Tamoxifen is now limited to 5 years of use based upon the latest recommendations from the NSABP and Dr. Fisher.

In 1990 at the *Adjuvant Therapy of Cancer VI Conference*, Geoff Weiss and Chuck Coltman summarized the "well-known outcome of the intergroup study of surgical adjuvant therapy of colon cancer using 5-FUra and levamisole." In this meeting, Drs. Wolmark, Pronzato, and Wong questioned the role of levamisole.

At the *Seventh International Conference on the Adjuvant Therapy of Cancer* (1993), Michael Seiden and Karen Antman were prophetic in recognizing that "the starting point for designing a potentially efficacious adjuvant regimen most frequently began with the definition of an active chemotherapy regimen." They reported the effectiveness of BEP in testes cancer and CMF and CAF in breast cancer and then noted, "however, the combination of 5-FUra and levamisole was not defined as an active regimen in metastatic colon cancer."

At the *Ninth International Conference on the Adjuvant Therapy of Cancer* (date to be determined), we expect to learn the role of high-dose chemotherapy with autografts in the adjunctive treatment of breast cancer, the value of taxol chemotherapy in early-stage ovarian and breast cancer, and that there has been a moratorium on studies of 5-FUra modulation. Hopefully, new combinations of 5-FUra with a camptothecin analogue in patients with cancers of the colon and rectum have demonstrated efficacy.